Nurses' Aids Series

PAEDIATRIC NU

NURSES' AIDS SERIES

ANAESTHESIA AND RECOVERY ROOM TECHNIQUES

ANATOMY AND PHYSIOLOGY FOR NURSES

EAR, NOSE AND THROAT NURSING

GASTROENTEROLOGICAL NURSING

GERIATRIC NURSING

MATHEMATICS IN NURSING

MEDICAL NURSING

MICROBIOLOGY FOR NURSES

MULTIPLE CHOICE QUESTIONS, BOOKS 1 and 2

NEUROMEDICAL AND NEUROSURGICAL NURSING

OBSTETRIC AND GYNAECOLOGICAL NURSING

OPHTHALMIC NURSING

ORTHOPAEDICS FOR NURSES

PAEDIATRIC NURSING

PERSONAL AND COMMUNITY HEALTH

PHARMACOLOGY FOR NURSES

PRACTICAL NURSING

PRACTICAL PROCEDURES FOR NURSES

PSYCHIATRIC NURSING

PSYCHOLOGY FOR NURSES

SOCIOLOGY FOR NURSES

SURGICAL NURSING

THEATRE TECHNIQUE

Nurses' Aids Series

Paediatric nursing

FIFTH EDITION

Margaret Duncombe
M.B.E., R.S.C.N., S.R.N., S.C.M.

Barbara F. Weller
R.S.C.N., S.R.N., R.N.T.

BAILLIÈRE TINDALL LONDON

A BAILLIÈRE TINDALL *book published by*
Cassell Ltd,
35 Red Lion Square, London WC1R 4SG

and at Sydney, Auckland, Toronto, Johannesburg

an affiliate of
Macmillan Publishing Co. Inc.
New York

First published 1961
Fourth edition 1974
Reprinted 1975, 1976
Fifth edition 1979
Reprinted 1980
Reprinted 1981

First Spanish edition 1963 (C.E.C.S.A. Mexico)
Second Spanish edition 1966
First Portuguese edition in process of translation 1977
(Publicacoes Europa-America Mira-Sintra)
First English Language Book Society (E.L.B.S.) edition 1979

ISBN 0 7020 0688 2

Printed in Great Britain by
Spottiswoode Ballantyne Ltd., Colchester and London

British Library Cataloguing in Publication Data

Duncombe, Margaret
Paediatric nursing – 5th ed. – (Nurses' aids series).
1. Pediatric nursing
I. Title II. Weller, Barbara Fiona
610.73'62 RJ245

ISBN 0–7020–0688–2

Contents

	Foreword to the first edition	vii
	Preface	ix
	Acknowledgements	xi
1	The healthy child	1
2	Infant feeding	17
3	Nursing the newborn	36
4	The low birthweight baby	50
5	Apparent and true abnormalities of the newborn	59
6	Children in hospital	96
7	Sick children at home	124
8	Diseases of the respiratory system	131
9	Diseases of the ear, nose and throat	156
10	The cardiovascular system	185
11	Rheumatic and collagen diseases	210
12	Diseases of the blood	225
13	Diseases of the alimentary system	239
14	Disorders of metabolism and absorption	292
15	Diseases of the endocrine system	312
16	The genito-urinary system	324
17	The nervous system	360
18	Diseases of the skin	395

19 Diseases of the muscle, bones and joints 404
20 Tuberculosis in childhood 421
21 Communicable diseases 428
22 Burns, scalds and accidents 438
23 Terminal illness and death in the children's ward 455
Appendix 1 461
Appendix 2 465
Index 469

Foreword to the first edition

In the early days of the treatment of tuberculous meningitis with streptomycin there was a 5-year-old boy who was cured of meningitis but who seemed to be a human 'write-off'—blind, deaf, spastic and mindless. It was the Ward Sister who persisted, got him to play with a string of little toys, and heard him say, fingering them in turn: 'One—two—three—four . . .' So he *had* a mind, and he has since been educated.

That was a great perception; that was Sister Duncombe, now Matron, and still as distinguished in mind as in manner. She is not interested only in the very young, but has similar intuitive understanding of the puzzled student nurse—floating perhaps between the Scylla of barrier nursing and the Charybdis of leaving a crying infant to cry alone.

Such humanity and depth of feeling combined with breadth of knowledge might suggest impatience with practical details, but Miss Duncombe is meticulous in nursing and has the common sense which is needed when a complex technical problem has to be pruned to essentials. She is just the person to write a thoroughly practical textbook (such as this one) on a sound basis of academic knowledge.

This is a book for nurses; for nurses training in children's hospitals or departments, for nurses who mainly look after adults but have children in their care, for sisters who teach nurses. There is another who is likely to want it too—the nurse who has left hospital for marriage and has a family of her own. All will find it reliable, interesting and delightfully illustrated.

PHILIP EVANS

Preface to the fifth edition

Once again, new techniques in nursing practice and advances in medical science have made necessary a new edition of *Paediatric Nursing*. The nursing of sick children is a definite specialty, with its own body of knowledge, and is not adult nursing applied to a young age group. In the United Kingdom we have a precious heritage in the part of the Register for those who wish to work with children, a heritage which *Paediatric Nursing* should help to support and preserve. Since the last time the text was revised and brought up-to-date, integrated schemes of training have become established and a new type of examination paper has been introduced by the General Nursing Council. A significant proportion of nurses who qualify to become registered sick children's nurses now do so on a post-registration basis and more candidates than ever before are coming forward to take the paediatric-based training for the Roll. All these factors have been borne in mind in producing this new edition. While the basic teaching and information needed by learners has been retained, the need of the state registered general nurse working for an additional qualification has not been neglected. Experience has also shown that many nursing officers and ward sisters wish to have a copy of *Paediatric Nursing* to hand. The new edition should be useful to them all. All the nurses who use this book will become aware of the fact that whatever their technical skills there is no substitute for tender, loving care in nursing sick children.

In this new edition additional space has been given to the emotional needs of children and the chapter on handicaps has been enlarged. Where there have been new developments, as for instance in renal therapy, the care of the low birth weight baby or intensive care, these have been included. The preventive aspects of paediatrics are stressed throughout, and the need for early recognition and educative treatment (developmental care) is emphasized in, for example, deafness and Down's syndrome. Much detailed revision has taken place throughout the book: to the illustrations; to the reading lists; and within the text greater reference has been made to the social aspects in relation to clinical conditions.

Care of the sick child extends beyond the hospital ward boundaries into the home, community and school. Children can never be nursed in isolation, but their care must be related to their environment. The child's family have the most important role in establishing the child's well being, and good liaison and teamwork between hospital and community of all professionals concerned in child care is essential to achieve this.

We hope that this new edition of *Paediatric Nursing* will continue to serve well those entrusted with the nursing care and welfare of sick children either in the community or hospital.

September, 1978

MARGARET DUNCOMBE
BARBARA F. WELLER

Acknowledgements

The authors are particularly grateful to friends and colleagues working with children for their advice and support throughout the preparation of this edition. Very special thanks are due to Dr C. Fison, until recently Medical Superintendent, The Royal Children's Hospital, Brisbane, Australia; Dr P. F. Benson, Reader, Paediatric Research Unit, Guy's Hospital, London; Miss S. Burr, Senior Tutor, The Queen Elizabeth School of Nursing, Birmingham; and Miss J. Saxton, Senior Tutor, The School of Nursing, The Hospital for Sick Children, London.

We are greatly indebted to Dr P. Evans for his previous help and for allowing us to retain the original foreword he wrote for the book.

Illustrations

We gratefully acknowledge permission to reproduce illustrations as follows: to Dr D. C. Morley for Fig. 2; to Cow and Gate for Fig. 3; to the *Nursing Times* and Dr H. B. Valman for Fig. 9; to the *Nursing Times* for Figs 11, 39, 51, 59 and 60; to the Institute of Child Health and the Hospital for Sick Children for Figs 40, 41, 43, 46, 50, 52, 55, 57, 65, 66, 67 and 68; to Harvey Miller & Medcalf for Figs 16, 30, 47 and 48 taken from *Baby Surgery* by D. Young and B. F. Weller; to Guy's Hospital Medical School for Figs 24 and 25; to Guy's Hospital Paediatric Department for Fig. 54; to the Institute of Dermatology for Fig. 62; to Keystone Press Agency for Fig. 18; to D. Young, Senior Lecturer, Royal Hospital for Sick Children, Glasgow for Fig. 38; to Central Office of Information for Fig. 49. Figures 8, 12 and 54 are taken from *Children in Health and Disease* by Brimblecombe and Barltrop published by Baillière Tindall, and Fig. 16, first published in O'Doherty: *The Battered Child*, Baillière's Medical Transparencies, by kind permission of Mr M. N. Saad and Professor N. O'Doherty.

1

The healthy child

THE NURSING of sick children is a far more complex and difficult task than many people would suspect. To deal successfully with children some knowledge of their health, growth and behaviour is necessary, for only then can deviations from the normal, such as are caused by sickness, stress and separation, be fully understood.

Many detailed studies of children have enabled paediatricians and psychologists to work out average standards of mental and physical development at any given age. But no two children are alike, and norms and milestones must never be taken too literally. Each child is an individual with his own pace of development which is influenced by many factors such as his constitution, his surroundings, his family, his opportunities for experience, the physical and mental care he receives and the emotional security he is able to achieve.

The average standards are known as norms or milestones. They should be familiar to those who deal with children in health and sickness, but it is important to realize that variations of up to 10 or 15 per cent below or above that standard may still be considered within normal limits. For that reason many paediatricians now refer to developmental progress as a percentile of the average, rather than use rigid figures. Sometimes a line is drawn running diagonally across the weight chart, which is meant to indicate the 'normal' gain of weight, but this is now frequently replaced by a shaded area covering from 30 to 45 per cent below and above the average line. This allows for variations without causing alarm, and stresses the point that steady progress is of far greater importance than conformity with an arbitrary standard. For example, values which are not exceeded by 10 per cent of all children are spoken of as 10 percentile; values which are not exceeded by 90 per cent of all children are spoken of as 90 percentile, and so on. Thus the range between the highest figure (90th percentile) and the lowest one (10th percentile) represents 80 per cent of the measurements taken.

Antenatal Development

Development begins at the moment of conception and is most rapid before birth and during the first 18 months of life. The tiny, helpless creature we see at the time of birth is a perfect little being, capable of carrying on a life of his own, though only a few moments before he was completely dependent on his mother for all his vital processes and needs. He now has to breathe to obtain oxygen, to supply his own warmth and to obtain his own food by making the effort of sucking. His physical, mental and emotional growth, three completely interdependent factors, will be helped in greater or lesser measure by favourable surroundings, loving parents, a healthy and secure home and adequate educational and social services.

It is possible to detect developmental errors and to anticipate obstetric complications which may lead to problems in the newborn. Good antenatal care is, therefore, of very great importance. Organized, early discharge after hospital delivery makes the detection of neonatal abnormalities even more urgent than it used to be. Some of these abnormalities are described in Chapter 5.

The Child at Birth

The average newborn infant may be expected to weigh approximately 3·4 kg (7½ lb.) and to be 50 cm (20 in.) in length. The *head circumference* is approximately 33 cm (13 in.), with a cranium which is disproportionately large compared with the face.

Anterior and posterior fontanelles are open, moulding may be present and the sutures can be felt. The limbs seem short in comparison with the body and the head and abdomen large, in comparison with the thorax. Subcutaneous fat is sparse, the skin looks red and inelastic and the hair is, as a rule, merely a fine, down-like growth. The nails are soft and are inclined to peel off. The eyes lack pigment and appear blue. Reaction to light is merely reflex. Hearing is present. The infant is sensitive to hot and cold. He responds to pain and hunger. Movements are mostly reflex.

The *respirations* are rapid at 40 breaths per minute and are frequently irregular in rhythm and in depth. The heat-regulating centre is immature and variations in the body temperature may be sudden and considerable. The *pulse rate* is in the region of 120 to 140 beats per minute. The systolic blood pressure readings are between 60 and 80 and the diastolic between 50 and 60 mmHg. The *haemoglobin* will be as high as 110 per cent (20–24 g/dl). When held out, there may be a reflex response of bladder and bowel movement. Bowels act three to four times per day. The first stools passed are meconium, changing after 2 to 3 days to soft, sour-smelling stools. Ninety to 120 ml (3 to 4 fl oz) of urine are passed daily.

The infant spends 20 to 22 hours a day asleep and rarely wakens except at feeding time. When awake, his movements are instinctive and reflex. The head turns towards the mother's breast in search of food. He can clasp his fist so tightly round an outstretched finger that he can be lifted up by it. If held in a 'standing' position, he will make walking movements and he will kick and withdraw his leg if it is pricked or pinched. Breathing and sucking are also reflex actions. He has not yet gained control of his *eye movements* and squinting is a common and quite harmless feature. *Hearing* is present from birth and the infant will react to sudden or strong noises by reflex movements or by crying.

The First Year

During the first year development is astonishingly rapid and some progress can be noticed daily by those in close contact with the child. The *weight* increases by some 0.170 kg (6 oz) a week in the first months of life, and the birth weight is usually doubled by the age of 5 months and trebled by the end of the first year.

At 3 Months. Weight 5 kg (11¼ lb). Head now normal shape and growing rapidly in circumference. Posterior fontanelle closed. Begins to balance head and to lift it off the mattress. Limbs now well covered, the face round, the skin elastic. Second growth of hair replaces the initial down. The eyes have their permanent colour. Has achieved some co-ordination of eye movement and fixes on objects and may notice new surroundings. Enjoys music, cooing and soft voices. Will accept or reject new tastes.

Takes notice, recognizes the mother, responds to her smile, smiles with pleasure. Plays with own hands and feet. Attempts to grasp rattles and soft toys. Sleeps 18 to 20 hours/24 hours.

Haemoglobin: about 85 per cent (10–13 g/dl). Pulse: 110 to 120 beats/minute, respiratory rate slowing down. Urine: 300 to 480 ml (10 to 16 fl oz) daily.

At 6 Months. Weight 7.5 kg (16½ lb). Eyes can follow people round; turns head to increase the visual field. Can determine direction of sound. Enjoys new tastes and takes solid food. Begins to masticate; drinks from a cup.

First teeth erupt (usually lower central incisors); carries everything to the mouth. Can hold objects in both hands. Grasps things deliberately (no longer reflex). Sits up, if supported. Has pleasure in rocking his body. Spine is very straight. Smiles back at familiar faces. Is capable of real laughter. Coos and babbles. Makes sounds involving the use of lips and tongue. Prepares for speech. Loves repetitive games, e.g. hide and seek by pulling shawl over the head.

Blood pressure: systolic 75 mmHg. Pulse rate 110 to 120 beats/minute. Sleeps 14 to 18 hours/day.

At the End of the First Year. By this time the weight will be about 10.5 kg (23 lb) the length 73 cm (29 in) and the head circumference 46 cm (18 in). The face and limbs are well covered with subcutaneous fat and there are dimples over the knuckles, elbows and knees. The skin is firm and elastic and no longer hangs in loose folds as in the newly born.

The toddler looks around freely, eats most foods with the family, masticates well and is beginning to feed himself. He has between eight and ten teeth (central incisors, four; lateral incisors, four; pre-molars, two to four). The hair may need its first cut and the nails are now strong and hard. The eyes, which in most babies are blue at birth, are now a definite colour and the child is capable of focusing and of deliberate co-ordination. Lachrymation is now fully established and crying is accompanied by tears. He sits up on his own and can move from one place to the other and becomes expert in rolling from back to front and by creeping, rolling and pushing himself along on his seat. He can pull himself up with the help of the bars of the cot or a chair and makes ready for the first steps which he is likely to achieve by 10 to 16 months.

During the latter part of the first year, the child enjoys movements and skills of many kinds by constant experimenting. He can bring thumb and forefingers together and pick up tiny objects. He loves tearing up paper. Most children can say several monosyllables, two or three proper words and imitate a variety of sounds.

The toddler goes through a negative stage and may be difficult with diet. When awake, the 1-year-old is incredibly active but he still needs 12 to 16 hours sleep a day. With careful routine may be dry by day, though relapses and regressions occur during difficult times such as teething or periods of sickness or separation.

Blood pressure: systolic 80 mmHg; pulse rate: 100 to 110 beats/minute. Respirations: 20 to 30/minute. Bowels opened twice a day, stools formed and getting darker. Passes 450 to 600 ml (15 to 29 fl oz) urine per day.

This rapid growth is not confined to physical growth. From the young infant who is wholly mother-centred, the young child has developed into a 1-year-old filled with curiosity and anxious to make contacts with others, provided strangers allow him to make their acquaintance slowly and approach him quietly. As experience is lacking the 1-year-old knows no fear and delights in a game with all sorts of animals and moving objects. He still needs cuddling and physical contact with a familiar person or object, and the majority of children at this age have a precious 'cuddly', a teddy bear or a soft doll.

The Second Year

Throughout the next year the young child remains greatly attached to his mother and seems lost and afraid if she is out of sight for long. He is both a possessive and a jealous little creature and it takes a mother's tact and love to achieve smooth acceptance if there is a new arrival in the family. Disturbances during that period are not merely due to jealousy but also to the fact that the child is still upset by changes in the daily routine and expects his food and daily activities to be as he has always been used to having them. 'Tomorrow' is a term that has no meaning and promises involving time have to be linked to familiar happenings such as 'after tea' or 'when Daddy comes home'. A full understanding of this dependence on the mother and on familiar routine, means that every effort should be made to avoid hospitalization or any other separation from the mother at this stage. Facilities for mothers of young children to be resident when hospital admission is inevitable, should always be provided. An imaginative and adaptable nursing staff will always find this possible, no matter how impossible it seems to find the necessary space. If for any reason a separation of mother and child is unavoidable every effort should be made to find a 'mother substitute' who can take her place temporarily.

Gradually the toddler develops greater independence and as he loves to imitate others, he makes the first attempts at dressing and feeding himself. These first attempts will be slow and messy, but this is an important stage in the child's development and those who deal with children have to learn to curb their impatience and accept delays or messy clothes. Play and other activities continue to be essential to his development, and media such as sand and water, climbing frames and bricks should be available for all children of this age. By the age of 18 months, most children can walk fairly steadily, turn corners without accidents and will begin to run. They love to go on simple errands, to fetch and carry and they are full of curiosity, ready to open everything within reach. The 18-month-old takes an interest in strangers, enjoys the company of other small children for short periods and loves animals. Given a cup of water to carry, he can do so without spilling for a short distance. The toddler loves stories, if confined to a small repertoire which he loves to hear over and over again and he gets very upset when a variant is introduced. Nursery rhymes are popular at this stage. The 2-year-old is often able to repeat parts of them. He even knows short ones by heart and delights in reciting them.

At 2 Years Many children can feed themselves and dress and undress with help. They are able to build a tower of bricks, turn pages of books and fold paper into small parcels. They play happily on their own, provided mother is close at hand. Sand, clay and water are favourite play materials. The 2-year-old can usually say phrases of three or four words, mostly expressing his needs and desires. He lives entirely in the present and mothering and affection are still very important.

Physically he has grown much taller with bodily proportions nearer to those of the fully grown child. He may be dry at night time. Weight: 11 to 12 kg (24 to 26 lb). Length: 76 cm (30 in). The anterior fontanelle should have closed. Head circumference: 48 cm (19 in). The first set of teeth is almost complete, twenty in all (central incisors, four; lateral incisors, four; pre-molars, four; canines, four; second molars, four). Blood pressure systolic: 80 to 90 mmHg. Pulse rate: 90 to 100 beats/minute. Respirations: 20 to 30/minute. Haemoglobin: about 75 per cent (13–16 g/dl).

After this, progress appears less rapid and milestones are less well defined and less striking. An important period begins approximately at the age of 3 to 3½ years. For the first time the child shows signs of *independence* and emancipation. He is no longer wholly dependent on his mother and at this stage he develops and exhibits a will of his own. *Temper tantrums* in response to frustration are common and unless the child is wisely handled this may prove an exasperating period for the family. Much trouble may be caused by restricting the child in his activities during the early years of development. Every child needs a suitable place where he can play unrestrictedly and be untidy and where disorder, sand brought in from the garden, or water splashed all over the floor while bathing the dolly, cause neither damage nor an indignant outcry from mother or nurse. Children's *clothes* should be serviceable rather than fussy and should be easily mended and washed when torn and soiled. Rompers and dungarees are most suitable for girls as well as for boys as they give adequate protection from cold and dirt, are hard wearing and easily laundered. Furthermore the bib and braces help to keep knickers, cardigans and socks in place. Shoes should allow ample room for the toes and should have a small heel. Sandals are suitable both for indoor and for outdoor wear unless there is some orthopaedic contraindication.

The *toys* should be strong and suitable for the child's age. The desire to experiment is a natural drive and toys which allow for taking apart and 'looking in' will encourage this urge and permit a certain measure of destructiveness which is natural in children. Such toys include ordinary boxes and tins, building bricks, strong wooden engines and trucks, soft animals and glove puppets. Sand and water and equipment which allows the child to imitate adult activities such as 'cooking', 'washing day', 'going shopping', 'playing at doctor' and dressing up, are particularly popular and can occupy children for many hours while teaching them a variety of skills. Whatever toys or play materials are given to the child, care must be taken to select ones that are safe. The colours should be fast and of a vegetable type, corners should be rounded and there must not be any sharp edges or nails on which the child could harm himself. If the toy can be taken apart, no part should be small enough for the child to swallow or inhale it or to push it up his nostrils or into his ears.

All children need to learn independence step by step. *Accidents* are miraculously uncommon when children are left to their own devices and it is essential that adults should be capable of watching them instead of stepping in and forbidding adventure with endless warnings to be careful. Constant nagging or cries of 'don't do this' or 'do that' cause children to become indifferent to them and eventually produce disobedience. Some parents expect standards of achievement and behaviour far beyond the child's developmental stage, and discouragement and indifference are bound to follow such an attitude.

Emotional Development

Children need love, sympathy and sincerity. Criticism should be of a helpful rather than a squashing character and at no time should parents mock their children's friends or their achievements, or the child may be discouraged from making friends and bringing them home. The ability to make friends and easy relationships is essential in a happy life and it should be fostered from the earliest days. The secure child is the one who is outgoing and capable of making friends; he is able to occupy himself and shows no fear of any natural situation such as being in the dark or being left alone for short periods of time. He is sure of his parents' love, and though most children go through a phase in which they imagine that their parents do not love them and want to get rid of them, these phases are of short duration and rarely have any serious significance.

Some children are 'too good', as if wanting to please their parents, of whose love they are not sufficiently certain. Alternatively, they may be clinging or always wanting to attract attention, for the same reason. Manifestations of such insecurity may take a variety of forms, such as naughtiness, food fads, fits of temper tantrums or jealousy, and may even contribute to starting attacks of asthma. Parents can be helped to understand the significance of such behaviour and many will be able to deal with them wisely and successfully simply by giving a little extra time and showing more than the usual interest in their child and in his activities.

Punishment, if given, should be severe enough to hurt, but should always be adjusted to the gravity of the offence and to the individual child's tolerance for punishment. It should neither be delayed nor allowed to continue for a long period and should be logically related to the offence committed. Once given, it should be forgotten. Children in hospital need rarely be punished and hitting children is strictly forbidden. Any disciplinary action should be taken only with the full permission and advice of an experienced ward sister, who frequently can cope with the situation in some far more satisfactory way than by punishment.

Occasionally parents are worried about their children's interest in their bodies. This interest is entirely natural and need not be discouraged. Questions about the differences in the bodies of boys and girls should be answered simply and without embarrassment. The same applies to questions about sex. To children these questions are not very different from any others they may ask and it is usually only the embarrassment and the 'hush-hush' attitude of the adult which suggests that there is something special or secret about them. The child who asks the questions should have an immediate and straightforward reply. He is unlikely to absorb more than he can understand, and a child who really wants to obtain information will gain it elsewhere if satisfaction cannot be obtained at home.

Thumb sucking. During normal development the child goes through a phase of putting everything into his mouth, including his thumb or fingers. Occasionally, it may be his forearm that he sucks or the corner of an old blanket. If the practice continues it is usually that either the child feels unhappy and insecure or is bored. The nurse should direct her attentions and those of the parents to relieving the child's fears, or finding some suitable occupation rather than using cross words or sarcasm to get the child to remove his thumb. If thumb sucking continues after the age of 6 years the alignment of the permanent teeth can be affected unless treated by an orthodontist.

Masturbation and body rocking, which gives pleasurable sensations of a similar kind, cause parents much anxiety. Frequently neither is of serious significance. The best way to deal with them is to keep the child well occupied and to make sure that he has sufficient activity during the day to ensure sound sleep at night. Tight knickers or pants should be avoided. Occasionally, however, masturbation may grow into a real problem and, when it is coupled with other signs of disturbance, a paediatrician or child psychiatrist should be consulted.

Food fads and refusal to eat are other difficulties which may make family life very trying. They often start when the child is very young and not infrequently begin, as it were, accidentally. On some odd occasion when he shows a lack of appetite the child may find out that an interesting amount of concern is caused. In no time the refusal of food becomes a weapon against his mother. By it he can attract attention, can witness her distress on his behalf, and may obtain the food he most enjoys. The answer to the problem is at the beginning. No child who is not otherwise showing signs of illness will ever come to harm if he is allowed to miss a certain dish or even a meal. He will soon get hungry, and if he is told that he has to wait for the next meal he will have no wish to repeat the performance. Apparent indifference on the part of the mother is not easy, but it is certainly the soundest way of dealing with the child on such occasions.

Many books have been written on the development of children, on their behaviour and their needs, but in this chapter some of the more common milestones and problems have been described and some suggestions made as to how best to deal

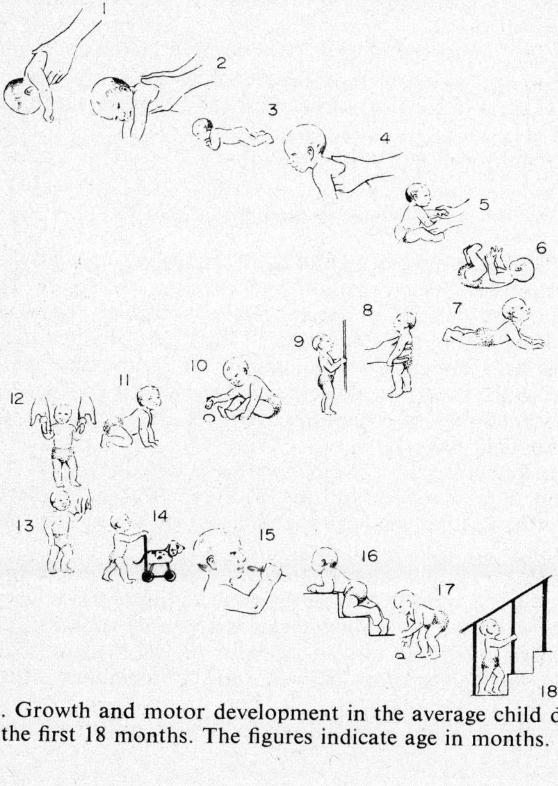

FIG. 1. Growth and motor development in the average child during the first 18 months. The figures indicate age in months.

with them. Only experience in handling children will give a nurse confidence and the more she learns, the more she will understand the great complexity of child behaviour and child care.

Summary

Although this summary has been compiled to help the student nurse working with children for a short time only, it is stressed once again that there is no universal 'norm' and that every child is an individual who develops and responds in his own way. Earlier or later development can be taken as a sign neither that the child is abnormally forward nor that there is necessarily any cause for anxiety.

The section on the normal development of the child and the summary on 'milestones' is the result of extensive studies by many experts in the field of paediatrics, psychology and education. There are many interesting books on these subjects which the student nurse will enjoy reading.

Safeguarding the Child's Health

Even before the birth of a child there are many services available which are designed to promote his health, to prevent disease and to treat defects at the earliest opportunity. Provision is made for the care and education of the physically handicapped and the deprived child. Although in hospital the medical social worker is the expert on these special services, it is of interest to know something of the facilities available and to have an idea of the wide field they cover.

Already before the child is born he is cared for by means of the antenatal services for his mother. Maximum health is assured by regular medical examination of the mother and by providing her with additional milk, vitamins and iron. Adequate National Insurance enables an expectant mother to cease work about 3 months before the expected date of delivery and to receive a maternity allowance for about 4½ months. A well-developed midwifery service cares for the mother and baby up to the tenth day after delivery and immediately after this the health visitor takes over. It is her function to promote the health and happiness of the whole family, and it is often the newly born infant who brings her into contact with each individual member of the household. Child health centres in every district hold regular clinics at which the infant's progress can be watched and guidance given. Whenever necessary the clinic doctors are readily available. Vitamins and dried milk are on sale, or are available free of charge under certain circumstances, and immunization programmes are carried out. Informal talks and demonstrations are given, a good deal of health education is undertaken, and the mother is taught how to live a healthy life and bring up children who too are healthy and contented. She may also be helped with household problems and with her weekly budget.

Mothers who have to go out to work can take their children to nurseries where they are cared for both physically and educationally up to the age of school entry. The *School Health Service* aims at supervising the child's health throughout school life. The object is to reveal defects which require attention and to refer the child to the family doctor and through him, when necessary, to the specialist for treatment. The *School Dental Service* supervises the child's teeth and can advise on conservative and corrective treatment. These services constitute a valuable follow-up of the child's health throughout school and right into early adult life.

Special Schools

Children with handicaps are also catered for. Those whose sight or hearing is too poor for them to be educated by ordinary means go to schools for the physically handicapped, e.g. those for the deaf and blind run by the local education authorities. Education for these children can start at the age of 2 years. Special arrangements are made for sufferers from cerebral palsy, for haemophiliacs and for children who are in any way crippled. Debilitated children and those suffering from chronic heart disease or chest infections and nervous illnesses, can be sent to special schools where extra rest hours, fresh air, physiotherapy and medical supervision are incorporated in the programme. The mentally handicapped go to schools for the educationally subnormal. Children who suffer from epileptic fits which either are so severe or occur so frequently that they have to be excluded from ordinary schools, are provided with special education. Any of these schools may be day or residential ones. Special school buses take these children from their homes to school in the morning and back again in the evenings. Finally child guidance clinics deal with those children who suffer from behaviour or other psychological disorders and schools for the maladjusted are also provided. Chronically sick children can be both nursed and educated in their homes and the deprived or illegitimate child is catered for by foster parents or adoption societies and voluntary agencies such as the Dr Barnardo's Homes. For the severely mentally handicapped training schools and sheltered workshops are provided.

While this list is by no means complete, it gives some idea of the many-sided care which assures maximum mental and physical health for our children and helps to produce citizens capable of supporting themselves and living happy and useful lives, not withstanding their difficulties.

Immunization and Vaccination

In Great Britain all immunization is voluntary and the Government relies on the effect of propaganda and health teaching by posters and through personal contacts from family doctors, health centres and schools. Good knowledge of the advantages and possible dangers of immunization and vaccination and a good personal approach will set the minds of most mothers at rest and convince them of the value of these protective measures for their children.

It is now possible to offer to children a substantial measure of protection against measles, diphtheria, whooping cough, smallpox, tetanus and poliomyelitis.

The necessary injections can be given either at the local child health clinics or by the family doctor. It is usual to give three injections, at the age of 3, 5 and 9 months to protect against diphtheria, tetanus and whooping cough. Most clinics now use the oral vaccine for poliomyelitis. This involves giving three doses, each of three drops, at intervals of about 4 to 8 weeks.

Enforcement doses of oral polio vaccine, diphtheria and tetanus vaccine are recommended when the child starts school.

It is useful to issue a card to every child which can easily be produced in case of an accident, showing an up-to-date record of tetanus immunization and reinforcing injections.

Smallpox vaccination if done in infancy can give protection for some years and lays a foundation on which to build up immunity by further vaccination later in life. In the United Kingdom routine vaccination of children against smallpox is no longer recommended because of the possible, if small risk of complications. These risks include post-vaccinial encephalitis in the very young infant and generalized vaccinia. Infants with eczema must never be vaccinated, nor should eczematous babies be allowed to be in contact with others recently vaccinated as they might develop eczema vaccinatum by such contact. Children who have been vaccinated, should be given enforcement doses, when they start school and at school-leaving age.

Vaccination against measles is carried out during the second year of life (measles is uncommon before the age of 12 months). It gives substantial measure of protection. One injection is sufficient and by that time immunization for diphtheria, tetanus and whooping cough will have been completed.

Diphtheria is now so little known in the United Kingdom that mothers who are ignorant of the terror of this disease frequently need some persuasion before they consent to immunization. This loophole in the immunization programme may lead to occasional outbreaks of the disease with tragic results.

Rubella. A live, attenuated vaccine is now available and is offered to young girls in one injection prior to the menarche. The dangers to the fetus, should a woman contract rubella during the first 3 months of pregnancy, are well known.

BCG vaccination against tuberculosis is not a routine procedure in the United Kingdom, but BCG (Bacillus Calmette-Guérin) is now available to infants exposed to tuberculosis and children who remain negative to tuberculosis tests at the age of 12 to 13 years. They can be given substantial protection for several years by BCG injection of live, attenuated bovine mycobacterium tuberculosis. This produces a benign type of tuberculosis and a relative immunity in the inoculated child (for further details see p. 422).

Further Reading

ILLINGWORTH, R. S. (1968) *The Normal Child; Some Problems of the First Five Years*, 4th ed. Edinburgh and London: Churchill Livingstone.

MITCHELL, R. G. (1970) *Child and Health*, 5th ed. Edinburgh and London: Churchill Livingstone.

WINNICOTT, D. W. (1969) *The Child, The Family and the World Outside*. Harmondsworth: Penguin.

2

Infant feeding

THE NORMAL infant approximately doubles his weight in the first 5 months of life and trebles his weight in the first year. In order to meet the demands of this rapid growth rate, the nutritional requirements of protein, carbohydrate, fats, vitamins, minerals and fluids must be met either by breast-feeding or by artificial feeding.

Breast feeding

All mothers should be encouraged to breast feed their babies for a minimum of 2 weeks and preferably for the first 4 to 6 months. Breast-feeding is nature's way of establishing close physical and emotional contact between mother and baby as well as providing all the nutritional requirements for growth and development. Other advantages of breast-feeding include the avoidance of hypocalcaemic tetany and convulsions, which may occur if the baby is fed on cow's milk. It is also reported that when epidemics of gastro-enteritis occur and such epidemics are by no means rare, the incidence of infection and mortality are lower in the breast-fed infant. In the developing countries breast-feeding offers the only chance of survival for many infants.

In order for breast feeding to be a success, it is important that the details of breast feeding are discussed with parents antenatally. Good teaching and patience on the part of midwives and health visitors will also be required during pregnancy and post-natally for breast feeding to become well established. This may take as long as 14 days, during which time the mother may become anxious and so worried as to give up the attempt.

Undue stress on the importance of breast-feeding may, however, cause feelings of guilt if the mother is unable to manage this for any reason. The nurse advising the mother should know the family circumstances and whatever the mother's choice of feeding she should be well supported with advice and guidance.

Management of Breast Feeding

In the management of successful breast-feeding, of first importance is a peaceful, confident attitude on the part of the mother. She should if possible feel unhurried and relaxed. Her position needs to be completely comfortable, and a low or easy chair with suitable footstool can be of great assistance in achieving this. The mother should hold the baby comfortably in her arm, but support from a pillow may be necessary to avoid fatigue.

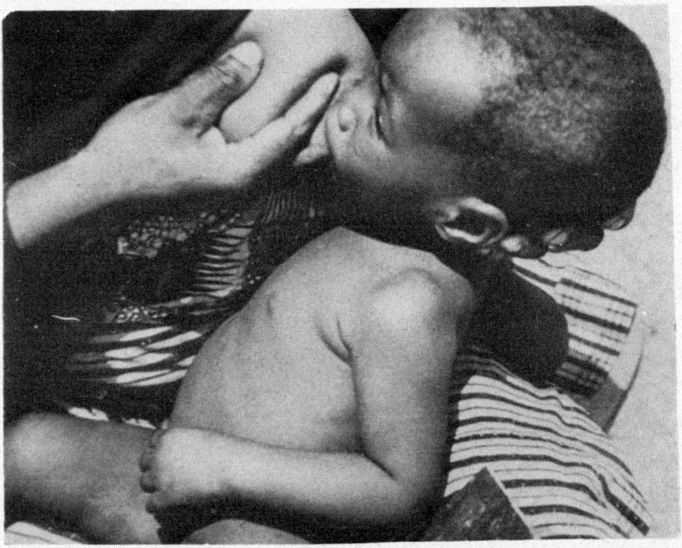

FIG. 2. Feeding position. The baby is held snugly against his mother with his head supported and his hands free. The nipple is guided by the fore and middle fingers (thumb and forefinger are also suitable) so as to prevent the breast falling over the baby's nose.

The baby must be allowed to play with the breast and nipple before starting to suck as this acts as an excellent stimulus to milk flow. A little milk squeezed from the nipple may cause a baby who is slow to realize that he is expected to suck to take the nipple into his mouth and start to feed. He should always be allowed to take the whole nipple and areola into his mouth or sucking may give the mother pain and cause sore nipples. The baby will also obtain less milk if he takes only the tip of the nipple into the mouth.

The baby should be put to the breast at regular intervals up to seven times in 24 hours from the age of 1 day, reduced to five times daily at the age of 2 months. If the baby is hungry after a feed a complement of an artificial feed may be given to satisfy him. Even a short period of breast-feeding is worth while.

Mothers with poor lactation can be helped by stimulating the flow of milk by hot and cold bathings before starting to feed, by breast massage, by adequate support from a good brassiere and by drinking plenty of fluids. Adequate washing and drying of the nipples will prevent them from cracking—a very painful condition for the mother which will interfere with successful breast-feeding. The mother's general nutrition and state of health may need some attention as conditions such as anaemia or inadequate protein intake will produce poor lactation and fatigue, making breast-feeding a burden instead of being one of the greatest experiences in a mother's life.

Artificial Feeding

If breast-feeding is not possible the artificial milk feeds given to the baby should approximate to the composition of breast milk as nearly as is practicable. The success of infant-feeding is assessed by the rate of growth. During the first few days of life the infant loses weight owing to the passage of meconium and urine, the drying of the umbilical cord and the poor feed intake during this period. But, by the end of a fortnight birthweight is regained. For the next 3 months the infant gains on average 170 g per week.

For the purpose of estimating the average feed requirements of a baby, it is necessary to know his expected weight, that is the weight he should be. It is useless to feed an underweight baby according to his actual weight as in this way he will never achieve his expected weight.

To Calculate Expected Weight of Infant

1. Take infant's birth weight.
2. After initial loss this should be regained by 10 to 14 days.
3. From 2 weeks to 3 months infant should gain 170 g per week.

Calorie* Requirements in 24 hours

	Per kilogram of body weight in 24 hours
Premature infants (up to 2.5 kg)	130–150
Underweight infants	130–140
Normal infants	110–120

Fluid Requirements in 24 hours

Premature infants (up to 1.4 kg)	250 ml
1.4 to 2.5 kg	220 ml
Infants over 2.5 kg	150–200 ml

Number of Feeds in 24 hours

Up to 1.4 kg	2-hourly feeds × 10
Up to 2.5 kg	3-hourly feeds × 7
2.5 to 3 kg	4-hourly feeds × 6
3 kg upwards	4-hourly feeds × 5

Example to Calculate Feed for Baby John

John's age	3 months
Birth weight	3.4 kg
170 g gain for (12 minus 2) weeks = 170 g × 10 =	1.7 kg
Expected weight is	5.1 kg

* Instead of measuring the energy value of foods in Calories there is a tendency to be correctly scientific and measure it in joules. Conversion is relatively easy if one remembers that approximately 4·2 joules = 1 calorie and 4·2 kilojoules = 1 kilocalorie (which is the large Calorie used in dietetics).

N.B. John's actual weight is 4.95 kg and so he is a little underweight.

(Remember that the aim is to feed to the expected weight for age.)

Calorie Requirements for Baby John

5.1 kg × 115 ml = 586 Calories in 24 hours

Fluid Requirements for Baby John

5.1 kg × 175 ml = 893 ml in 24 hours

Number of Feeds in 24 hours

4-hourly × 5 = 180 ml per feed
Each feed containing 120 Calories
30 ml contains 20 Calories

(Calculations taken to the nearest whole number.)

Artificial feeds should in making up, be reconstituted to equal (as far as possible) the calorific value of human milk (20 Calories per 30 ml).

Choice of Artificial Feeds

In this country there are many types of artificial feeds available and all, except a few, derive from cow's milk.

The percentage composition of human milk and cow's milk compare as follows:

	Human milk		*Cow's milk*	
Protein	1.5	casein 0.5 lactalbumin 1.0	3.3	casein 2.7 lactalbumin 0.4 lactoglobulin 0.2
Fat	3.8		3.8	
Carbohydrate	7.0 (lactose)		4.8	

The chief difference as shown between human milk and cow's milk is the fact that cow's milk contains six times as much casein as does human milk. Cow's milk therefore is likely to cause large indigestible curds to form in the infant's stomach. Although this could at least partly be remedied by diluting the milk, this would also mean diluting all the other constituents as well.

In order to make cow's milk suitable for babies the milk should be modified to achieve the following changes:

A reduction in the excess amount of casein;
A breaking up of the casein so as to render it more easily digestible;
A reduction in the amount of fat;
An increase in the amount of carbohydrate to the amount contained in human milk.

The usual methods of modifying are:

Heating to boiling point to make the casein curd more digestible and finer;
Dilution with water;
Drying the milk to produce a milk powder;
Skimming the milk (up to 80 per cent of fat can be skimmed off after the milk has been allowed to stand for some time);
The addition of sugar to increase the carbohydrate content.

Dried Milk. There are certain advantages in using dried rather than fresh cow's milk or condensed milks. Dried milk is easy to obtain and easy to store, less liable to bacterial contamination, simple to make up and constant in composition and the drying process has already modified the milk. With some preparations sugar has to be added. There are various dried milk preparations to choose from; but basically they are either:

1. Half-cream milk;
2. Full-cream milk;
3. Preparations of dried milk where the cow's milk has been altered to make it more like human milk, so that it contains less protein and more sugar than untreated cow's milk.

For the young infant up to the age of 6 months, a small but definite risk of hypernatraemia and neonatal tetany associated with the use of unmodified milks is identifiable and undisputed. The risk results from their high concentrations of phosphate and sodium. The risk is greatest in the first weeks after birth and gets progressively less with age. The risk is also increased if for any reason the baby is dehydrated.

Proprietary brands of modified baby milks suitable for feeding to infants under 6 months old include:

Cow and Gate Baby Milk Plus;
Cow and Gate Premium Baby Food;
C & G V Formula;
Osterfeed;
Ostermilk Complete Formula;
New Improved Formula Ostermilk 2;
S M A Gold Cap;
S M A Liquid;
S M A Regular Powder.

They are available to hospitals in a ready to feed form under the same brand names with the exception of New Improved Formula Ostermilk 2 and S M A Regular.

It is important always to remember that feeds should never be given in greater concentration than full strength (each reconstituted 30 ml = 20 Calories) as there is a risk that the level of sodium chloride in the blood will increase excessively with consequent danger of injury to the brain.

If sugar is being added to the feed this should be reduced if the baby has loose stools or a sore anus until the condition has improved. If the baby, however, is constipated demerara sugar may be added for its aperient value instead of granulated sugar.

Crying often implies thirst or over-heating rather than hunger; thirst is better quenched with boiled water than additional milk. Never give cereals to the young crying baby; it may be necessary to add up to 30 per cent more water to a feed (or give separately as water) before the baby's thirst is satisfied.

Evaporated Milk. Evaporated milk is easy to buy and to mix, but it is bulky for the mother to carry from the clinic or the shop. Once the tin has been opened it is liable to bacterial contamination and its use is not advisable in homes where the standard of domestic hygiene is poor. It should not be given to infants under the age of 6 months.

Fresh Cow's Milk. Fresh cow's milk is bulky and will not keep long without refrigeration especially during the summer months. It is also easily contaminated with pathogenic bacteria. Digestive disturbances are more common than if the baby is fed on modified milks. For these reasons the use of fresh milk is inadvisable unless there is absolutely no alternative available.

If fresh cow's milk has to be used it should be boiled and cooled rapidly. During the first few months diluted milk in gradually increasing strengths should be offered until the baby is able to digest full-strength milk, usually by the age of 5 to 6 months. Vitamin additions must always be given, and the deficiency of iron in cow's milk made up by the introduction of a weaning diet at the age of 4 to 6 months.

Whatever the mother's choice of artificial milk preparation following advice and help from the nurse and doctor, she should understand thoroughly how to prepare and mix the feed. It is never advisable to change from one preparation to another unless there is good reason. Frequent changes are likely to cause digestive disturbances in some infants and should never be advocated in the treatment of colic, teething, vomiting, diarrhoea or failure to thrive, without medical advice.

Other Basic Dietary Needs of Infants

Iron. This mineral is stored in the liver of the fetus from the thirteenth to fortieth week of the pregnancy and is usually sufficient for the baby until he takes a weaning diet containing iron. However, in a premature infant the liver store of iron is often much less than in the full-term infant, and therefore it is advisable that iron supplements are given to all premature infants after 3 to 6 weeks of life.

Iron can be administered orally and is best given in the first 30 ml of a feed in a separate bottle, to ensure the full amount of iron is taken, even if some of the remaining feed is left. Many dried milks and some evaporated milks have additional vitamins and iron, care should be taken not to give added vitamins in excess of the essential daily dose, or a serious state of hypercalcaemia may occur.

Recommended Daily Vitamin Supplements

Vitamin A	2000 International Units
Vitamin C	20 to 25 mg
Vitamin D	400 International Units

The vitamin A and D preparations in the form of oily drops should be put either directly onto the tongue, or on the outside of the teat before the baby starts to feed, since, if added to the feed, the oil will coat the bottle and the infant will fail to get the vitamins intended for him.

Vitamin C may be given as orange juice, rose hip syrup, blackcurrant juice or as ascorbic acid tablets. The juices should be diluted with the recommended amount of boiled water and given between feeds. The use of sweetened comforter feeding bottles, reservoir feeding bottles and dummies that have been dipped in vitamin C syrups should be avoided as there is evidence to suggest that this practice is related to dental caries in very young children.

Vitamin additives should be given from the age of 2 weeks and should be continued for at least 2 years.

The Milk-Room or Feed-Kitchen

Children's hospitals and units usually have a special room set aside for preparing artificial milk-feeds.

As feeds are made up in bulk and therefore the risk of bacterial contamination is very real, scrupulous attention should be given to the cleanliness of this room. The ventilation must be efficient and safeguards taken to prevent the entry of flies and bluebottles. No one should be allowed into the milk-room whilst feeds are being prepared. Gowns and headwear to cover all the hair should be worn by those making up the feeds.

The room should be so planned that all bottles and equipment required are cleaned and sterilized before the feeds are prepared. Feeds are then normally prepared to cover a 24-hour feeding schedule. As feeds are being prepared in larger quantities than in the home both the dried powder and the sugar should be carefully weighed before mixing with measured amounts of sterile water. The milk mixture is then divided into individual bottles, labelled, pasteurized (or autoclaved) then refrigerated until required.

Preparation of an Individual Feed

After setting out the utensils required, i.e. spoon, whisk, spatula, graded glass measure, funnel, mixing-bowl or jug and a small strainer, on to a clean Formica-type surface the nurse should again wash her hands.

The milk powder according to the amount required is measured into a bowl. The measure provided by each manufacturer is correct for that particular product only and should not be used with other brands, since there are small differences between the measures. A measured amount of sugar is then added and boiled water is poured from the glass measure a little at a time into the bowl whilst stirring vigorously to avoid lumps forming. The amount is then strained carefully via a funnel into the bottle which is then capped.

The Ready-to-Feed Concept

Recent years have seen the introduction of pre-packed feeds ready for use. Many hospitals have found the use of these feeds economical, much more convenient and labour saving as their use avoids the need to staff milk-rooms for routine bulk-feed preparation.

Most hospitals using this method use one brand of feed only to avoid confusion. The pre-packed feed is available in half-cream and full-cream strengths and usually provided in disposable 120-ml bottles. Sterile screw-type teat units are provided to fit the top of each bottle (Fig. 3). Although these teat units can be disposed of after each feed, in practice it is more economical for each infant to keep his own teat unit. In between feeds the teat is placed in a solution of hypochlorite, the teat can then be replaced as necessary or disposed of when the infant is discharged home.

The feed of one or two bottles according to the infant's requirements are taken to the cot-side with the special bottle-opener which should be boiled daily. The bottle top is removed and the teat unit screwed on to the bottle and the correct volume

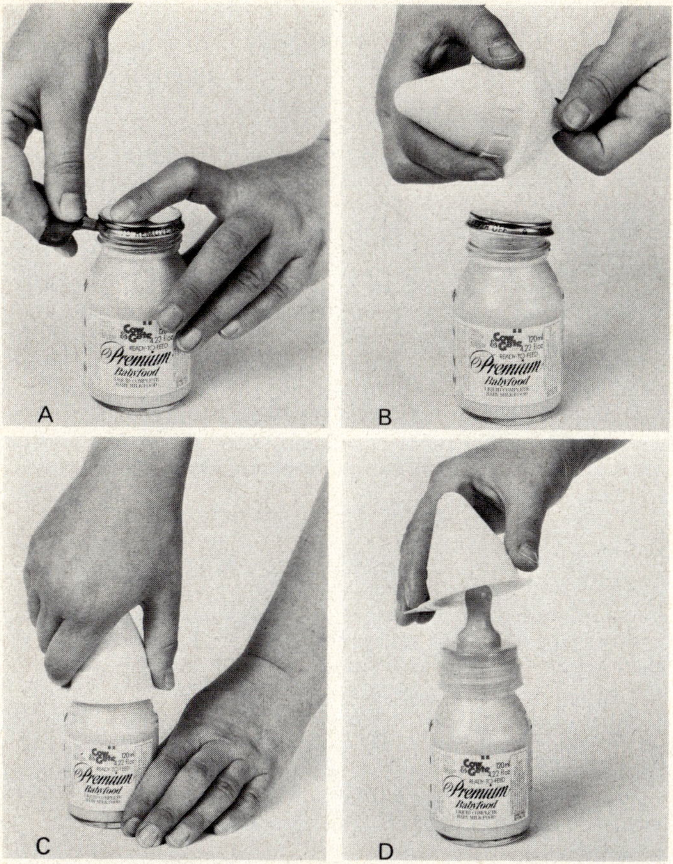

FIG. 3. Sterile pre-packed feeds. (A) Shake the bottle thoroughly and loosen the cap by twisting the opener provided below the rim. Do not remove the cap completely at this stage. (B) Hold the retaining ring of the teat unit firmly through the cover. Strip the paper seal from the base and continue to hold the retaining ring firmly without removing the cover. (C) Lift the cap from the bottle and screw on the teat unit in a clockwise direction until the unit is tightly in place. (D) When ready to feed, remove the plastic cover from the teat unit taking care that the fingers do not come in contact with the teat. If the feed has been heated check the temperature by shaking a few drops on to the wrist. Any unused portion of the milk feed must be disposed of with the bottle.

fed to the infant as ordered. The teat unit is then removed, rinsed under cold water and cleaned with salt, then returned to the solution of hypochlorite in a small plastic container. The remaining feed is discarded, the bottle rinsed and returned to the ward kitchen where it is stored in an empty feed carton. Sterile pre-pack feeds can be fed at room temperature, or can be warmed before the top is removed.

Sterile pre-pack feeds can be kept for 3 to 6 months at room temperature.

For infants requiring very small feeds when it would be wasteful to use the 120-ml bottles, these can be prepared in the milk-room where 25-ml feeds can be pipetted automatically into special miniature bottles. Some maternity units use the 'Redifeed System', this method allows the nurse in the ward area using a portable unit to obtain small measured feed quantities. This completely enclosed mixing and dispensing system reduces the risk of bacterial contamination from external sources.

Bottles

There are many types of bottle obtainable but the most commonly used is the upright, heat resistant glass bottle. The upright type is easy to store and to handle, but it is not always easy to clean. The wider neck type of upright bottle has the advantage that it is easy to fill and much more easily cleaned although it is more expensive. The boat-shaped bottle is not so readily available now, but its advantage is that this can be flushed through easily in the cleaning process. Plastic bottles are also available with narrow or wide necks, but these tend to discolour after several weeks of use and look unsightly.

Teats

It is often a good idea to experiment with teats to find the one to suit the particular infant's needs best. A strong rubber teat is good for babies who suck strongly and is obtainable in three sizes of hole: small, medium and large. The softer teat with airflow is helpful for babies with a poor sucking reflex but has only one size of hole which may need enlarging and the teat becomes flattened if the sucking is too strong. Long-lasting silicone teats are available that fit any sized neck bottle but these have the disadvantage of being expensive.

Nurses in training should never tamper with holes in teats, as only an experienced person knows the optimum size of hole and rate of flow for each baby. If a hole requires enlarging it should always be done with a heated needle and never by using scissors which ruins a teat and causes the feed to flow too quickly and therefore risks choking the baby.

Sterilization

The sterilization of equipment can be carried out by boiling, autoclaving or immersion in a hypochlorite solution, e.g. Milton 1:80 for $1\frac{1}{2}$ hours. But the success of any of these methods is entirely dependent upon thorough cleanliness before sterilization in order to completely remove all traces of milk curd and fat.

Bottles will be easier to clean if each one is rinsed after use and filled with cold water. The use of hot water for this purpose will congeal the milk protein and make the bottle very difficult to clean, teats should also be rinsed immediately after use and some cold water squeezed through the holes.

Later the bottles can be washed using a soapless or detergent cleaner, hot water and a bottle brush and then sterilized. Teats should be rubbed inside and out with salt to remove any milk deposits, thoroughly rinsed in cold water before sterilizing.

If the hypochlorite method of sterilizing is used, it is important to remember that the solution must be changed every 24 hours. There is no need to rinse the solution off equipment, bottles or teats before re-use.

Feeding the Infant

Whenever possible the baby should be taken out of the cot for feeding, and held, comfortably wrapped, in the nurse's arms. He should have been changed recently and the napkin placed in a completely covered receptacle or plastic bag. The hands should be washed again before feeding commences.

Feeding time should be used as an opportunity for cuddling and physical contact which plays an important part in any infant's development but is particularly important for the baby deprived of his mother if she is unable to be with him.

The bottle should be held at a sufficiently steep angle to keep the teat constantly filled with milk and so prevent the baby from sucking in air. He should be allowed to bring up wind at least once during a feed, but babies who are sick often need to bring up wind very frequently often before starting as well as during the feed.

The teat should, if possible, be the one the baby is accustomed to, and the hole should be of a size which allows him to take his feed without much effort, and yet does not deliver the milk so quickly that he chokes. It is sometimes a good idea to ask the mother to bring the teat she uses at home. Inadequate holes can cause a baby to tire before completing the feed and so he refuses the last few millilitres, or swallows air by sucking hard without effect. Colic, vomiting and restlessness result.

When using an upright bottle it may be necessary to twist the bottle and teat while the baby is sucking, in order to allow air to enter and replace the milk, though many babies will let go from time to time and so prevent a vacuum forming, thus solving the problem for themselves.

Babies who are too eager or are underfed tend to gulp the first 60 ml or so, a habit which is likely to result in vomiting. A feed of 30 ml of boiled water before the milk formula is given, or an increase in the milk-feed are two ways of solving this problem. Failure to bring up wind, and excess crying due to hunger or discomfort between feeds may cause air swallowing with distension which may in turn cause vomiting.

A blocked nose can cause quite serious difficulty in feeding and can be one of the most commonly missed reasons for refusal of feeds. The nasal passages may be cleaned by inserting a wisp of cotton wool in the anterior nares, so inducing sneezing, alternatively nasal drops may be prescribed for a short time. Any baby with a blocked nose will take feeds more easily by spoon, as he is unable to breathe adequately with a teat in his mouth.

Bringing Up Wind

It is important to help the baby to bring up his wind, if unnecessary regurgitations, vomiting and colic are to be avoided. The baby should be sat on the nurse's lap, his head and body well supported, or alternatively laid over the nurse's shoulder and his back either rubbed or gently patted. This is comforting to the baby and appears to help in obtaining the desired effect. The principle is of course that of the air bubble which rises in a bottle. All babies swallow air when crying or feeding, and the nurse should not be satisfied until the baby has had at least one good eructation. Babies who cry a lot should be allowed to bring up wind before starting to feed.

Complementary Feeds

Complementary feeds are those offered after breast feeds when these are insufficient. The baby may have been test-weighed to estimate the amount to be offered or he may be offered about two-thirds of his requirements and allowed to please himself.

The technique of sucking from the breast is very different from sucking from a bottle. Many authorities prefer spoon- rather than bottle-feeding when complementary feeds have to be given. The feed should not be sweetened as there is the danger of the baby preferring the artificial feed to the less sweet and less readily obtained breast milk.

Supplementary Feeds

Supplementary feeds are given to replace one or several entire breast feeds per day. This may be done to rest the mother's nipples or because the mother is temporarily absent or indisposed. Once more the feed should be given by spoon in preference to a teat.

Some Feeding Difficulties

Vomiting

There are some babies who vomit more readily than others and this must always be investigated as the small baby can very quickly lose essential water and minerals and become dehydrated.

When describing a vomit, the nurse should always state whether it was forcible or effortless, and when it occurred in relation to the feeds. She should describe the appearance of the vomit, the presence of curds, blood or mucus and the apparent stage of digestion.

There are very many causes for vomiting in infancy, some of which are directly related to feeding including failure to bring up wind adequately, sucking from a teat with too small a hole, gulping a feed too quickly, finger sucking associated with air swallowing. Once pathological causes for vomiting have been excluded the nurse should advise the mother how to remedy any other cause.

Regurgitation and Posseting

This should not be confused with vomiting. In these babies a small amount of the feed is returned as he brings up wind or between feeds. It is rarely of importance, but is often a sign that a little too much feed is being offered.

Ruminating

Ruminating is a very tiresome condition which is difficult to control. The ruminating baby is as a rule 1 to 3 months old, alert, intelligent, and overactive. He appears to enjoy the taste of the regurgitated feed which he brings up in mouthfuls and which he moves around his mouth as though he is 'chewing the cud'. This habit can be very persistent and considerable amounts of nourishment can be lost through it.

The feeds should be thickened with 'Nestargel' which is of particular benefit in this condition and the baby should be placed in a 'Baby Sitta' for 24 hours a day as this will make it less easy for the baby to vomit. Sedation such as chloral should be given at least ½ hour before feeds. Mobiles and other coloured objects should be placed near the baby for him to see easily and to touch, in order that he can be occupied and feel less frustrated and not need to resort to rumination.

Weaning

There are quite considerable differences in the approach to weaning from one society to another, some authorities advocate the introduction of a weaning diet at the age of a few days, whilst others may leave it until much later. The most satisfactory is to introduce mixed feeding at the age of 4½ to 5½ months or when the baby weighs about 7 kg and is no longer satisfied with only milk feeds.

The common practice of introducing a mainly cereal diet is to be avoided as this results in the baby becoming overweight, flabby and often prone to chest infections. Obesity in infants has been shown to lead to obesity in older children and adults.

Additions to the diet should be tried for 2 to 3 days before a further addition is tried, and if the baby obviously dislikes the taste after a few days, the addition should be omitted and tried again later. If the baby is unwell, no new foods should be introduced for fear of upsetting his digestion until he is quite well again.

The additions to the diet should be given with a spoon, and the amounts gradually increased, with a corresponding decrease in the milk-feed. Because of the very poor iron content of milk, iron-containing foods such as eggs, meat, peas and beans should be included in the diet. As the baby becomes accustomed to the mixed diet the times of the feeds can be altered to fit in with the household meal-times if these are most convenient for mother.

There is a large selection of canned foods especially prepared for a weaning diet, but although these are convenient they are expensive and there is no real substitute for freshly cooked food. If canned food is used, but the whole amount not consumed at the one meal, the can or jar should be covered and kept in the refrigerator.

It is important to increase slowly the size of particles from fine pureed mixtures to more lumpy meals in order that the baby gets accustomed to dealing with lumps in his mouth. If for some reason weaning is not achieved over this period, the child may refuse to tolerate any lumpy foods up to the age of 3 to 4 years. At the age of 5 to 6 months a rusk or crust can be given as the baby enjoys biting it when teething.

Suggested Diet for Baby of 6 Months

On waking	Orange juice. Rusk.
08.30 to 09.30 hours	Breakfast: Cereal, Farex, Twinpack. Hen's egg, lightly boiled (only the yolk given), or crisply fried bacon. Bread and butter. Milk 120 to 150 ml to drink from a cup or feeder.
12.00 to 13.00 hours	Finely minced meat, fish, liver or grated cheese with vegetable puree (made with the aid of a Turmix machine or Mouli-mixer) a little mashed potato, and a nourishing gravy or white sauce with fish or cheese. Pureed fruit, custard or milk-pudding. Water or orange juice to drink.
During the afternoon	Biscuit or rusk, milk if desired.
17.00 to 18.00 hours	Farley's Rusk or cereal or custard and jelly. Bread and butter with honey, Marmite or seedless jam. Biscuit or sponge cake (sponge cakes made for trifles can be bought and cut into fingers and are useful as they do not crumble). Full milk-feed (from a bottle or cup).
22.00 to 23.00 hours	Milk-feed from a bottle until such time as the baby no longer wakes for this.

Suggested Diet for a Toddler 16 Months

Breakfast	Cereal or porridge with milk. Toast and butter. Scrambled hen's egg (the whole). Cup of milk.
Mid-morning	Orange juice.

Dinner	Minced beef, mashed potato with mashed carrots. Stewed fruit (without stones) and custard. Water to drink.
Tea	Cheese savoury (with macaroni). Fish with bread and butter. Cake (plain) or biscuit. Milk to drink.

Further Reading

CLOSE, S. (1972) *The Know-How of Infant Feeding,* 3rd ed. Bristol: John Wright & Sons.

GUNTHER, M. (1970) *Infant Feeding*. London: Methuen.

MACKEITH, R. C. & WOOD, C. (1977) *Infant Feeding and Feeding Difficulties*, 5th ed. Edinburgh & London: Churchill Livingstone.

ROBERTS, F. P. (1968) *Breast Feeding*. Bristol: John Wright & Sons.

STANWAY, A. & P. (1975) *Breast is Best*. London: Pan Books.

3

Nursing the newborn

NURSING NEWBORN babies is a great responsibility at all times but even more so when they are premature, feeble or sick. Changes in the infant's condition may be extremely sudden and of urgent importance, and the nurse must be observant and capable of fine judgement and swift action when caring for these babies.

To be a really good baby-ward nurse, considerable knowledge and great experience are essential, coupled with the keenest powers of observation, alertness, integrity and gentleness. Only the nurse who knows the normal, can appreciate the often slight, but always important, deviations from it and she needs to be the kind of person who will always stop and enquire thoroughly into the reason for such a change. Speed may be life-saving in infancy and even an hour's delay in seeking medical aid or advice may entail disaster. Initiative, too, is a great asset in dealing with sick babies and may often save a life. On the other hand an experienced baby nurse knows that masterly inactivity may sometimes be the most appropriate way of dealing with a sick baby. This applies in particular to the immature infant and to cerebral babies. Neatness and toilet routine may be of secondary importance to undisturbed rest and doing too much may be as fatal as neglect.

General Points

For the nursing of sick babies the cot should be large enough to allow for all procedures to be carried out with ease and for adequate observation of the infant without necessarily coming close up to the cot. No baby under the age of 1 year should be given ordinary pillows on account of the danger of suffocation. Small firm pillows may be built up armchair fashion in special cases or where orthopnoea is present. The head of the mattress can also be raised by placing a pillow underneath it, or the head end of the cot can be raised on specially designed hooks. The majority of babies are best nursed lying flat. At the head end the bottom sheet can be protected by a piece of plastic sheeting covered by a small pillowcase. This is neat and allows for easy and frequent change of linen if it becomes soiled by mucus, secretions or vomit. Babies who have to be nursed in an upright position can be helped by a rolled-up napkin placed underneath their thighs like a knee pillow. If this is slipped under the macintosh and napkin the baby is sitting on, with the distal end doubled around it, the baby will be effectively prevented from slipping. Young babies should always be allowed as much freedom to move around and kick as is compatible with their condition.

Nurses working with sick babies soon learn the significance of their cry. The causes may be manifold, for example hunger and thirst, loneliness, fear of the dark, discomfort from cold or heat, colic, teething, excessive wind, tight clothing or a soiled napkin. The cause should always be found and dealt with. It is erroneous to contend that it is good for a baby to cry for long periods and the danger that a bad habit will be formed if the baby is picked up when he cries, has probably been exaggerated. Some authorities maintain that, if the child is given the security, comfort and love he is asking for at the infant stage, he will grow into an easier, less demanding personality in later life. Research and experiments have also shown that the close bond between mother and child which is necessary to the mental health and happiness of every human being, is established in the first days after birth. The mother has been said 'literally to fall in love' with her baby in the first 2 or 3 days, a process which cannot be delayed or it will never really take place. The seriousness of having to deprive a baby of this experience for reasons of illness or prematurity cannot be over-estimated. Mothers have been known to be unable to establish the same feelings for their sick or premature infants nursed in special units as for their other children with whom they have been able to have regular physical contact soon after birth. The conclusions to be drawn from these findings are obvious and it is for the nurses to see that such a situation is avoided if at all possible.

Taking an Infant's Temperature

Every infant must have his own thermometer. Infants may have a very low temperature and in these cases special low reading thermometers are used. They record temperatures as low as 29.4°C (85°F). Thermometers with short, rounded bulbs are supplied for taking rectal temperatures. Oral and skin temperatures are not usually suitable for infants. They have little subcutaneous tissue and friction from slight movement may give a false reading. Infants are of course too young to have the thermometer placed in the mouth. If a skin temperature is taken, this is best done in the groin after carefully drying the skin. Occasionally it is convenient to leave the thermometer in the groin while feeding the infant. When taking a rectal temperature the anal region is cleansed and dried with a swab and the bulb of the thermometer carefully inspected and then lubricated with some petroleum jelly applied on a piece of old linen (thermometers should preferably not be dipped into the lubricant as the bulb might break; this might go unnoticed because of the petroleum jelly covering). A broken bulb can cause painful abrasions in the rectal mucosa. The baby should be lying on his cot or on the nurse's knee, his legs are raised, the thermometer inserted and the buttocks held together with the thumb and fingers either side, the thermometer being steadied between the first and second fingers as one would hold a cigarette. Alternatively the baby can lie on his side. Once the child is over one year old it is undesirable for psychological reasons, to take temperatures rectally.

Taking the Pulse

Both pulse and respiration are taken while the infant is asleep or resting and before he is disturbed or the cot-side lowered. In small infants it is often difficult to feel the radial pulse. Alternative methods are: feeling the pulse over the temporal artery immediately in front of the ear or over the external iliac or the femoral artery in the groin, or to count the pulsating movements of the fontanelle.

Bathing a Sick Baby

In the United Kingdom most babies are bathed on the mother's or nurse's lap. Everything should be prepared and conveniently arranged before the baby is disturbed. A plastic and a Turkish towelling apron, reserved for each individual baby, are worn to protect the nurse's gown and uniform.

The bath temperature should always be checked with a thermometer and the water should be approximately 40°C (104°F) when first prepared. It will have cooled to 37.2° to 37.8°C (99° to 100°F) by the time the baby is ready to be lowered into it. The hot water tap should be movable and should swing to the side to avoid water dripping on to the baby.

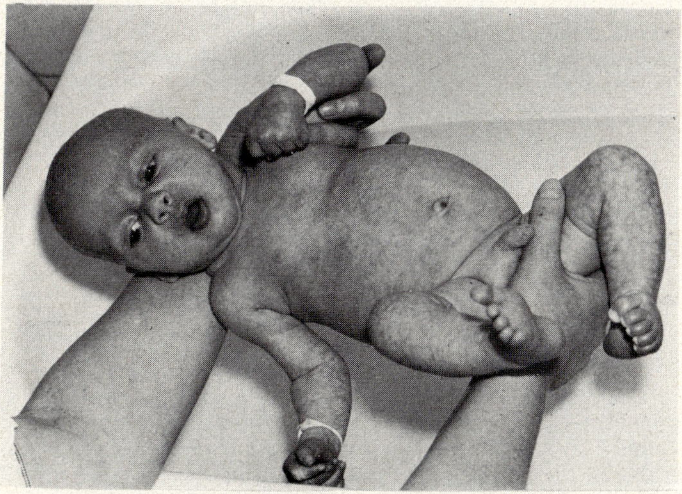

FIG. 4. A good way of holding a baby while lowering him into his bath.

After taking the pulse and respirations the baby is lifted from his cot, his clothes taken off and a bath towel securely wrapped around him. After washing her hands the nurse swabs his eyes with sterile cotton wool and water from within outwards, using each swab once only. In some country areas where the water supply is of doubtful purity, a bowl of boiled water should be ready for swabbing the eyes. The face is then washed, and dried with plain water and cotton wool. None of the orifices, such as mouth, nose or ears, are cleaned. Should special cleansing be necessary, this is considered a treatment and not part of the daily toilet. Next the head is washed, holding the baby over the bath water. The scalp should be made thoroughly wet before applying soap and then thoroughly rinsed, as soap left on the hair is a common cause of seborrhoeic dermatitis. On account of the wide open fontanelle the washing and drying should be done with great care and gentleness. The napkin is next taken off and the infant's buttocks washed. He is placed on a clean square of non-absorbent cotton wool or cellulose while his temperature is taken. Care is taken not to expose the baby unnecessarily. In hospital, babies are frequently weighed daily and this is now done, though the scales will have been tested before disturbing the baby. Returning the baby on to her lap, the nurse now soaps him with her own soapy hands, carefully including all skin folds and the palms of the baby's hands. Weak or sickly babies are best not rolled on to their stomachs too often, as milk is easily regurgitated. The back can be soaped by raising the shoulders and the buttocks in turn. As both the nurse's hands and the baby's body are slippery he must be very securely held when lowering him into the bath (Fig. 4). Care should also be taken not to allow the head to drop backwards. Babies should enjoy their bath and should be allowed a few moments kicking time in the water.

In lifting the baby back on to her lap the nurse may roll him *towards* herself into the prone position. (This is the only time the child should be rolled.) The skin is well dried. A soft towel should be available and dabbing movements are preferable to rubbing the infant down. It is preferable to avoid the use of talcum powders in the care of young infants.

The vest and previously folded napkin are now placed over the infant's back before he is turned over. In doing this the towel is brought out and the baby comes to lie on the dry apron. The baby is now dried in front and again great care should be taken to dry the skin folds thoroughly. The remaining clothes are then put on and the nails and hair attended to. The total procedure should take no more than 15 minutes.

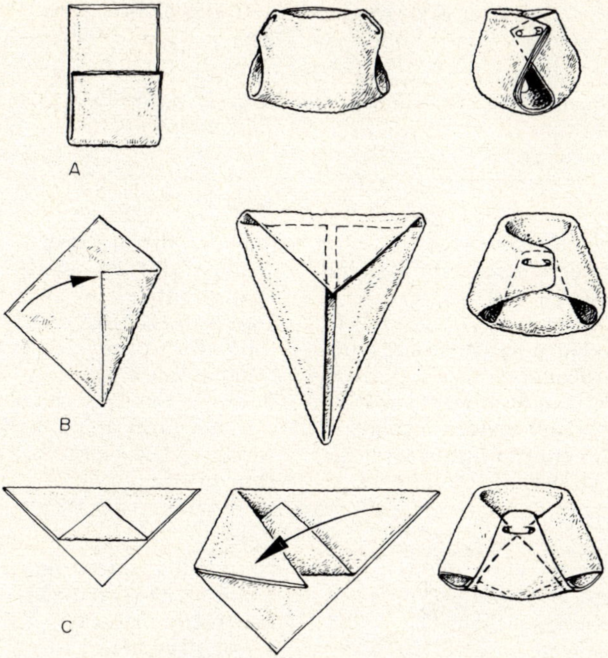

FIG. 5. Various ways of folding napkins.

Increasingly, disposable napkins are being used, with some types special pants are worn. Whatever the type or method of putting the napkin on in all cases the safety pin should lie horizontally in order to minimize any risk of injury should it accidentally become undone (Fig. 5).

When discharging a baby home the mother can be told that a daily bath is desirable but not essential and that it might well be omitted at her discretion should the only room available not be well heated at times.

Sore buttocks in the newborn may originate from a variety of causes, the most common of which are frequent loose stools, 'strong' ammoniacal urine, excessive fat in the feeds, careless or

List of Requirements for Bathing a Sick Baby

For the nurse

Plastic apron. Towelling apron.
Special gown.
A table or special trolley for requirements.

For the bath

Bath thermometer.
Water temperature initially 40.6°C (105°F).
Pure soap.
Boiled water in sterile container.
Sterile cotton wool swabs.
Zinc and castor-oil cream.
12.5 cm (5 in) squares non-absorbent cotton wool.
Rectal thermometer with moist and dry swabs and lubricant.
Two buckets or receivers with lid, for soiled clothes and napkins.
Baby scales protected by tissue paper and a napkin.
A pair of fine nail scissors.
Hair brush.

For the baby

Bath towel.
Vest and open gown.
Woollen jacket.
Bootees.
Napkin and safety pin.
Small blanket or shawl.
In exceptional cases mittens (see page 61).

For dressing the umbilical cord if not left exposed

Sterile pack for umbilical dressing.
Sterile cord powder.
Crepe bandage.

In most cases the cord is 'tied' with a metal clip which needs no cover and is usually removed after 36 hours.

infrequent toilet and changes of napkins, inadequate rinsing of napkins after washing them in detergent, and unduly sensitive skin. Frequently the distribution of the rash gives a clue to the cause. A urine-soaked napkin will cause a widely distributed rash not only over the genitalia but spreading up to the abdomen and the sacrum and down to the thighs, while the skin folds and the natal cleft may be left unaffected. On the other hand, loose or fermented stools cause soreness of the perineum, around the anus and the back of the scrotum.

Intertrigo is a variant of napkin rash, which causes much soreness particularly in the groins and flexures. Intertrigo may also appear in the folds of the neck and is as a rule seen in fat and ill-kept babies. The soreness is caused by contact of two moist skin surfaces which are cut off from the air and gradually infected. Careful hygiene and drying and the use of dusting powder is the only treatment required.

The *treatment of sore buttocks* varies according to the preference of those in charge and to the cause of the soreness. Dietary errors should be investigated and corrected. Ammonia dermatitis may be due either to a low fluid intake which is readily put right, or to decomposition of urine when in contact with stools and intestinal bacteria. Frequent changing and careful toilet is the best remedy. The practice of sprinkling boracic powder on napkins to prevent 'burning' from ammonia produced by the decomposition of urine is dangerous. When boracic acid is absorbed, e.g. through broken skin, it is cytotoxic and may cause convulsions, diarrhoea and extensive rashes. Roccal (benzalkonium chloride 1:5000) and NappiSan products, used in the washing of nappies, assist in the prevention of sore buttocks, but the best way both to prevent sore buttocks and also to cure them is by regular washing with plenty of water, adequate drying using a soft towel and dabbing movements, and the use of a good plain dusting powder. Petroleum jelly or zinc oxide cream, either plain or containing castor oil, may be applied. Babies suffering from gastro-enteritis are best protected by the application of tulle gras to prevent contact of the stools with the skin. In many cases it is a good plan to expose the infant's buttocks. If this is done, the infant should wear bootees and may have the feet lightly restrained by ankle restrainers. A small blanket covers the feet, another one the body of the infant, while the buttocks are left exposed, resting on a napkin. Draughts are kept off by the use of a bed cradle. Whenever possible the healing properties of sunlight should be utilized.

The Stools of the Newborn Infant

The stools of the newborn infant are at first dark green to black in colour with a shiny appearance and viscid consistency and are known as *meconium*. After 1 to 2 days they gradually change to lighter ones and are then called *changing stools*. The stools of breast-fed babies are a golden mustard colour and of soft consistency. They have a characteristic, slightly sour smell. From one to six stools are passed each day.

The stools of infants fed on any type of cow's milk (whether fresh or dried) are pale yellow, larger in bulk and more formed than those of breast-fed babies. From one to three stools are passed daily. The stools of infants should always be carefully observed for much can be learned from their colour, odour, frequency and consistency. Changes occur readily and may be caused by slight deviation from health, change of the usual feed or amount of fluid intake, or by medicines. When putting up stools for inspection (see Fig. 6) it must be remembered that

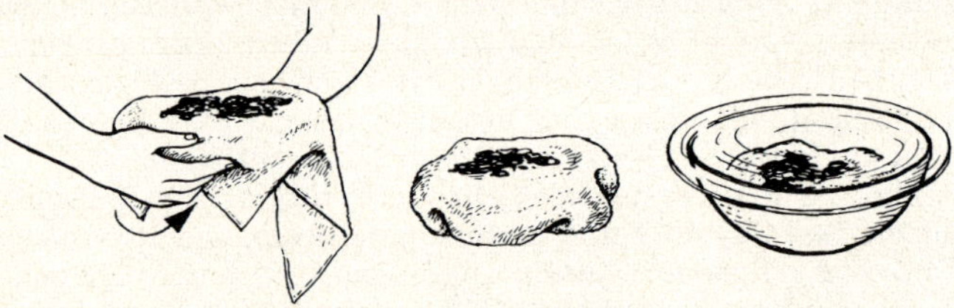

FIG. 6. Preparing a soiled napkin for inspection.

they change colour quickly on the surface. To get a true picture a stool may first have to be broken up.

It sometimes happens that a newborn baby fails to pass meconium in the first 24 to 36 hours. This is an important abnormality and must be reported at once as it may be due to a variety of serious causes such as imperforate anus, meconium ileus and atresia of the bowel.

The Temperature of the Newborn Infant

It is often difficult to maintain a stable temperature in the newborn because the heat-regulating mechanism is still poorly developed and the body surface is large in proportion to the body weight. During the first days it is not uncommon to find a rise in temperature known as *dehydration fever* in cases where the fluid intake is inadequate owing to the slow establishment of lactation. Boiled, plain water or glucose water should be given. Infants do not always respond to infection with a rise of temperature so that absence of pyrexia need not exclude an acute infective condition.

The Weight of the Newborn Infant

Variations in weight are usual and undue importance should not be attached to stationary weight or to slight, occasional losses. A contented baby who sleeps and feeds well, whose colour is good and whose skin looks healthy need not be weighed daily or even weekly. Much anxiety—one of the causes of poor lactation—could be avoided if scales were less frequently used.

Prevention of Infection in Neonatal and Sick Infants' Units

General Points

The younger the child the greater is the risk, from infection, to his immediate and subsequent health. Many of the infections prevalent in infant wards have lost some of their terror since the advent of antibiotics. But undue faith in antibiotics and general complacency are never justified where sick children are concerned, and each time infection and cross-infection occurs, nurses and others in contact with the children should try to discover where a fault in technique may have occurred. These remarks about the newborn may be taken to apply also to older children, although both technique and dangers are modified as the older child has greater resistance to infection. Barrier nursing and general preventive technique must always be of the highest standard when dealing with children whose resistance is already lowered by illness.

At birth the infant possesses few antibodies and the process of building these up takes several years. Some passive immunity is passed on from the mother, as for instance immunity to measles; on the other hand many antibodies, for instance those of whooping cough, do not cross the placental barrier. Infants have, in addition, a poor heat-regulating mechanism and exposure to cold easily causes chills with an attendant lowering of resistance to attack by pathological organisms.

Staphylococcal infections are a particular danger in the new-born, who easily picks up the infection from adults who are carriers (such as the mother, medical and nursing staffs) or from other infants who act as carriers.

Cubicle Nursing

Ideally, sick babies under 1 year should be nursed in separate rooms or cubicles. These should be light, well ventilated and free from draughts. The temperature and humidity should be even and easily regulated. The flooring should have a smooth, easily washed surface and sweeping and high dusting should be done with an efficient vacuum cleaner, lined with a strong paper bag. Dusting should be done with a damp duster and each cubicle or nursery should have separate cleaning materials.

The number of staff allocated to infants' and children's wards is usually high, in order to make a wise allocation of duties, and isolation of infected babies a reality. The number of people in contact with each individual patient should, however, be cut to a minimum, though this should never mean exclusion of the mother. Any person approaching the young, sick child must be free from infection, and the highest standard of personal hygiene, integrity and health is essential for sick children's nurses and medical staff. Where masks are worn, the technique must be absolutely faultless and masks must cover both nose and mouth effectively. They must never be touched. (To take off a mask when talking to a superior is a sign of irresponsibility rather than of courtesy.) When finally taken off, only the strings of the mask should be handled. Masks should be changed every hour and the supply of clean masks should be virtually unlimited. The hands should be washed each time a mask is handled.

Gowns should be used properly and there should be two gowns for use with each infant. These should always be worn when more than the nurses' or other persons' hands come into contact with the baby or any part of his equipment and bed linen (Fig. 7).

Equipment required for toilet purposes, cleaning, treatments or feeding should be reserved for the individual infant. Some such articles are thermometers, washing utensils, powders, creams, towels, stethoscope, tape measure, pencils for charting frequent observations (other charts should be kept outside the cubicle), sphygmomanometer cuffs, and pulsometers. Medicine bottles and bottles containing vitamin preparations should either be handled before entering the cubicle or kept for the individual infant. The empty bottle is disinfected before returning it to the dispensary.

Equipment common to several babies, such as weighing scales and their weights, should be adequately protected using fine tissue paper. They should be thoroughly cleaned at least once a day.

Ideally, three pedal bins should be provided for every cubicle. One for used napkins, one for used clothing and one for bed linen. Where removable lids are used they should always be laid down with the inner side uppermost to avoid contamination of the floor by the soiled side of the lid.

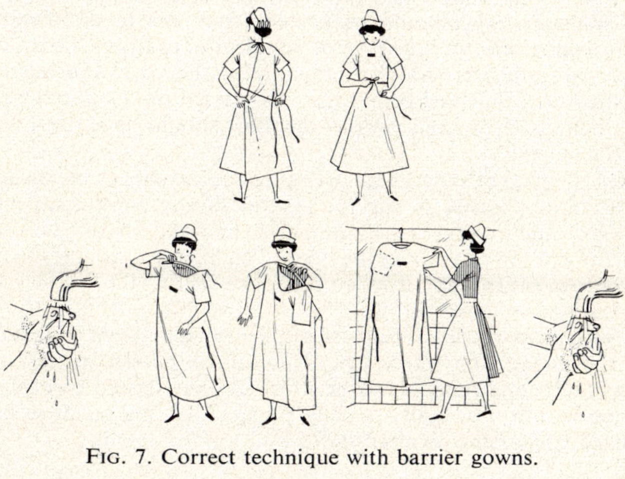

FIG. 7. Correct technique with barrier gowns.

Infectious Babies

Cubicles of infants suffering from infections should be supplied with separate brooms, dust pans, dressing drums and feeding utensils. None of these should be returned to the common storage places, kitchen or milk-room until they have been thoroughly disinfected. In all children's wards crockery and cutlery are boiled after they have been washed. Occasionally sterilization in a solution of electrolytic sodium hypochlorite (Milton solution 1:80 for 1½ hours) can conveniently be substituted for boiling, but since Milton solution corrodes metal, plastic spoons should be used. Similar precautions are taken with washing bowls, tooth mugs, bed pans and pots. When carrying infected equipment, such as bed pans from a cubicle, one hand should be kept clean to touch door handles. Each cubicle should have its own cleaning cloths, mini-mop and bucket.

There should be a liberal supply of soft 'paper wipes' for use as handkerchiefs, and paper bags should be available for their safe disposal by burning and for the safe disposal of all dressings. Disposable plates, beakers, knives, forks and spoons are ideal when carrying out cubicle and other barrier nursing.

Children's toys should be passed from one to another as little as possible, and the toys of infants and toddlers should be reserved exclusively for the individual patient and thoroughly washed or disinfected before they are passed on. Children who are liable to drop their toys on the floor should have them tied to the cot-sides.

On the patient's discharge the entire cubicle should be washed down and allowed to air for several hours. Mattresses and pillows unless covered by macintosh material should be sent for fumigation or aired in the open. The blankets, which should be cotton rather than woollen ones, are sent to the laundry to be boiled.

Napkins and soiled linen should never be allowed to remain in the cubicle or ward. They should be placed in covered receptacles and removed without delay. They should be washed in the laundry, by staff specially engaged for the purpose, not sluiced by nursing or ward staff.

Further Reading

BATES, S. (1971) *Practical Paediatric Nursing*. Oxford: Blackwell Scientific.

CRAIG, W. S. (1969) *Care of the Newly Born Infant*, 4th ed. Edinburgh & London: Churchill Livingstone.

VULLIAMY. D. G. (1967) *The Newborn Child*, 2nd ed. Edinburgh & London: Churchill Livingstone.

4

The low birthweight baby

BY TRADITIONAL, international standards, a baby weighing 2.5 kg ($5\frac{1}{2}$ lb) or less at birth, has always been termed premature. Many babies with a low birthweight, although thought to have been born at or near full term, are wrongly placed in this category. The proper term for them is dysmature, low birthweight babies or small-for-date babies. These infants are at greater risk than truly prematurely born babies and need as much careful and skilled observation and care as premature ones. Both categories are therefore discussed together in this chapter. Infants weighing below 0.9 kg (2 lb) are unlikely to survive but the chances of survival increase in direct proportion to their weight.

The nursing of these babies is a responsible and exacting task and only a brief outline can be given in the pages of a small text book. Approximately 40 000 babies are born prematurely each year in Great Britain. Much research is going on to determine whether prematurely born babies may eventually be expected to reach normal standards and recent reports suggest that past fears may have been greatly exaggerated. It would seem that, all other things being equal, premature infants are likely to have reached satisfactory standards by the age of 4 years.

All human beings need love, physical contact and a sense of security. The low birthweight baby is no exception. As soon as he is independent of continuous oxygen therapy, even if only for a short time, he should be taken out of his cot and nursed. If this is done under first-class nursing conditions the benefit to the infant greatly outweighs the slight risk involved. Nurses caring for premature babies must be exceptionally patient, gentle and observant and should have real devotion and interest for this type of work as much of the responsibility for the infants' health and survival falls on the nursing staff.

Meticulous attention to every detail of observation and technique is essential if a success is to be made of premature baby nursing. The essentials of 'cubicle nursing' are set out in Chapter 3, p. 46 and these apply also for the nursing of low birthweight babies although in their case any carelessness in technique may lead to even more serious consequences than in the nursing of stronger babies. Hand washing, the use of a disinfectant barrier cream such as chlorhexidine (Hibitane), correct mask technique and absolute integrity with regard to personal hygiene and health are essentials. As few people as possible should be allowed to go near the baby (but those few must include the mother) and the infant should be handled as gently and infrequently as is compatible with reasonable care. Fatigue must be avoided by measures such as tube feeding and

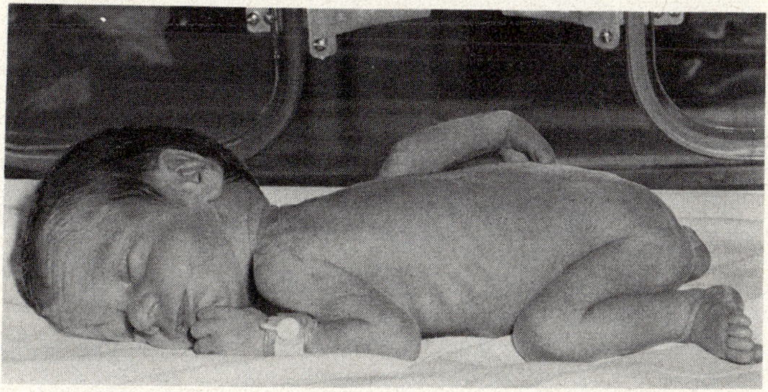

FIG. 8. The normal posture of the premature infant.

by supplying a constant atmosphere, adequate in oxygen, humidity and temperature.

The premature or immature infant presents a number of characteristic features (Fig. 8). His head is large in comparison with the body, the skin is wrinkled and the nails are soft and short. Insulation is poor due to the absence of subcutaneous fat and to the fact that the baby's body surface is proportionately large. Both heat-regulating centre and cough reflex are poorly developed. The body temperature may at first be as low as

32.2°C (89.8°F). The baby may be so feeble as to be unable to expand his lungs or, if the lungs have been expanded, to keep them adequately inflated (*primary and secondary atelectasis*). Due to the general immaturity of the respiratory system the gaseous exchange may be inadequate leading to carbon dioxide retention, respiratory acidosis and low pH. Because of these physiological changes the baby will have greatly increased respirations. These will be shallow and irregular. Coupled with drawing in of the soft chest wall at every breath, this will contribute to the frequency of cyanotic attacks and periods of apnoea so often a problem with these babies. Exhaustion and asphyxia may eventually prove fatal.

In order to enhance safety and to facilitate supervision by the nursing staff, a special 'mattress' known as 'apnoea alarm' is sometimes used. Should breathing stop for a significant length of time, an alarm is set off which alerts the nurse.

Physiological jaundice is more common in the immature baby and is usually more severe and prolonged than in babies born at term. Careful monitoring of serum bilirubin levels must be performed to avoid the danger of kernicterus developing. Recently it has been shown that the use of ultraviolet light reduces the serum bilirubin level. Phototheraphy units are now available that can be easily placed over any incubator or cot. During this treatment the eyes must be kept firmly bandaged to prevent damage to the retina. At frequent, regular intervals and away from the light these bandages should be removed for a short period—it is often most convenient to do this during feeding. The bandages should always be removed and the phototherapy unit switched off when the mother visits.

Intracranial bleeding, or bleeding into the intestinal tract and lungs on the slightest provocation is common, probably due to some abnormality in the clotting properties of the blood. Vitamin K therapy, often necessary in premature babies, is discussed on p. 68.

In the first 2 weeks of life the renal tubules are still immature and unable to cope with the high phosphate load present in cow's milk. Blood calcium levels may therefore fall below the safe level of 2.25 mmol/litre (9 mg/100 ml) causing twitching and even convulsions. Calcium gluconate given first intravenously and then orally, will counteract this complication.

Hypoglycaemia may occur spontaneously due to poor glycogen storage in the liver or in those infants born to diabetic mothers. It is one of the earliest abnormalities a nurse must watch for. Hypoglycaemia may cause cyanotic attacks, convulsions, a high pitched cry and apathy and may lead to brain damage and even death. Serum levels should be estimated 4-hourly with 'Dextrostix' on a blood sample obtained from a heel prick. Treatment should be instituted as a matter of urgency as soon as the serum glucose level falls below 1.1 mmol/litre (20 mg/100 ml) in the low birthweight infant. Frequent feeds are given as well as 10 per cent glucose via scalp vein infusion. Steroid therapy may be necessary. Tests are continued until the serum glucose level is stable at the normal range. Prevention is better than cure, and to avoid hypoglycaemia, early and frequent feeding should be commenced and chilling avoided.

All babies should be examined carefully by a specialist in neonatal care as soon as possible after birth. Prematurely born and low birthweight babies born at term are at even greater risk than normal weight, full-term babies and the tests which help to assess these infants should be applied with the greatest care and expertise. These tests can only be listed here, but nurses dealing with neonates should make it their responsibility to learn the details and understand their significance.

Briefly these tests include the following:

The Moro reflex test
Wrist and ankle flexion
The scarf sign
Heel and ear manoeuvre
Plantar creases
Posture
Head rotation.

General Care

The general care of low birthweight babies follows the lines indicated by their physiological characteristics and their implications. The infant should be kept warm but must never be overheated. Both oxygen requirements and general metabolism are reduced when the temperature is low and these babies often do very well even when their body temperature is as low as 33.8° to 35.5°C (93° to 96°F). A special low reading, 29.4°C (85°F) thermometer is used. If they are nursed in an incubator (Fig. 9), the incubator temperature may be kept at 32°C

(90°F) in order to maintain the infant's temperature at 35° to 36.6°C (95° to 98°F), or if nursed in a cot, the cot temperature can be maintained at a maximum of 32.2°C (90°F) by means of well protected hot-water bottles kept well away from the baby. A useful routine to achieve this is to have three hot-water bottles suspended in pockets in the canvas cot sling and to change one every hour in rotation. The room is kept at a temperature of 21° to 27°C (70° to 80°F). Because these infants lose comparatively much moisture from the large skin surface and through rapid breathing, and because their initial fluid intake is likely to be low, the room humidity should be as high as 60 to 80 per cent, checked by means of a special hygrometer. When an incubator is being used this is easy, but if the baby is nursed in an open cot, the room humidity may have to be raised by using a steam kettle or fine spray nebulizer. Babies who are cyanosed or have repeated periods of apnoea have to be given oxygen. The doctor may intubate the baby and give the oxygen via an endotracheal tube. Alternatively the oxygen may be given intermittently via a mask of the polythene bag type at 0.5 to 1 litre/minute. When oxygen is needed for short periods, until respirations are established after birth, 1 to 2 litres are delivered by means of an incubator. Oxygen must always be given in the minimal effective dosage and for the shortest possible period and if given for any length of time, withdrawn very gradually when no longer needed. The danger of causing blindness from retrolental fibroplasia should always be borne in mind (see p. 85).

The feeble respirations of low birthweight infants can be aided by changing their position every 3 hours, by occasionally slipping a hand beneath the back and gently lifting the thorax so expanding the chest wall, and by nursing the infant naked to avoid impeding the respiration by the weight of clothes. In positioning babies, care must be taken to avoid any kinking of the trachea and no feeble baby should ever be allowed to lie on his back lest he inhale mucus and saliva. The careful use of a mucus extractor is often indicated as both secretions and regurgitated feed are liable to be inhaled. At feeding time the head of the cot is raised but it is lowered during cyanotic attacks and when the airway is being cleared. When a feeble infant requires to be resuscitated, the process should include gentle clearing of the air passages from mucus, feed or liquor and an ordinary mucus catheter may be used to do this. Sometimes the tongue has to be brought forward with a pair of fine tongue forceps of the double pointed type. In severe cases endoscopy is performed and suction carried out under direct vision. A suitable laryngoscope and sucker should always be kept in readiness. Sometimes an airway is secured by performing nasotracheal intubation and by using a mechanical ventilator to maintain respirations. *Artificial respiration* is sometimes needed after clearing the air passages (see p. 54).

The *daily toilet* is reduced to a minimum, as all handling which is not strictly necessary should be avoided. The infant need be weighed only once or twice a week and unless each baby has a pair of scales of his own, the weights and the scales are carefully protected with tissue paper to prevent any risk of cross-infection.

Use of Incubators

Infants of low birthweight or in need of special care should if possible be nursed in an incubator (Fig. 9). The modern incubator is designed to control the environment for the infant and

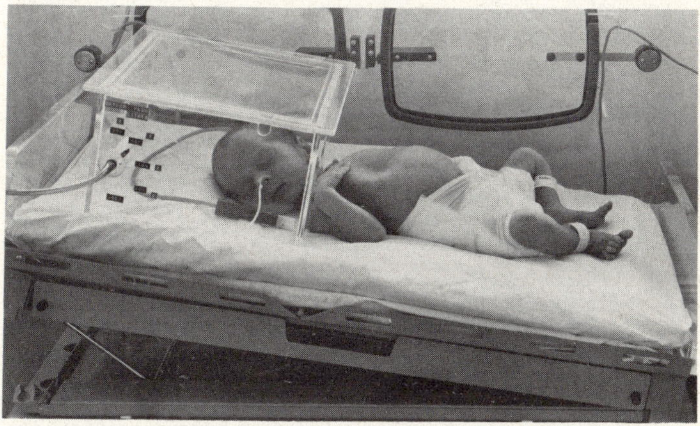

FIG. 9. Premature infant in incubator with head box.

facilitate care without exposing the infant to drastic changes of temperature. Using the incubator will enable the nurse to maintain an environment of moistened filtered air at a controlled temperature set for an individual infant's needs. The oxygen concentration should be carefully monitored to ensure that the level does not rise above 30 per cent concentration.

Special devices are incorporated to set off an alarm system if the incubator becomes over heated.

Incubators should be well maintained and cared for in order to ensure efficiency. When in use the humidity chamber should be replenished daily and the inside of the incubator cleaned with a damp disposable cloth. The incubator should be changed every 5 to 7 days for maintenance and to prevent possible infection.

If the infant cared for in the incubator has an infection, disinfection will be needed after use. Routinely incubators after use should be switched off, chamber drained and all parts washed with hot soapy water and dried. If possible the incubator should be exposed in the fresh air and sunshine for a few hours before re-use after cleaning.

Feeding the Low Birthweight Infant

The feeding of the low birthweight infant has to be varied according to the need of the individual and the methods of the paediatrician and the sister in charge. Great experience is required to find the right balance.

The first feed should be given within 3 hours of birth unless the infant is being fed intravenously. Some paediatricians prefer this first feed to be of 5 per cent dextrose. If the infant is strong enough to suck, he should be put to the breast or bottle-fed. Small frequent feeds are given, gradually increasing the interval between feeds as the infant progresses.

It must be remembered that these small infants tire rapidly and it is a mistake to persevere with bottle-feeding for too long. It is far better to divide the feed and allow a period of rest between each half. Before feeding commences the head of the cot or incubator mattress should be raised and the infant placed on the right side, as in this position regurgitation is least likely to occur. Occasionally the nurse will need to stimulate the sucking reflex for the infant who is a bit lethargic and this is best done by either applying gentle pressure under the chin or by pressing the teat down on to the tongue. The bottle teat should never be twisted in the mouth as this may cause abrasion of the mucous membrane and so predispose to thrush.

However, if the infant is unable to suck, feeding should be via a catheter (polyvinyl English size 4), which for the very small baby is usually left in position between feeds. This catheter should be changed every 5 days and if still required replaced with a new one inserted through the other nostril. Interrupted catheter feeding is an alternative method which is generally used for larger infants (see p. 287). Tube-feeding should always be used in preference to a Belcroy feeder, pipette or spoon, as there is less danger of inhalation. All tube feeds must be given slowly with great care and throughout the procedure the baby must be watched carefully for choking and inhalation. If this occurs the baby must be tilted head-down, the catheter pinched, withdrawn and the pharynx cleared using suction.

The Choice of Food

Every effort should be made for these infants to receive breast milk, but if this is impossible, feeds of one of the modified dried milks should be given as these are less likely to cause neonatal tetany or hypernatraemia (see p. 22). Frequent changes of feed should be avoided as these small infants tolerate such changes badly. If a change is necessary it should be achieved slowly taking several days, so that the baby can adjust to the difference in taste and composition. The low birthweight infant requires at least 130 calories/kg/24 hours to be reached by the age of 1 week. Water miscible preparations of vitamins A and D should be started at the age of 1 week (400 i.u. vitamin D, 4000 i.u. vitamin A) together with vitamin C (40 to 50 mg daily). Iron supplements should be given from the age 1 month.

In the case of very small or immature infants it is necessary to progress from one stage of care to the next in graded phases until a satisfactory point of development has been reached and before discharge home can be achieved. As soon as the baby has reached the stage of gaining weight steadily, when he appears to be making uninterrupted progress and when he weighs about 2 kg (4½ lb), steps are taken to wean him from the special care and conditions of the premature baby unit. He will already have been moved from the incubator or Sorrento cot to a normal cot and he may now be moved into a 'cooling off' room (10°C, 50°F) or to a sheltered corner of the general nursery. It will then be possible to allow the mother to take a greater part in her baby's care. She may be taught to bath him, to give him his feeds from an ordinary bottle and to nurse him for longer periods than before. If progress remains uneventful and the mother seems competent, the baby can usually be allowed home when he has reached 2.25 kg (5 lb) in weight.

Further Reading

CROSSE, V. M. (1976) *The Pre-Term Baby*, 8th ed. Edinburgh & London: Churchill Livingstone.

5

Apparent and true abnormalities of the newborn

IN THE FOLLOWING section an attempt is made to describe briefly some of the abnormalities which may be seen in an infants' ward of a hospital for sick children or in a maternity unit. In some cases their significance and treatment are discussed in this section; for others, treatment and nursing care are dealt with in more detail in later chapters.

The parents of children born with apparent or true abnormalities will need help in coping with this stressful situation. Inevitably the shock of learning that their child is suffering from a physical or mental handicap or a progressive illness, must be very great and much time and sympathy is needed to help the parents come to grips with the situation. They will ask many questions from a variety of people. In hospital the doctor and senior nurse should be the only ones to discuss the parents' problems with them initially. Later medical social workers and others responsible for handicapped children will assist the parents to get maximum help from the various organizations experienced in these special problems (see p. 461).

Most parents will ask the question 'Why **our** child' or 'What have **we** done to deserve this?' They may wish their child to die. These feelings are natural and parents need to be reassured and helped to understand them. They should be encouraged to express and discuss their feelings. Parents of handicapped children are often over-protective or they may reject them, and they need deep understanding and continued guidance to avoid extreme situations of this kind.

Babies who have undergone a difficult birth, have suffered from an infection in the perinatal period, have been difficult feeders, those with a history of genetic disorders, low birthweight babies and neonates whose mothers are known to be drug addicts, are among those who need particularly careful observation and nursing. This is best given in special-care nurseries, by nurses and midwives especially trained and interested in this special branch of nursing. Prompt recognition and treatment of abnormalities can be assured in this way and the equipment can be of the highest standards and most modern designs. This can make all the difference to the future of the baby. Close liaison with the health visitor will not only ensure continuity in the care of these babies, but may also mean that the detection of clinical problems, which often first present in the first weeks of life, will not be delayed. Certain tests are now carried out as a routine; a typical example is the Guthrie test, done on the eighth day to exclude phenylketonuria (see p. 297).

The newborn infant has recently undergone tremendous stress during the process of birth and this may sometimes result in more or less serious damage. Asphyxia at birth probably accounts for a large proportion of spastic and mentally subnormal individuals. Likewise, great changes have taken place in the physiology and mechanism of the body within a short space of time and in some instances the process may have remained incomplete or be faulty. Abnormalities might well be more frequent than they actually are.

The *skin* of the newborn is covered with a wax-like substance, the *vernix caseosa*, which serves as a lubricant, heat preserver and protection for the skin. Few authorities now favour bathing a newly born baby before the sixth or seventh day; left untouched the *vernix caseosa* dries off in scaly flakes. '*Stork beak marks*' as they are commonly called, are areas of red staining on the eyelids, the nape of the neck and the edge of the hair line. They are quite harmless and usually disappear within a few days of birth. Small white spots may cover the nose. These minute, blocked sebaceous glands known as *milia* are very common and disappear spontaneously after a short time.

The *scalp* tends to be scurfy. Daily toilet includes washing it with a bland soap followed by very thorough rinsing. In some cases the application of sodium bicarbonate (one teaspoonful to a pint of water), gentle massage with olive oil or a shampoo with 1 per cent cetrimide solution assists in getting rid of excess scurf. Generally speaking the skin should be left alone as much as possible. When washing or drying any part, gentle, dabbing movements are preferable to rubbing. The oral and nasal orifices should never be cleaned as part of the daily toilet. A wisp of cotton wool touching the margin of the nose suffices to make the baby sneeze and so clear his little nose, should this be necessary.

The *finger nails*, which at first are very soft, should be cut straight across if they grow too long and the infant may also be prevented from scratching himself by little cotton mittens which can be changed carefully each day. The use of mittens must, however, be considered carefully as it has happened that a loose cotton thread inside the mitten has become wrapped round a finger, resulting in gangrene and loss of a phalanx. The *umbilicus* must be kept dry from the time of birth. It is usual to apply a metal clip and then to leave the umbilicus exposed. The healthy cord stump should dry up after 24 hours and fall off within a week. It is important to realize that a moist umbilicus is an ideal breeding ground for sepsis and that the direct communication between umbilicus and liver in the newborn may be the path of a most serious spread of infection and generalized septicaemia. *Sweat rashes* and '*woollie rashes*' are common in infants and should be treated by careful hygiene. In some cases it is best not to allow wool next to the skin.

The *colour* of the healthy newborn baby is a raw, bright red. Abnormal colouring includes pallor and cyanosis due to neonatal anoxia; a grey, ashen appearance due to severe shock or generalized infection; a yellow tinge due to physiological jaundice and a dark orange tinge caused by haemolytic disease, obliteration of the bile duct or severe jaundice of the newborn, due to prematurity.

Physiological Jaundice

Physiological jaundice occurs in about 50 per cent of babies and is caused by liver insufficiency and by the liver's inability to metabolize bilirubin broken down at a rapid rate during the first days of life. This condition can usually be expected to clear spontaneously within the first week of extrauterine life. Jaundice due to this cause is never present at birth and jaundice present at that time or appearing during the first 2 days of life is due to other, more serious causes. The jaundice caused by congenital obliteration of the bile duct appears much later and is of progressive intensity. Another serious condition causing jaundice is haemolytic disease of the newborn. Both these conditions are discussed in detail later in the text (see pp. 68 and 83).

Enlarged Breasts

Enlarged breasts are seen fairly frequently in newborn babies, and girls may have a vaginal discharge similar in mechanism to menstrual bleeding. Both these conditions are caused by maternal hormones still present in the infant's circulation. They require no treatment, but must be reported to the doctor or sister in charge.

Post-Natal Convulsions

Convulsions in the neonatal period are alarming and can be of great significance. The causes include: difficult delivery, intracranial haemorrhage, septicaemia, urinary tract infections, biochemical abnormalities (such as low blood serum-calcium levels in artificially fed babies) and drug withdrawal symptoms in babies whose mothers are drug addicts.

Minor Head Injuries

Cephalhaematoma. Cephalhaematoma is one of the common injuries to the infant's head which may occur in the case of vertex (head first) deliveries. A swelling may appear on the first or second day after birth. It is due to a sub-periosteal haemorrhage caused by birth trauma. As may be expected the swelling is limited by the suture lines to any one of the cranial bones. It should be left alone and requires neither drainage nor aspirating, although it takes some weeks before it disappears. Very occasionally it may be an indication of a bony fracture.

Caput Succedaneum. Caput succedaneum is another of these harmless injuries. The presenting part is subjected to severe pressure during delivery. Oedema of the soft tissues may result and is present at the time of birth but will resolve within a matter of days. Unlike the cephalhaematoma, the swelling is not confined by the suture line, when it occurs on the skull.

Moulding of the Head. Moulding of the head may be marked and may not disappear for some time. It is caused by the overlap of the cranial bones at the suture lines, one of nature's ways of adapting the size and shape of the skull to its passage through the birth canal. Considerable temporary asymmetry may thus be caused.

More Serious Head Injuries

Precipitate, premature or difficult labour may be the cause of intracranial injury.

Intracranial Injury. Intracranial injury is usually serious and may lead to cerebral palsy, hydrocephalus, mental handicap, epilepsy or death. Infants who have suffered such injuries are limp and apathetic, their colour is ashen grey and their respirations irregular and shallow. They are often restless and have a wrinkled, worried facial expression and seem constantly wide awake. Other important signs include nystagmus, twitching, convulsions, rigidity, a high-pitched whining cry and an unstable temperature. The fontanelle may be tense and bulging. Occasionally these symptoms are present at birth but improve within the first 24 hours only to reappear with greater severity after a further 24 to 48 hours. Once feeding has started this is often noticed to be slow; the infant sucks feebly and the powers of swallowing are impaired. As a result the baby fails to thrive. Vomiting and cyanosis are not always present but when they do occur are warning signs of severe injury with a poor prognosis.

Treatment. Infants suspected of, or known to have sustained intracranial injury need absolute quiet. They are not taken out of their cot, toilet attention is reduced to a minimum, noises and sudden lights must be excluded and medical examinations are as restricted as possible. Inhalation pneumonia is prevented by keeping the air passages clear with the help of a mucus extractor and by raising the head end of the cot. Feeding may not be attempted for 12 hours and tube-feeding may be deemed safest and least tiring for the infant.

Sedatives such as chloral hydrate 30 to 60 mg ($\frac{1}{2}$ to 1 gr.) 4-hourly or phenobarbitone 8 mg ($\frac{1}{8}$ gr.) 4-hourly may be prescribed. Diazepam 0.5 to 1 mg may be given if convulsions occur. With care, recovery may be complete but prognosis must always be guarded and a special watch is kept over such children for the first year or 18 months.

Subdural Haematoma. Subdural haematoma is a somewhat later manifestation of intracranial injury. The baby may at first appear to be normal, but fails to thrive, becomes difficult with feeds, and eventually convulsions and other signs of intracranial pressure, such as a bulging fontanelle or an enlarging head and irregular breathing may become apparent. The haematoma is close to the dura and may lie over any part of the brain, though a common site is over the cerebrum. Treatment consists in aspirating the haematoma, usually through the coronal sutures lateral to the angle of the fontanelle. The blood-stained fluid obtained varies in appearance according to the length of time it has been present. For the purpose of the treatment the infant's head has to be shaved. He is wrapped securely in a blanket and the head steadied by the two hands of the nurse held over the sides of the face and skull, presenting the fontanelle towards the doctor. Successful treatment carries a hopeful prognosis.

Other Injuries

Local Nerve Injury. Local nerve injury may be caused by forceps or by any other abnormal delivery. *Facial paralysis* is clearly seen when the infant's mouth is pulled towards the unaffected side in the act of crying. Nursing measures include careful feeding, keeping the skin around the mouth and in the folds of the neck healthy (with vasogen ointment), in spite of the constant dribble of saliva, placing the child on the affected side to avoid saliva reaching the permanently open eye, and protecting the cornea with lubricating eye drops (e.g. castor oil drops). This type of paralysis may be expected to clear within the first month.

Erb's Palsy. Erb's palsy is a nerve injury affecting the brachial plexus. The limp arm is internally rotated with the elbow. The hand is partly closed and the palm directed backwards. The arm should be rested in a position which relaxes all the affected muscles. This is easily achieved by pinning the baby's cardigan sleeve to the bottom sheet with the humerus at right angles to the body and forearm pointing upwards, the hand lying beside the head (Fig. 10). Alternatively a light splint is used to maintain the correct position. Recovery is usually complete though

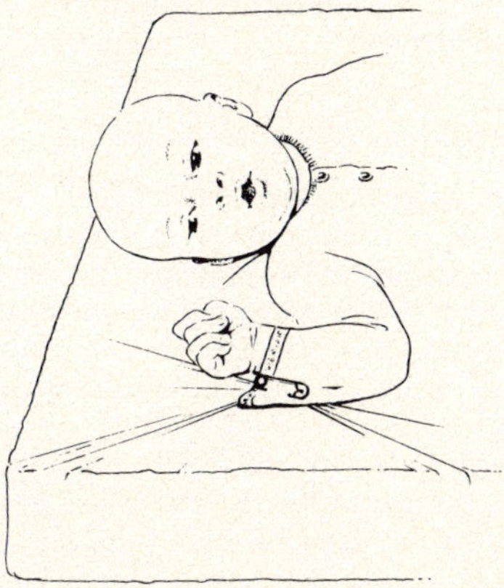

FIG. 10. Position for arm in Erb's palsy.

passive movement or massage may be needed for several weeks or months.

Injury to the Sternomastoid Muscle. Injury to the sternomastoid muscle is occasionally caused by difficult labour. A small tear may result in bleeding and exudate which, after a matter of days, causes a noticeable, firm but painless swelling. The only treatment needed is passive movement of the head to avoid fibrosis and resulting torticollis.

Fractures. Fractures are as a rule not of a serious nature as the bones unite easily and in a good position with a minimum of treatment. The bones most commonly affected are the clavicle and humerus. A pseudo-paralysis or reluctance to move the arm may be the first sign of such injury.

The Newborn Baby of Drug Addicts

Babies born to mothers who are drug addicts, are liable to suffer from withdrawal symptoms which have to be treated in a similar way to those in adults. Nurses should be alert to the possibility of this condition. Good history taking will highlight such a possibility. It is interesting to note, that these babies all seem to 'chew their fists'.

Conditions of the Respiratory System

The newly born baby breathes exclusively through his nose, and nasal obstructions may have to be overcome by gentle cleansing or the instilling of nasal drops. It is frequently sufficient to insert a wisp of cotton wool into the anterior nares, so causing the baby to sneeze. A blocked nose is a common and often missed cause of slow or reluctant feeding even in healthy infants.

The respiratory system of the newly born baby is immature and respiratory failure is by far the most common cause of death in the first few days of life. Inhalation of meconium, blood or mucus causes aspiration pneumonia, and this is virtually present at birth. In order to prevent inhalation as far as is possible, a mucus catheter is used to suck out the mouth and pharynx as soon as the head has been born.

Respiratory Distress Syndrome

In respiratory distress syndrome the surfactant which normally lines the alveoli is diminished or absent and therefore the alveoli collapse resulting in atelectasis. A fibrinous exudate may then form known as the hyaline membrane. The incidence of this syndrome appears to be increasing but if the infant can survive 2 to 3 days, there is an increase in surfactant and recovery takes place. Affected infants are most commonly pre-term and usually lie quietly appearing 'greyish' and apathetic. Respirations are rapid and shallow and an expiratory grunt is often heard, periods of apnoea and cyanosis may occur. The body temperature tends to be low.

Treatment and Nursing Care. These infants should be nursed naked in an incubator with high humidity. The infant will require sufficient oxygen to prevent cerebral damage from hypoxia and yet avoid the possibility of retrolental fibroplasia. Levels of oxygen given throughout treatment must be carefully monitored. In order to eliminate cyanosis it may be necessary to give a continuous high concentration of oxygen and the best way to give this is by the use of a transparent plastic box which fits over the infants head (Gairdner head box). This allows a high concentration of oxygen to be given with a relatively low flow rate. The infant should be disturbed as little as possible with nursing procedures kept to a minimum. Feeding will be through an in-dwelling nasogastric tube. The infant should be nursed on an apnoea monitor mattress and his position changed at regular intervals. When nursed in the prone position the chest should be raised to facilitate the drainage of mucus and to ensure that the abdomen is lower than the chest thus avoiding pressure on the diaphragm. It is most important that the airway is kept clear by using suction. Regular micro-Astrup analysis of blood chemistry will reveal any acidosis which should be corrected with intravenous sodium bicarbonate together with glucose. Some paediatricians prefer to use THAM (Tris-hydroxy-methylaminomethane) in severe cases. If the infant still fails to breathe normally, artificial ventilation is indicated. More recently, Continuous Positive Airway Pressure (CPAP) has been used most successfully for these infants in some centres.

Nursing Care and Treatment Summary

1. Carefully planned (minimal) nursing care
2. Control of oxygen administration

3. Correction of abnormal blood chemistry
4. Careful feeding
5. Maintenance of respiration, possibly with mechanical assistance
6. Prevention of infection.

Haemorrhagic Disease of the Newborn

Occasionally a baby may suddenly vomit blood or pass a melaena stool or blood-stained urine, or may be found to be bleeding from the nose, vagina or umbilicus. The bleeding occurs without warning and is most common from the third day onward. The cause is lack of vitamin K, which in turn causes hypoprothrombinaemia and an abnormally long prothrombin time.

Treatment by giving vitamin K (1 to 2 mg by intramuscular injection) must not be delayed, commonly used preparations being phytonadione (Konakion) and Vikastab. Fibrinolysis or fibrinogenolysis are other conditions which may cause bleeding.

Occasionally a small vomit of altered blood or a melaena stool are caused by the baby swallowing blood as, for instance, during birth or from the mother's cracked nipple. It is for the doctor to decide and confirm the cause of any such signs of bleeding and the nurse must report them promptly and save the abnormal stool or vomit for medical inspection.

Haemolytic Disease of the Newborn (Rhesus Incompatibility)

Neither Rh-positive or Rh-negative individuals normally have anti-Rh antibodies in their serum, but if an Rh-negative woman bears an Rh-positive child or fetus she may develop anti-Rh antibodies. With future pregnancies these antibodies can pass via the placenta into the fetal circulation causing the red cells to haemolize resulting in anaemia and jaundice of the newborn infant.

All Rh-negative mothers of Rh-positive babies are now given anti-D gamma-globulin within 36 hours of delivery to prevent rhesus incompatibility problems with future pregnancies.

However, if Rhesus incompatibility does occur the principal manifestations are:

1. Still birth or death within a few hours, associated with hydrops fetalis;
2. Icterus gravis;
3. Congenital anaemia.

Newborn infants with anaemia and jaundice resulting from rhesus incompatibility must be treated as soon as possible after birth with an exchange transfusion.

Hydrops Fetalis

Infants with this condition are grossly oedematous and anaemic and the placenta shows pathological changes. The condition cannot be treated once it has occurred.

Icterus Gravis

The infant is either born jaundiced or becomes so in 24 hours. Jaundice may become intense producing kernicterus if serum bilirubin rises above 20 mg %. Kernicterus causes straining and degeneration of the brain cells. If the infant survives he may suffer from deafness, cerebral palsy or mental handicap.

Congenital Anaemia of the Newborn

Congenital anaemia may be present at birth and be severe, or it may develop within the first two weeks of life and be of a mild type (see also familial thrombocytopenic purpura, p. 237).

Exchange Blood Transfusion

In anticipation of severe disease, a blood specimen is taken from the cord at the time of birth and examined in the laboratory. The cord is not tied in the usual manner but is kept moist by wrapping damp, sterile gauze around it, while tests are carried out. If there is evidence that the bilirubin level is reaching dangerous proportions, or if the cord haemoglobin is less than 150 g/litre an exchange blood transfusion is given. The umbilical vein, still patent at this stage, is used to introduce a plastic cannula. With the help of a four-way tap and syringe, 20 ml of blood at a time are withdrawn and replaced by Rh negative blood. Alternatively the blood can be of the baby's own group or group 'O'. It should always be fresh blood. The procedure is continued until approximately 80 ml of blood per pound of body weight have been exchanged. (The total volume of blood of a 3.2 kg baby (7 lb) at birth is approximately 300 ml.) The infant is securely immobilized on a firmly padded board or a pillow and it is important to ensure that he is kept warm throughout the procedure, and allowed to rest when the transfusion has been completed. Appropriate antibiotics may be given. Vitamin K, 1 mg, may be ordered and sometimes calcium gluconate is given to counteract the effect of the citrate in the donor blood. A specimen of the last blood withdrawn is sent to the laboratory for estimation of the haemoglobin and serum bilirubin levels. To avoid clotting in the apparatus, heparin in saline is syringed through it at each withdrawal and injection of blood. (Saline 100 ml to heparin 1000 units.) Throughout the transfusion a careful watch is kept on the heart action and on the blood chemistry. One millilitre of a 10 per cent solution of calcium gluconate may be injected after every 100 ml of blood has been transfused, as a precaution against convulsions or sudden collapse. Following the transfusion, the level of serum bilirubin is carefully watched in case it should rise again to dangerous levels, necessitating a second transfusion. Haemorrhage from the cord and sudden changes in temperature may occur after exchange transfusion and call for vigilance on the nurses' part.

Oedema of the Newborn

Severe anoxia and respiratory distress, infections such as septicaemia, excess chilling, prematurity, congenital heart disease with cardiac failure, and faulty feeding may all cause oedema in the newborn. This is often difficult to assess and the carefully kept weight chart is of great value. The oedema is not necessarily of the pitting type, as in adults, but the fluid accumulation in the tissues causes the extremities to take on a rounded appearance while the skin may be unusually pale and shiny with a rubbery sensation when touched. Oedema is postural and marked in the dependent parts or on the side on which the infant is lying. Treatment is according to the cause. It should be appreciated that salt retention automatically causes fluid retention. Hartmann's and other solutions containing salts are consequently not given unless diluted nor is cow's milk, which has a comparatively high salt content.

Cold Baby Syndrome (Sclerema)

Cold baby syndrome occurs as a rule in the first month of life, in premature babies, babies who suffer from severe heart disease, infection or cerebral birth injury. Of all hypothermic babies admitted to hospital 42 per cent are due to inadequately heated rooms at home.

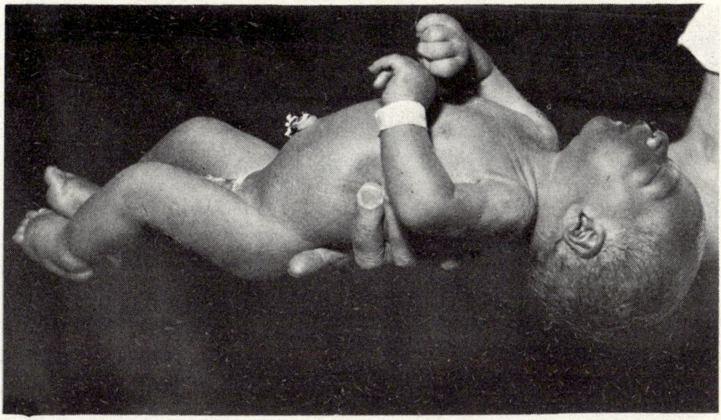

FIG. 11. Baby with 'cold injury' showing the generalized rigidity characteristic of this syndrome.

The infant's colour may at first be bright pink and this may give a deceptive impression of excellent health; the colour soon changes to a grey pallor. He is reluctant to feed, drowsy and slow to react to external stimuli. The entire baby is rigid (Fig. 11). Oedema may be present and urinary output is low. The skin is cold and hard to the touch and the rectal temperature registers between 26.4° and 32.2°C (80° and 90°F), or even less. The low reading thermometer should be inserted into the rectum for a distance of at least 2.5 cm (1 in) and left in position for 2 full minutes.

Treatment. Admission to hospital is usually necessary. During transfer the baby is placed in a 'silver swaddler' which can be improvised from previously warmed household tin foil. In order to prevent overheating and to make it possible to observe the breathing, part of the chest is left exposed. The baby is often best nursed in an incubator at a temperature 1° to 2° above his own; rapid overheating may prove fatal. The baby should be handled as little as possible. Food is not well tolerated. During the process of re-warming the baby, metabolism is increased and this in turn increases the need for glucose, in addition to normal feeds which will need to be given via a nasogastric catheter. Oxygen will be required initially whilst respirations are shallow. An antibiotic is usually prescribed to combat any infection.

Improvement is steady and rapid in the majority of cases and the baby may be expected to recover completely from the cold syndrome although the underlying condition may yet have to be treated.

Infections in the Newborn

Infections occur readily in the newborn as the infant has little resistance and few antibodies. It is often difficult to notice the early signs of infection in the neonate. Frequently there is no rise in temperature, pulse or respiration and only the most experienced nurse would notice a disinterest in feeding or a minor change in colour as being of importance. Sometimes there is merely an unaccountable change in the baby's previously good condition, but this change should be a warning that the paediatrician should be consulted. Osteomyelitis, pneumonia, urinary tract infections, meningitis and gastro-enteritis are not uncommon and are frequently secondary to a blood stream infection, particularly due to *Escherichia coli* (bacterium). Infection at this age presents an atypical picture and can be easily missed if experience is lacking. Often a serious infection is associated with very vague signs. The infant may merely become reluctant with his feeds or become lethargic and limp. A fall in temperature may be the first sign of an infection and the temperature may even remain subnormal for the first day or two. His colour may be grey and ashen, jaundiced or cyanosed, and every possible irregularity of respiration and pulse rate and volume may be registered.

Meningitis is typically associated with a bulging anterior fontanelle but even this may be absent or possibly reversed if loss of fluid from vomiting or diarrhoea has caused dehydration.

Pneumonia. Pneumonia may be present without any sign of dyspnoea or cough, and *convulsions* are common. Alternatively there may be high fever and a hot, flushed skin.

Urinary Tract Infections. Urinary tract infections are particularly common in the neonatal period and these infections often recur. Investigations are usually carried out to exclude congenital abnormalities of the urinary tract.

Skin Infections. Skin infections, however slight, should be treated with care in order to avoid a spread of the infection or generalized septicaemia. With the advent of modern drugs many skin infections have lost their severity but occasionally a particularly resistant strain may still cause serious disease. The skin is easily damaged in young babies and small pustules and paronychia should be treated immediately and the patient isolated at once. For instance pemphigus, a bullous septic skin eruption, caused by *Staphylococcus aureus*, continues to carry a poor prognosis, despite treatment with penicillin, antibiotics and cortisone.

Down's Syndrome (Mongolism)

Down's syndrome occurs about once in every 600 births. The cause is genetic, as these children have 47 chromosomes instead of the normal 46. All these children are mentally handicapped, usually with an I.Q. range 35 to 55, although very occasionally mongols have been found to have I.Q.s up to 70.

Mongol children are short in stature with small round heads, the eyes which slant upwards and outwards with epicanthic folds give the face its characteristic mongoloid appearance. They have large protruding tongues and dentition is often delayed. There is general hypotonicity, posture is poor and often these children have a tendency towards obesity. The shoulders are round, the chest flat and the abdomen protuberant, often with an umbilical hernia. The hands are characteristically broad and short with a deep palmar crease, short thumb and a small curved fourth finger. Some of these children have additional physical handicaps such as heart lesions, deafness, poor sight and are often troubled with recurrent respiratory infections.

Most mongol children love music and dancing and are great mimics who benefit from the type of education which encourages them to learn the skills of living. Although they may never learn to read or write, they can learn to become self-confident and lead happy useful lives. Some adolescents are able to obtain jobs in the community usually in repetitive routine employment. Hospital care is necessary for some of these children but the majority are able to stay with their families who will need long-term support from the health and social services. The parents of all these children should be offered genetic counselling if they are considering further additions to the family. A woman over the age of 40 has a 1 in 100 chance of having an affected child and a woman of 21 years, 1 in 2000.

Congenital Anatomical Abnormalities

Many congenital abnormalities can nowadays be treated surgically. A list of the more common types is of interest and some knowledge of them may lead to keener observation in a maternity or medical paediatric ward.

The head. Microcephaly, hydrocephaly, oxycephaly, naevi, choanal atresia.

The eye. Buphthalmos, congenital cataract, strabismus, microphthalmia.

Ears. Absence of the pinna or meatus. Congenital deafness. Bat ears.

Mouth. Cleft lip (hare lip), cleft palate, micrognathia (congenital smallness of the lower jaw).

Alimentary tract. Pyloric stenosis, oesophageal atresia, tracheo-oesophageal fistula, hiatus hernia, Hirschsprung's disease, imperforate anus, congenital obliteration of the bile duct, meconium ileus, rectovaginal fistula.

Bones. Osteogenesis imperfecta, spina bifida, achondroplasia, syndactyly, talipes, congenital dislocation of the hip joint, missing bones.

Thorax. Diaphragmatic hernia, congenital heart disease (with or without cyanosis).

Abdomen. Varieties of hernia, exomphalos.

Genito-urinary tract. Horse-shoe kidney, double ureters, hypospadias, epispadias, rectovaginal fistula, pseudo-hermaphroditism, hydrocele, undescended testicles, ectopia vesicae.

Central nervous system. Cystic spina bifida (meningocele, myelomeningocele), anencephaly, microcephaly, hydrocephaly and a variety of conditions which may be responsible for cerebral palsy.

Naevi or Birth Marks

Naevi (singular: naevus) consist of a localized cluster of dilated blood vessels (Fig. 12). There are various types of naevi, some of which are present at birth, others appear some months later. Of the different types most disappear spontaneously but others persist. Some naevi are very extensive and may disfigure an entire side of the face or cause considerable enlargement of the tongue associated with difficulty of speech, eating and breathing.

Treatment. Treatment is by means of irradiation, diathermy and surgical excision. The nursing care of patients treated by deep X-ray therapy or radium is given in Chapter 16 (Wilms's tumour page 357).

One type of naevus which can be expected to disappear spontaneously is known as strawberry or cavernous naevus. This type of naevus, which usually appears only several days after birth, is liable to grow considerably at first but rarely causes serious trouble or haemorrhage. After the first year of life the naevus tends to shrink and gradually regresses completely leaving a flat, paper-like scar by the age of about 5

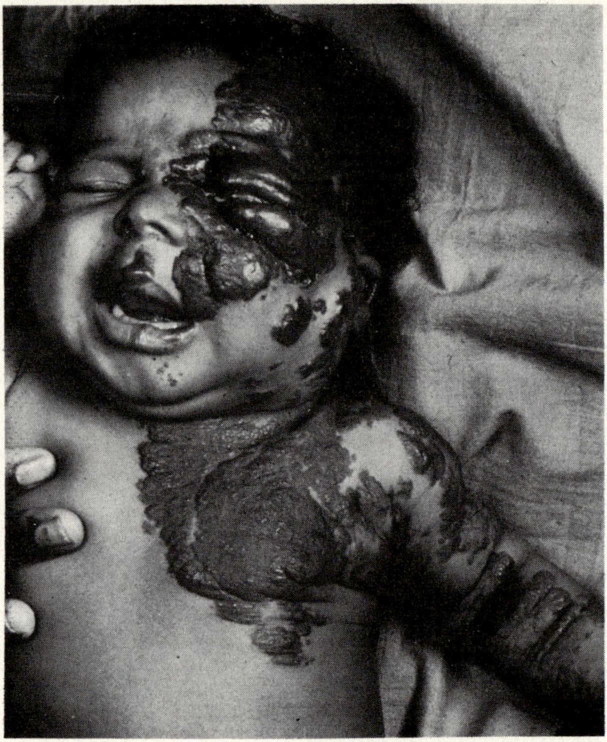

FIG. 12. Cavernous haemangioma.

years. No treatment should be given for such a naevus but much tact will be needed in persuading the mother to accept conservative treatment for her disfigured child. In contrast to this naevus, those known as 'portwine naevi' stay for life. Excision and grafting is usually the treatment of choice.

Diaphragmatic Hernia

Some babies are born with a defect in the diaphragm (usually on the left side). As a result abdominal organs such as stomach and intestines, and sometimes even the liver, rise into the thoracic cavity. The heart may be displaced to the right and, since the lungs cannot expand normally, cyanotic attacks occur. If an attempt is made to relieve these by giving oxygen via a mask, the oxygen may enter the stomach causing further distension. The procedure is therefore a dangerous one and must be avoided. Early and accurate diagnosis is life saving and must never be delayed.

Treatment. Treatment consists of intubating the baby and giving oxygen via an endotracheal tube. An emergency operation is carried out without delay. A laparotomy (or occasionally thoracotomy) is performed, the intestines returned to their proper position and the defect in the diaphragm repaired. The operation may prove difficult if the abdominal cavity has not developed adequately before birth, due to the displacement of its normal contents. A gastric tube is left in position and for the first 2 or 3 days the stomach is aspirated at frequent intervals. After-care is similar to that for any other cases recovering from thoracic surgery, but the baby is often sat up in a 'hiatus hernia chair to maintain an upright position for several weeks following operation.

Hiatus Hernia

Hiatus hernia is a special type of diaphragmatic hernia. The abnormality is caused by a defect in the muscles forming the diaphragm so that these do not fit closely around the distal end of the oesophagus and part of the stomach is pulled through the opening into the thoracic cavity. Sphincter control is impaired and there is a constant reflux of gastric secretions and food into the oesophagus. As a result the baby starts regurgitations within a week of birth. As time goes on he vomits mucus, food and even blood soon after feeds and later at any time. He fails to gain weight as much food is lost in this way and if the condition is not corrected, ulceration of the lining of the oesophagus results. The milky vomit may become streaked with blood. In time the oesophagus becomes scarred, and stenosis, shortening and fixation develop at the distal end. Regurgitation is worst when the baby is lying in his cot.

The diagnosis is confirmed by a barium swallow and radiographs but sometimes this procedure has to be repeated once or twice before the condition is proved. Oesophagoscopy may be performed in some cases.

Treatment. Treatment in mild cases consists of keeping the baby constantly in an upright position and this position should be maintained day and night and even when the baby is bathed or nursed. In this way the stomach is kept below the diaphragm and vomiting made more difficult by force of gravity. It may help to thicken feeds with Nestargel or with Benger's. Feeds should be given slowly. Mild cases are likely to improve when a solid diet can be started. Severe cases which are not likely to respond to postural therapy are best treated by surgery.

Operation for repair of hiatus hernia. Thoracotomy is performed and the stomach reached through the left side of the chest. The organ is replaced in the abdominal cavity below the diaphragm, the hiatus stitched closely around the oesophagus and the defect in the muscle repaired. The chest is then closed and after-care is similar to that of any case of thoracic surgery. As soon as his condition permits the child is, however, returned to his hiatus hernia chair and the upright position maintained for several more weeks. Recurrence is common and for that reason optimism with regard to permanent cure should be restrained.

Abnormalities of the Oesophagus and Trachea

There are a number of variants of the abnormalities of the oesophagus and these may or may not involve the trachea. They are best understood by studying Fig. 13.

1. Tracheo-oesophageal fistula without associated atresia of the oesophagus.
2. Oesophageal atresia, i.e. the oesophagus is not continuous but neither end communicates with the trachea.
3. Oesophageal atresia with associated tracheo-oesophageal fistula.

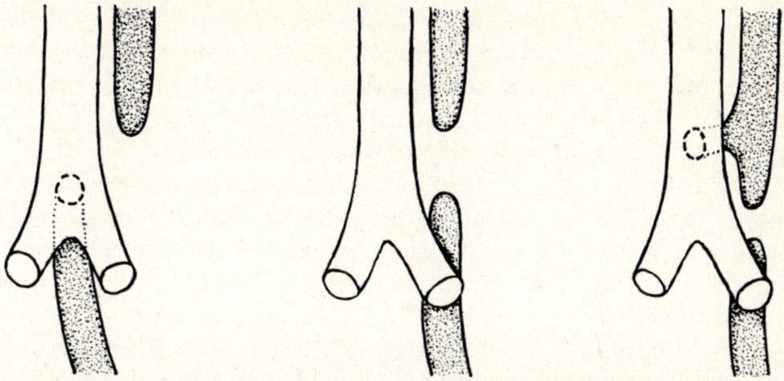

FIG. 13. Common varieties of tracheo-oesophageal abnormalities.

These abnormalities occur most commonly in low birth weight babies. There often is a history of hydramnios during pregnancy. Symptoms vary according to the abnormality.

1. In the case of tracheo-oesophageal fistula not associated with atresia of the oesophagus, gastric reflux will cause inhalation of secretions and of hydrochloric acid from the stomach into the trachea causing ulceration of the mucous lining.
2. As neither saliva nor oral fluids can pass into the stomach the blind pouch of the proximal end of the oesophagus soon fills up and spills over, causing coughing and choking as fluid enters the lungs. Inhalation pneumonia results.
3. When atresia associated with a communication between oesophagus and trachea is present, there is again obvious danger of reflux and inhalation of secretions and any feed that might be given.

In all cases, coughing and choking occurs from birth and this should alert the nurse. Frequent, gentle aspiration will prevent inhalation until a diagnosis can be made and operation carried out to rectify the abnormality. It is unwise to lower the head end of the cot, as this would encourage reflux of secretions and the contents of the oesophageal pouch or stomach, as the case may be. In those cases in which there is a communication between trachea and oesophagus, air enters the stomach and intestinal tract, causing abdominal distension. This in turn, may cause breathlessness and reluctance to feed. Diagnosis is confirmed by passing a radio opaque catheter; radiographs will show how far the tube has passed and outline the abnormality present. Diagnosis and treatment in all instances are a matter of urgency and should be carried out within the first hours after birth. Basically the repair consists of anastomosis of the two blind ends of the oesophagus and division and closure of the fistula. The approach in the case of a simple fistula is often via the neck while the more complex abnormalities require thoracotomy.

If the proximal and distal ends of the oesophagus are too far apart to be brought together, a graft to bridge the gap is necessary. The graft may consist of some inert material or may be taken from the patient's own, intestinal tract. Occasionally it is necessary to do the repair in two stages. In that event the proximal end of the oesophagus is brought to the surface at the base of the neck and through it secretions are discharged. A 'sham feed' of clear fluid is given at the same time as gastrostomy feed, so that the infant associates sucking and swallowing with the pleasure of a full stomach. This makes it easier to establish normal feeding when reconstruction of the oesophagus is completed. A gastrostomy is established through which the child can be fed. Later when the structures are larger and the infant stronger, extensive surgery is undertaken. Even the simplest repair of such a severe abnormality within hours of birth, is a serious matter and very careful and experienced nursing care is required. The usual points which apply to the nursing care of any cases undergoing thoracotomy are described in Chapter 10 (p. 200).

Post-operatively the baby should be handled as little as possible and it is convenient to use an incubator in which temperature and humidity can easily be adjusted and the plane tipped so that the foot end can be raised to treat shock and the head end raised during feeding, without disturbing the baby.

If a one-stage repair has been possible, a trans-anastomotic fine tube will be left in situ for several days and the first oral feed given will be a few drops of sterile water to test the adequacy of the anastomosis.

If feeds have to be given through a gastrostomy tube, they are given very slowly to avoid distension. The funnel should be held close to the baby's mouth and not raised more than about 2.5 cm (1 in) above it, so that the feed flows very gently and also to enable gas to escape when necessary. Special care is given to the skin surrounding the gastrostomy opening and to the mouth. For details of the nursing care of thoracotomy patients see Chapter 10.

Excess saliva and excretions may have to be aspirated several times a day by suction, both before and after operation. An intravenous infusion will be set up as soon as diagnosis has been confirmed and by this means hydration is maintained and the electrolytes regulated. There is a danger of disturbing the body chemistry due to loss of essential fluids via vomit, gastric and pancreatic secretions and excretions. Penicillin is given to prevent chest infections. Gentle vibration of chest and back and postural drainage are started as soon as the condition is recognized and continued post-operatively.

Neonatal Duodenal Obstruction

Duodenal obstruction in the neonate is due to narrowing or absence of the duodenal lumen or to a membrane across the lumen.

There often is a history of hydramnios in pregnancy and other abnormalities may be present also.

Signs and Symptoms. Vomiting starts within 4 hours of birth and the vomitus may contain bile. The baby is usually small for dates. The abdomen below the diaphragm is distended while the lower abdomen looks empty and flat. There may be visible gastric peristalsis.

The typical radiograph shows a 'double bubble' the one in the stomach, the other in the dilated duodenum, proximal to the obstruction.

Treatment. Even though intestinal obstruction calls for emergency treatment the infant has to be carefully prepared. A nasogastric tube is passed and any gastric contents aspirated, an intravenous infusion is set up, blood taken for grouping and electrolyte assessment in readiness for transfusion and the urine tested. The patient is likely to be shocked and handling should be gentle and reduced to essentials and he should be protected from exposure to cold and draughts.

At operation. The site of the obstruction is sought and a short-circuit gastro-enterostomy or resection of the stenosis and anastomosis of the normal segments performed.

Post-operatively. The infant requires the usual care given after any major operation. The intravenous infusion is continued until hydration and electrolyte balance are satisfactory and oral feeding has been established. Gastric aspirations with a syringe are continued until only a few millilitres are aspirated every few hours. Any strain from distension on the anastomosis should be avoided. Alternatively a gastrostomy may have been done and a fine tube introduced alongside the gastrostomy tube through the anastomosis into the small gut. Initial feeds are given through this tube at approximately 1 ml/minute. The prognosis is as a rule a good one. Feeding is commenced when the aspirate has almost stopped and bowel sounds can be heard.

Ano-Rectal Abnormalities

Imperforate Anus

The first examination of every baby must always include careful inspection of the perineum, but even if this is omitted failure to pass meconium must always arouse suspicion that an abnormality may be present. The deformity may be superficial or deep. The anus may merely be hidden by skin which covers a normal rectum and sphincter or the opening of the anal canal may be displaced forward on the perineum. In more severe deformities the rectum forms a fistula, which in the male communicates with the urethra and in the female with the vagina. In that case there is a gap between the anal dimple seen on the perineum and the blind end of the bowel.

Anal Stenosis

Some babies are born with anal stenosis. This abnormality is not recognized on first examination but the baby will pass toothpaste-like stools and will be seen to strain at defaecation. Treatment consists in performing dilatations and giving laxative drugs.

According to the abnormality signs and symptoms will vary. If the condition is missed, the three typical signs of obstruction, vomiting, abdominal distension and complete constipation, will develop in the case of severe stenosis or absence of an anal opening. If there is a moderate degree of stenosis, stools are passed but they are shaped like toothpaste and the baby will strain on defaecation. If the anal opening is displaced, meconium will appear in an abnormal position.

Diagnosis is made by thorough inspection, by digital examination and by radiographs. The baby is held upside down under the X-ray screen and this causes intestinal gases to rise to the apex of the blind pouch. A marker is placed over the anal dimple and the distance between this and the apex measured. In this way a concise diagnosis can be made and the distance between the blind end of bowel and the perineum determined.

Treatment depends on the type of abnormality. Very briefly: anal stenosis is treated by dilatation and laxatives; hidden anus with normal rectum, by incision of the covering membrane and dilatation; anal opening on the perineum but in a forward displaced position, by incision of the perineum and stitching of rectal mucosa round the new opening, followed by dilatation over a period of months. Recto-urethral and rectovaginal fistulae require major surgery and the creation of temporary or permanent colostomy (see p. 284).

Congenital Atresia of the Bile Duct

In spite of the fact that atresia of a bile duct is congenital, symptoms may be at first either missed or mistaken for physiological jaundice. Contrary to the jaundice in the physiological variety, the jaundice in case of obliteration of the bile duct fails to improve and the baby becomes more deeply jaundiced until he is almost olive colour. The urine and saliva are stained with bile and the stools are grey, clay coloured or white, the liver is enlarged and firm. The obstruction to the normal flow of bile is due to a complete block or absence of a segment of the common bile duct, so that bile cannot pass through it, although a small amount of bile can escape together with the succus entericus.

Diagnostic laparotomy is performed to pinpoint the site of the atresia and to take a liver biopsy. If a gall bladder is present, a radio-opaque substance is injected and this will outline the anatomy of the biliary tract under X-ray (Cholecystography).

If a bile duct of adequate size is present surgery, which aims at anastomosing it to a loop of bowel, is performed. Complications, such as breakdown of the anastomosis, leakage of bile and attendant excoriation of skin and post-operative bleeding due to delayed clotting time despite pre-operative cover with vitamin K, are common.

If operation is not possible, the jaundice gradually deepens, liver and spleen enlarge and cirrhosis of the liver develops. The abdomen becomes grossly distended, the veins of the abdominal wall are engorged and ascites develops. Death takes place within two years.

Ophthalmia Neonatorum

Any purulent discharge from the eye within 21 days of birth is notifiable, irrespective of the cause. The commonest causative organisms are staphylococcus and gonococcus.

Ophthalmia neonatorum once accounted for a high proportion of blindness in children, but nowadays owing to adequate prophylaxis and treatment with antibiotics, eye infections rarely have serious consequences. Symptoms vary from slight oedema of the eyelids, inability to open the eyes and presence of frank pus, to changes in the eye itself.

Infants with 'sticky eyes' should be nursed with strict precautions against spread of infection and should be carefully isolated from other babies with a special nurse attending them. In severe cases sterile normal saline irrigations are carried out every ½ hour, to remove accumulated pus. Appropriate antibiotic ophthalmic ointment is prescribed. If drops are ordered the following routine may be followed: one drop is instilled every minute for the first ½-hour, then every 5 minutes until all discharge disappears (usually a further hour) then ½-hourly until the swelling subsides (usually another 8 to 12 hours) then every hour for 12 hours, and every 2 hours for another 24 hours after that. This treatment is modified according to the wishes of the doctor. If one eye only is affected, the infant should be nursed on the affected side to prevent discharge from running over the bridge of the nose into the healthy eye. The baby's arms must be effectively restrained to prevent him from touching his eyes and so spreading the infection.

If the infection persists blockage of the lacrimal duct should be suspected.

Squint (Strabismus)

It is normal for the baby's eye to wander independently during the first few weeks of life. If one eye persistently turns inwards or outwards in relation to the other, a squint is present. The mother should never be told that the child will grow out of it but the advice of a paediatrician and ophthalmologist must be sought. It is important that treatment is carried out early and persistently if an amblyopic or lazy eye is to be avoided. Vision finally becomes fixed about the age of 8 years, so that any visual defect at that age is permanent and correction of a squinting eye will only result in cosmetic improvement. Rarely eye deviation in the newborn is due to a tumour in the eye or to toxoplasmosis.

Retrolental Fibroplasia

Retrolental fibroplasia is caused by excessive oxygen therapy which may result in vascular and retinal changes and the formation of an opaque membrane behind the lens. There is no known cure for the condition. Prematurely born infants are most likely to be at risk. Now that the cause of this kind of blindness is known, it is possible to prevent it by limiting and monitoring the use of oxygen.

Treatment of Abnormalities of the Newborn

Methods of giving oxygen to infants include polythene mask, incubator, ventilator, head box and oxygen tent. The advantage of incubators lies in the ease with which infants can be observed and nursed, the easy adjustment of the flow of oxygen, humidity and temperature, and the adjustment of posture by tipping the plane on which the infant is lying.

Intravenous and Blood Transfusion

The reasons for which intravenous fluids and blood are given to children are essentially the same as for adults, but the technique varies and the responsibility of looking after the patient during intravenous therapy is far greater owing to the small amounts and structures involved.

Splinting for Intravenous Therapy. When a limb is used adequate splinting is essential and this is a highly skilled procedure, as immobility must be achieved without compressing important blood vessels. The splint should be well padded and covered in order to make it waterproof. For an infant, the splint need be only about 7.5 cm (3 in) wide but the length should be sufficient to allow for it to support a loop of tubing. This takes the weight off the tubing and makes it possible to adjust the position of the needle in the vein by suitable padding (see Fig. 14). This method also minimizes the vibrations caused by restlessness or movement of the bottle which in turn helps to cut down inflammation within the vein. If the internal saphenous vein is used, the splint should reach from the fold of the buttock to some 25 cm (10 in) beyond the toes or if a vein in the arm is used, from the head of the humerus to some 25 cm (10 in) beyond the fingers. The foot and ankle are rotated externally and immobilized on the splint by lengths of 2.5 cm (1 in) adhesive strapping passing across the heel just below the knee. In this way pressure on important blood vessels is avoided. If the antecubital vein is used, the arm is rotated externally and three lengths of strapping applied: one across the palm of the hand, one just below the antecubital fossa and the third high up on the arm and across the bony prominence of the shoulder. In either case a firm bandage and cotton wool are applied to give added immobility, but a space of some 5 to 7.5 cm (2 to 3 in) is left uncovered so that the condition of the limb can be watched. A pad of foam sponge can be used to prevent foot-

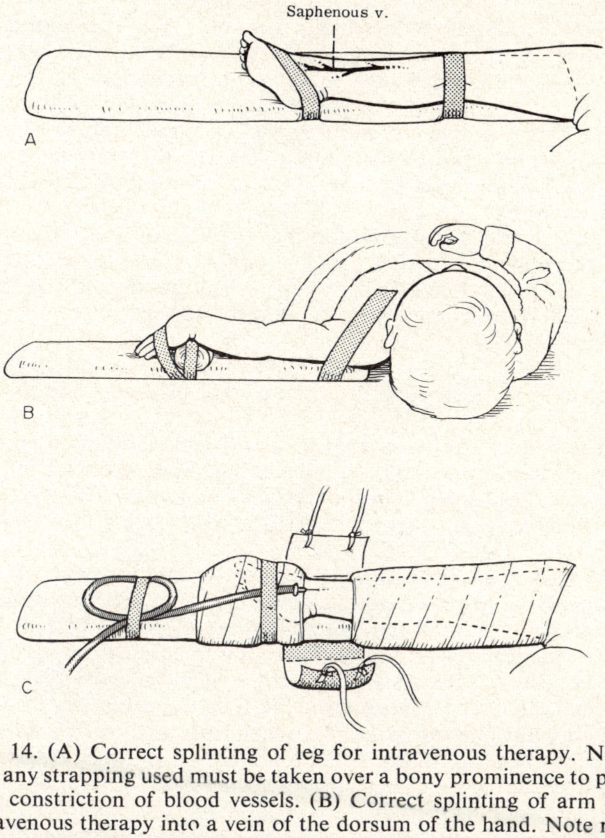

FIG. 14. (A) Correct splinting of leg for intravenous therapy. Note that any strapping used must be taken over a bony prominence to prevent constriction of blood vessels. (B) Correct splinting of arm for intravenous therapy into a vein of the dorsum of the hand. Note roll of foam sponge to prevent wrist drop. (C) A space is left between bandages for convenient and frequent inspection. The tubing is stabilized on the extra length of splint. This minimizes the movement and vibration and reduces risk of thrombosis or spasm of the vein.

drop or an over-extension of the elbow. The splint should be firmly tied to the bed to ensure immobility.

Good splinting is essential, not only for the successful running of the intravenous drip infusion, but also because it enables the nursing staff to move the patient up and down the cot or to lift him out for feeding or weighing. In order to make this possible an extra length of sterile tubing should always be attached to the adult giving set. Moving the patient at regular intervals is one way of preventing hypostatic pneumonia.

Care should be taken to see that the limb and splint are not twisted and that neither groin nor tubing are kinked or constricted. It is a good plan to have a bed cradle over the limb, to facilitate inspection and to support the weight of the bed clothes.

In newly born sick babies, the umbilical vein is sometimes used in an emergency despite the danger of portal vein thrombosis.

The veins most commonly used with young children are the internal saphenous and the antecubital veins, but with infants the superficial scalp veins or the veins on the back of the hand are often very satisfactory (see Fig. 14B).

Procedure. Unless a superficial vein can be used, it will probably be necessary to cut down to a vein. The instruments are similar to those used for adults, but mosquito forceps and fairy Spencer Wells artery forceps and scissors replace the larger instruments. As the operator's slightest movement may prejudice his success in entering the vein, it is often wise to place the instruments on a sterile macintosh and towel, on the patient's bed, in front of the doctor. The patient may be given a sedative and a local anaesthetic, such as procaine in a 1 or 2 per cent solution.

The usual needles or cannulae are often replaced by a Braunula or similar intravenous needle. The needle can be inserted into the vein unhandicapped by the weight and movement of the rubber tubing. With a child's small veins this can be of considerable advantage. Once the Braunula needle is tied into position, the tubing and adaptor, with the fluid dripping through it, can be inserted into the cannula without difficulty.

The junctures may be made watertight by the application of a little sterile petroleum jelly.

Polythene tubing with a special needle and adaptor is used in some hospitals and often makes it unnecessary to cut down, even with very young infants. Alternatively, there are cannulae, 'Trocaths' which can be introduced into an open vein up to a considerable length without using a needle or splinting. For exchange transfusions the newborn infant is bandaged to a T-splint and the umbilical vein is used for transfusing by means of polythene tubing.

Intravenous paediatric infusion sets are now made of polythene and are disposable. A second chamber is incorporated into the tubing and this can be filled with the amount of fluid which is intended for the following hour. This is a valuable safety device. As various types of infusion apparatus deliver drops of different size, it is essential to check on the instructions on the infusion set in order to know exactly how much fluid the baby is getting.

Young children and infants need constant nursing attention while intravenous therapy is in progress. The rate of the drip in the drip chamber should be checked with a watch every quarter of an hour and the amount given and absorbed should be charted. As the amounts given are very small, accuracy is essential. There are now automated infusion units available which allow far greater control, monitoring and correction of the infusion rate.

Children's veins easily go into spasm when manipulated and circulation is slowed down if the infant is cold. It is important to keep the child and especially the limb warm. Even if the doctor is certain that the needle is securely in the vein, a little time may elapse before the flow becomes established and the nurse can assist by applying warmed cotton wool to the limb. Sometimes the clip regulating the drip is left open for a while to encourage the flow. Great vigilance is then required as the vein relaxes and the circulation improves, since the fluid may commence to flow freely and too large amounts of fluid may reach the patient. A nurse should remain with the patient until a regular flow has been established.

In children's wards intravenous infusions may be difficult to maintain but it should be possible to have the same infusion running for 4 to 6 days. The following points may help in maintaining a regular flow.

If the flow slows down, the nurse should make sure that there is no kink in either the limb or the tubing. She may take off the bandage to make sure it has not become too tight on account of oedema. The limb should be warmed with warm cotton wool or bottles filled with hot tap water and each protected by two covers. The limb may be moved or elevated and the nurse should ensure that the patient is not restless. Gentle massage of the limb may improve both warmth and circulation. Occasionally it helps to raise the intravenous container on its stand.

If these procedures fail, a senior nurse or sister may take down the dressing and make sure that the needle is still in the vein and that its tip is not pressing against the vein wall. A slight twist of the needle may start the flow once more. If none of these measures prove effective, the house officer should be informed and in the meantime a tray prepared in anticipation of his needs. He may want to inject a saline, procaine 1 per cent or sodium citrate 3·8 per cent solution into the vein and the necessary equipment should be ready for him. The injection is intended to relax the vein.

If blood is to be given, it will have been cross-matched and grouped in the laboratory, but the doctor with the nurse should check the label against the patient's record sheet. The amounts to be given in a specified time will be stated by the doctor but will rarely exceed 10 to 15 ml per 600 g of body weight in all.

During prolonged intravenous therapy Intralipid (fat emulsion compound) may be given to provide a large number of kilocalories. Care must be taken that the recipient set is changed before and following administration of this solution. Vitamin supplements, electrolyte solutions or drugs must not be added as large fat particles will form. Aminosol, a mixture of amino acids may also be given to provide essential protein for body growth and metabolism. Aminosol and Intralipid may be administered simultaneously through a Y-shaped connection.

Intravenous therapy is never without hazard. Vigilance is necessary to notice sudden shivering or rigor, restlessness or pyrexia, at the onset. The nurse should tighten the clip at once and stop the intravenous drip before informing the doctor. The

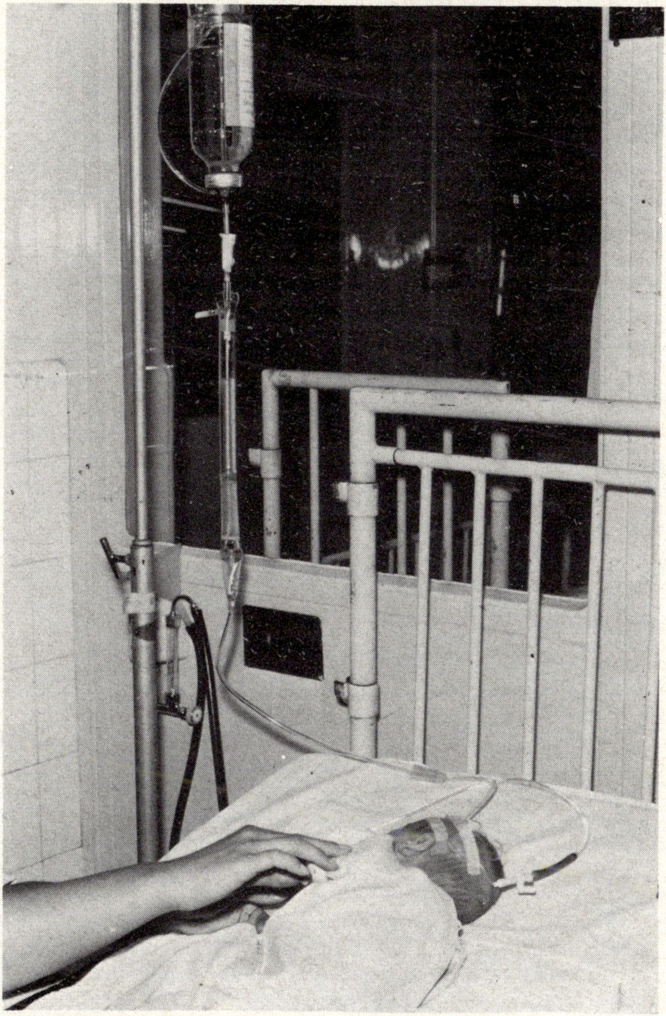

FIG. 15. Scalp vein infusion in a young infant following surgery.

reaction may be due to a blood clot, an air embolus, overloading of the circulation, or blood incompatibility. Phenergan or adrenaline may be ordered to counteract transfusion reaction. Long-term complications include wound infection, deep vein inflammation and transfusion jaundice.

Scalp Vein Infusion. For a scalp vein infusion, the infant's head is shaved over the parietal bone and an assistant holds the head securely. Once the needle is in position, it may be secured by strapping or by plaster of Paris approximately 7.5 cm (3 in) in width (Fig. 15).

Subcutaneous Infusion

Fluids are given by the subcutaneous route when there is an urgent need to rehydrate a patient or to restore the electrolyte balance of the body in cases where it is expected that the patient will soon be capable of taking adequate fluids by mouth or while a difficult intravenous infusion is being set up. This procedure may be used with pyloric stenosis, with patients suffering from shock, when there is pre- or post-operative need for rehydration, and sometimes when the apparatus and skilled care needed for giving fluids by the intravenous route are not available.

Two methods are commonly used:

1. The fluid is given by syringe and needle (when the amounts given are limited to approximately 30 ml at a time);
2. The fluid is given over a period of hours by the drip method (when up to 600 ml can be given in 24 hours).

Isotonic solution of saline or Hartmann's solution are commonly used. Hyaluronidase (Hyalase) is given to assist absorption.

Hyalase is supplied in powder form 1500 units per vial. This is mixed with saline 2 ml and one vial each injected into the rubber tubing about 2.5 cm (1 in) above the needle, or given as a subcutaneous injection. The Hyalase may be repeated after 6 hours if absorption is unsatisfactory.

The usual sites for giving subcutaneous fluids are: the outer aspects of the thigh; the abdominal wall; and the chest wall over the pectoralis muscle. The procedure is a strictly sterile one and is usually carried out by the nursing staff.

Subcutaneous Infusion by the Drip Method into the Thighs. The apparatus needed includes a dressing trolley, a syringe and needle, a vacolitre of fluid to be given, the subcutaneous set, ankle restrainers, bootees, and a good light blanket or shawl. The subcutaneous set consists of tubing, a Y connection, three gate clips, a drip chamber, two needles 2.5 cm (1 in), narrow strapping, and two vials of Hyalase.

When the apparatus has been assembled the air is expelled from it and the drip (approximately 60 drops/minute) is adjusted with the help of the clip on the centre piece of tubing. The infusion sites are cleaned and the needles are inserted subcutaneously. They are secured with strapping and covered with a small dressing.

During the procedure it may be necessary to discontinue the infusion on one side or the other by adjusting the clip on that side. Although the site is bound to swell, the area must never be allowed to become cold, white, shiny or hard and for this reason frequent inspection is essential. A fluid balance chart must be kept.

Non-accidental Injury

While the following paragraphs describe a syndrome which cannot strictly speaking be called an abnormality of the newborn, the syndrome is of very great importance and may be mistaken for one of the conditions just described. 'Battered babies' can be any children up to, and even past, the toddler stage.

It has been increasingly recognized over recent years that some young children suffer repeated injury at the hands of their parents. The nurse should always remember that the reasons are very complex. Young parents in an overcrowded home and short of money may feel it to be the last straw when faced with a constantly crying child and give vent to their feelings. The nurse should never judge but attempt to understand and support the parents whilst at the same time protecting the child.

Many such children appear well cared for and loved, and the assault by one or other of the parents appears due to momentary loss of control and usually ceases when the child reaches the age of 2 years. Other children may present with profound physical and emotional neglect. Often the bruising and haematoma are obvious but occasionally rib and other fractures are detected by radiographs, taken for other reasons; and the parents may give no history of previous injury.

If the doctor or nurse has any doubt about the cause of the injury the following recommendations were made by the British Paediatric Association in 1966.

1. The child is admitted to hospital for appropriate treatment;
2. A detailed medical history is obtained with all the possible information about the family from the family doctor and the health visitor;

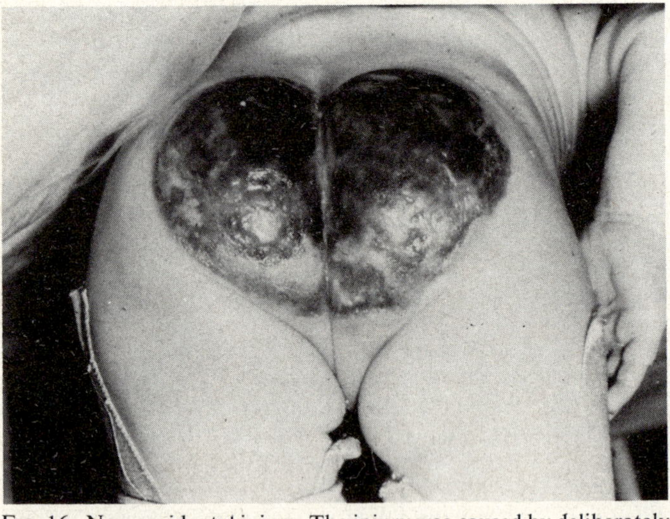

FIG. 16. Non-accidental injury. The injury was caused by deliberately immersing the child's buttocks in boiling water.

3. When all information is obtained the paediatrician should have a personal interview with the parents. If the evidence of inflicted injury is scanty, on discharge of the child the medical social worker should liaise closely with the family doctor and health visitor in order that supervision and social support can be given to the family to prevent further episodes and family breakdown. If the evidence is more definite the consultant should advise the parents that he is informing the Director of Social Services and that meanwhile the child will be kept in hospital. If the parents insist on taking the child home the paediatrician will explain that he will inform the police in order that a warrant can be obtained from a justice of peace to ensure that the child is kept in hospital or other 'safe place'.

This last action needs only to be resorted to in a minority of cases. Most consultants agree that it is best through the use of the psychiatric services and social agencies to concentrate on family rehabilitation and avoidance of further child abuse.

Further Reading

BLAKE, F. G., WRIGHT, F. HOWELL & WAECHTER, EUGENIA H. (1970) *Nursing Care of Children*, 8th ed. Oxford: Blackwell Scientific.

D.H.S.S. (1975) *Non-accidental Injury to Children*. London: H.M.S.O.

HARRIS, F. (1972) *Paediatric Fluid Therapy*. Oxford: Blackwell Scientific.

YOUNG, D. & WELLER, B. F. (1971) *Baby Surgery*. Aylesbury: Harvey, Miller & Medcalf.

6

Children in hospital

WHENEVER POSSIBLE the mothers of children under school age should be encouraged to be resident or stay with the sick child for as many hours as she can spare. A good nursing staff will however ensure that no mother feels compelled to spend so much time at the hospital that visiting becomes a worry. Pressures at home and the emotional security of her other children may be equally important as those of the sick child. No mother should be allowed to feel guilty if she does not spend all day in the ward and it is up to the good nurse to make parents see the opportunity for unrestricted visiting in the right perspective.

Resident mothers in particular are almost bound to worry about their husbands and any other children left to fend without her, or about a job they might lose by being absent.

Happy relationships between parents and staff develop readily if mothers are resident and the mother's contribution to the emotional well-being of her child is an invaluable asset to his mental health as well as to the job satisfaction of the staff. Much misery and future psychological difficulties may be prevented. Fathers too, should visit as much as possible.

Parents will need help in coping with the stressful situation of seeing their child sick or suffering pain. They may also be unfamiliar with hospital routine and even simple procedures they see carried out may, to them, seem traumatic or repulsive. It is also not easy for a mother, used to being in full charge of her child, to share this care and her authority with that of a nurse who to both of them is a stranger and who may, inadvertently make the mother feel inadequate or embarrassed in the hospital surrounding. Fear of the outcome of an operation may change the parents' manner temporarily. They may withdraw or alternatively become very demanding. On the other hand, nurses may feel observed and criticized by experienced mothers

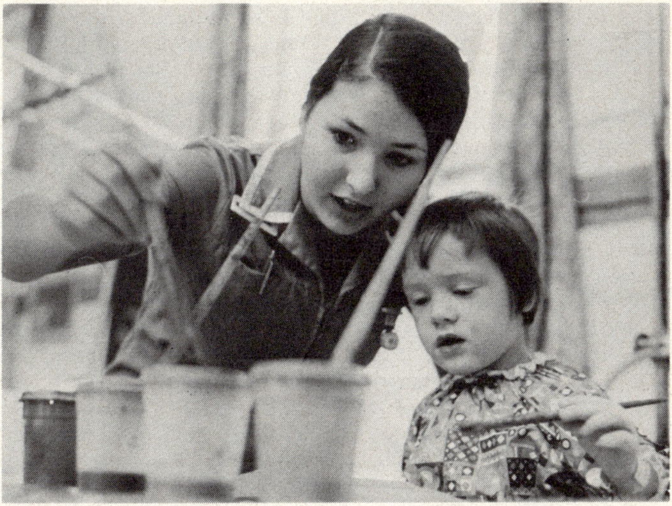

FIG. 17. Painting whilst confined to bed can be fun and absorbing for the young patient.

and either avoid them and their children, or become dictatorial and aggressive. The reaction of parents and the way in which nurses can help them in case of incurable disease or handicap is discussed in Chapter 23.

All these emotions add greatly to the stresses in a children's ward but if understood, make paediatric nursing all the more challenging and interesting. The young nurse will, in fact, be gaining experience in handling adults which is very important and helpful to her in her future career.

Young nurses dealing with children for the first time may well be puzzled by the problems arising from their behaviour. They will understand them far better if they consider them in relation to the child's family and social background. Children in the same way as adults are the product of their country, their district, their educational and social environment, their daily pursuits and contacts; but what applies to the adult applies to children in a far greater degree. The younger the child, the more dependent will he be on his mother or his mother substitute. It is important to realize that in many families the grandmother means as much to the young child as his mother, and that she often looks after him during the mother's absence at work. This should never be forgotten when visiting is considered. In addition, the pre-school child is defenceless and immature both in body and mind. He cannot express himself clearly. He has not yet learned to be adaptable and to make easy social contacts, and he misses his usual routine, his diet, familiar streets and familiar faces, occasionally beyond endurance. His emotional development is still immature and he lives in the present, incapable of understanding a tomorrow. He has a lively imagination and readily interprets what he sees and hears into frightening fantasies. He is very sensitive to the tone of people's voices, to their gestures and to the expressions on their faces and may read fearful and alarming things into them. Doctors and nurses should always bear this in mind when talking about a child in a ward or out-patient department.

Hospital Routine

Hospital routine may be deeply disturbing to children. To many of them being put to bed in the daytime implies punishment. This should be considered particularly with children admitted from a waiting list or merely for investigations. They do not feel ill and to put them to bed on admission can only add insult to injury and serves no useful purpose. Many children share a bed at home and few are used to cot sides after the age of 2 to 3 years. To sleep alone in a high, white bed, surrounded by bars can in itself be a disturbing experience.

The *newly admitted child* may never have seen people dressed in nurses' uniform and to some, hospital doctors and nurses have in the past been used as threats. It frequently happens that children are drawn to the ward cleaners, presumably because they wear less unfamiliar clothes and, in the case of a local hospital, talk the dialect to which the child is used.

Children are very dependent on a familiar routine, and no other person can imitate precisely the way in which the mother would set about the daily toilet or the dressing and undressing routine. This may lead to distress as well as protest. Children are readily labelled as having food fads. But here again, the child is used to certain foods, cooked and served in the way favoured by his mother at home. Family menus are very repetitive and only rarely will hospital diet be anything like the meals to which the child has been used.

Using a pot may be a worrying experience to a child who at home is used to going to the lavatory. Occasionally children fail to use the pot when given one, only to wet or soil themselves a few moments after it has been taken away. This is rarely due to naughtiness and should be treated with understanding. It is often helpful to place the pot on a piece of macintosh on the floor where it is easier to balance than in bed, and where the child may feel more secure. To balance the pot in bed requires some skill and the child will inevitably tighten up his muscles including those of the bladder and anal sphincters. For that reason the child may be unable to use the pot but as soon as he comes off it and is able to relax, he wets and soils himself.

The nurse should try to appreciate fully what this new experience of coming into hospital means to both mother and child and, whenever possible, should have a chat with the parents of the child she will be caring for and find out as much as she can about his habits and his home background. The following questionnaire is designed to assist nurses in finding out as much as possible about the newly admitted child and is particularly helpful in hospitals where 'patient assignment nursing' is practised, and for children below the age of 5 years.

Questionnaire Used for Children under 5 Years of Age

Name of patient. . . . .
Age last birthday. . . . . Birthday. . . . .
By what name is the child known?. . . . .
Names of other children in the family:
Brothers. . . . . Ages. . . . .
. . . .
Sisters . . . .
. . . .
By what name does he call his granny?. . . . .

Milestones:
Does he sit up without support?........
Can he feed himself without help?........ (does he use a spoon, fork or knife)........
Does he drink from a bottle or cup?........
Does he go to a nursery school?........
Does he go to a day school?........
Does he go to an ordinary or special school?........
What is his usual bedtime?........
Does he sleep alone? (*a*) in a pram?........
(*b*) in a cot?........
(*c*) in a bed?........
With whom does he share a bed?........
Does he take a favourite toy, dummy or 'Bye-Byes' to bed with him?........
Has the child brought this article with him?........

Toilet Training:
Does he wear a napkin?........ by day?........
by night?........
Are his toilet habits well established?........ still very new?......
Does he use a pot?........
What does he say if he wants to pass water?........
What does he say if he wants to have his bowels open?........

Diet:
Is his appetite good?........
Is his appetite capricious?........
What is his favourite dish?........
What is his favourite beverage?........

Occupation:
What types of toys does he like best?........
Does he watch television regularly?........
What is his favourite TV programme?........

Has he ever been away from home?........
Has he ever been separated from his mother?........
state reason........
Has he ever been to hospital?........ state reason........
at what age was this?........
Any special points of interest:

What is the child complaining of?........
(any pains, deformities, etc.)........
....
Does he know why he has come to hospital?........
....
Does he know how long he is likely to stay?........

Note for the child's 'own' nurse:
Admission to hospital and separation from the family (the mother in particular) may be a frightening and even harmful experience to young children. By knowing as much as possible about your patient you can help to minimize the trauma and give a feeling of security to both child and mother. If you wish, you may take further case notes on your patient and keep this questionnaire for your personal files after the child has been discharged.

The medical social worker and health visitor can do much to give added information and they are always happy to be called in to help. It is often possible to adjust hospital routine and procedures in certain ways and an imaginative, interested nursing staff can do much to mitigate the trauma of a hospital admission. Those nurses who are used to dealing with adults will have to take particular trouble in adapting themselves to the nursing of sick children.

It is now generally accepted that the mental welfare of the child in hospital is as important a consideration as the physical welfare. The very young child who has never been separated from his mother for any length of time, is at a complete loss for at his age she is the one who not only interprets the surrounding to her child, but also acts as buffer between him and the world. To have this security taken away suddenly must obviously be a very great shock and one which for many children, is more than they can properly cope with.

In some cases it is quite impossible for the mother to be with her sick child. It is then important to give the child a 'mother substitute' in the person of a nurse, play leader or other member of the ward team who can give a reasonable degree of continuity of care. The child who is faced with a variety of nurses, will feel lost and bewildered, a situation which may well result in serious consequences to his emotional well-being and development. To give a child a mother substitute (and this person has to remain the same throughout the child's stay if she is to be effective) is particularly important in the case of long-stay patients. It is also desirable to have family grouping, i.e. children of all ages and of both sexes within a ward and in hospitals where a child may spend a lifetime (e.g. in hospitals for the mentally handicapped) children should be cared for in individual units with a routine as near to family life as their condition will permit.

When Mother is Resident

The facilities provided for mother to stay with her child in hospital vary considerably from a chair at the bedside in which mother sleeps to an especially designed unit. The importance of this accommodation is that separation of child from the mother can be avoided at a difficult time for both of them when the child is in need of medical care.

Whenever mother is resident she should be made to feel welcome and introduced to other resident mothers in the ward by the nurse. The ward routine with details of doctors' rounds should be explained and the need for any special arrangements such as when mother may use the bathroom and where to make the occasional cup of tea. Mother should also be told that if she wishes to go out for a short period, perhaps shopping, she should inform the nurse in charge of the ward.

Mother should be encouraged as far as the child's condition allows to take part in the care of her child, helping to maintain fluid balance charts, giving medicines and assisting with washing and feeding. In some circumstances mother can be a very able assistant when holding her child for an injection or dressing giving support and encouragement. Mother often feels anxious and guilty when her child is in hospital and by allowing her to take a positive part in the care and treatment for her child will do much to allay these apprehensions.

The ward sister who knows the mother and family well should decide how much care each parent can give. Some mothers are able to do more than others but whatever part mother plays she will need support, guidance and information in the active partnership with the nurse for the care of the sick child.

The Surgical Ward

Children admitted to a surgical ward may need particular consideration. It often happens that they have been on the waiting list for some time and that they feel perfectly fit and are unaware of any abnormality which requires surgery and treatment. In these cases it is always important to take some time over explaining to the child in simple words that a certain treatment or operation will be undertaken. If the result is likely to be painful such as a sore throat following tonsillectomy, or immobility, such as may follow an orthopaedic procedure, the child should be carefully warned. Truthfulness towards children is always rewarded by trust and co-operation.

Elective surgery should be carefully planned so that admission at periods when the child is already under stress from other causes may be avoided. Whenever possible such operations should not be planned between the ages of 9 months and 3 years, at a time when the child starts schooling, when a new baby is expected while the child would be in hospital, or when there has been recent serious illness or a death in the home.

Children, like adults, are inclined to associate their own illness with illnesses they have heard discussed by adults and it is not uncommon for a child to have serious fears and fantasies for that reason. Children also resent and fear the loss of organs or parts of their bodies and can be seriously disturbed by the thought that a part of their body such as the tonsils have been 'thrown in the dustbin'. It is often a good plan to reassure the child by saying something to the effect that this part of his body was no longer needed and that he would get on without it even better than before. Fears of this kind are rarely expressed, but a good nurse should recognize the child who is in need of such reassurance.

Children are sometimes told that the operation will take place while they are asleep. Unless careful distinction is made between the usual sleep and this special one 'which is quite different from any other' a child may try to keep awake at night in self-defence, as it were, against the operation.

Long periods of starvation and the giving of enemata or purgatives before operation are quite unnecessary and may even be harmful. Any routine of this kind is outmoded and should not be carried out unless there is a specific reason for it.

The premedication should preferably be given to the child by his own nurse, whom he knows and trusts. Vallergan (trimeprazine) 3.0 mg/kg body weight is a useful pre-operative sedative. The patient should go to the theatre asleep or at least in a state of drowsiness. He should be allowed to hold his favourite toy. It is often possible to give the drug which will send the patient to sleep some time before giving the atropine if this is to be given by injection. Even though the injection may arouse the child, it is rarely remembered and in the majority of cases the child settles down to sleep again almost at once.

Surgical after-care in children calls for acute powers of observation and for fine judgement. Changes occur rapidly and delay in taking action or seeking advice may be serious. Changes in the blood chemistry, loss of blood, lack of oxygen and dehydration are all badly tolerated and young children become very toxic and disturbances in the renal function occur easily. On the other hand children recover more rapidly than adults. They rarely need to maintain a special position and can usually be allowed to adopt whatever position they find most comfortable. The absence of anxiety about themselves usually causes children to relax better than adults and muscular pain and tension rarely prevent a child from free movement, as they might do in the adult. Most small children will be ready to run around the ward the day after such operations as herniotomy or circumcision.

Bandages and splints require careful watching and very occasionally it may be necessary to restrain the patient's hands to prevent him from removing them. Bandages should be secured with adhesive tape or with a few stitches with needle and cotton rather than with safety pins.

A good nurse should never forget the parents' anxiety. She should see that they get the most accurate information they are able to understand about the child, the operation and the length of stay in hospital. In most instances it is both desirable and possible to allow the mother to stay with her child when the pre-medication is given and until he goes to sleep and to be at the bedside when he regains consciousness. Whenever possible the sister or staff nurse should personally speak to the parents the first time they enquire after the operation and so give them the maximum reassurance about their child.

The acutely ill child admitted to hospital is especially pathetic. He is not only feeling ill or in pain and incapable of understanding why all this is happening but, also, at a time when he would most need her, he is often deprived of his mother and everything that is familiar to him. A great deal can be done to lessen the distress.

Some hospitals have delightful little books or comics which tell mother and child about the hospital and what is going to happen there. Ignorance is one of the greatest causes of fear and the better informed the mother, the more she can help her child and impart her own confidence to him.

Visiting

Unrestricted visiting can make separation of mother and child more bearable and nurses should actively encourage parents to make full use of the facilities offered. Some parents are reluctant to visit because they think their child will cry when they have to leave. The nurse can explain to them that this is only to be expected, and that it is quite natural and far less harmful for the child that he should cry and be comforted than to feel abandoned, because the parents do not visit. Visiting can be made flexible so that fathers can slip in on their way to work and mothers come when the other children can be cared for by a kindly neighbour. The freer and the more extensive visiting can be made, the happier the ward. Occasionally, too, visitors other than the parents should be allowed. This applies particularly to a well-loved grandmother and to the child's own parish priest. Ward prayers and Sunday school are other links with a familiar routine which are appreciated.

Many mothers are eager to help with the nursing care of their child and enjoy giving him his bottle feed or a meal. Thus the mother gains in confidence and understands what is being done so that it is often possible to discharge the child far sooner than used to be the case when visiting was restricted to once a week. It should be the aim of every sick children's nurse to achieve early discharge rather than to keep a child in hospital unnecessarily.

Not infrequently nurses themselves are tempted to become possessive and to assume the mother-role with their young patients. The nurse's wisdom, tact and skill are needed in handling this kind of situation, and the more mature the nurse, the more likely is she to succeed in striking the right balance for the good of all.

Contact with Home

Occasionally children cannot be visited, perhaps because they have come from a considerable distance. Arrangements should be made to keep up contact with home in every possible way. Examples of this are: daily postcards or parcels from home, telephone calls between mother and child, photographs of members of the family to be kept on the child's locker, school and evening prayers. Any such link with home will make the stay in hospital less traumatic.

Children of 18 months or older may still be used to a *dummy* or a bottle feed last thing at night. However much a nurse may disapprove, she must resist the temptation to criticize the mother or to break the child of the habit at this particular time. The time of sickness and separation is not the one for breaking a habit which may give much needed comfort. On the contrary, a good nurse who is unable to comfort a toddler, might try a bottle or dummy on her own initiative. Sick children regress, and mothers sometimes do not disclose that their child is still used to a dummy or bottle feed, as they fear criticism from the doctor or nurse. The same applies to the child's favourite toy. It is a link with home and however dirty and worn or unattractive, the child should be encouraged to bring it with him and to keep it while in hospital. Hurry is always misplaced in a children's ward; the nurse who picks up a baby abruptly, or forgets to talk to an infant during feeding time, or leaves him crying merely because it is not changing time, is not a good nurse.

Play

Play is a fundamental part of every child's inheritance through which he develops physically, emotionally and intellectually. It is through play that the child explores his environment, communicates and learns; there is no dividing line between work and play. Toys are the tools of play. Throughout childhood the child plays, at first through contact with his mother, then on his own and later with other children of his own age. With play, the child expresses his feelings and fantasies and thereby learns to cope with the reality of everyday life. Play has these same values for the sick child and the need increases with being in hospital away from his home and family (Fig. 18). During

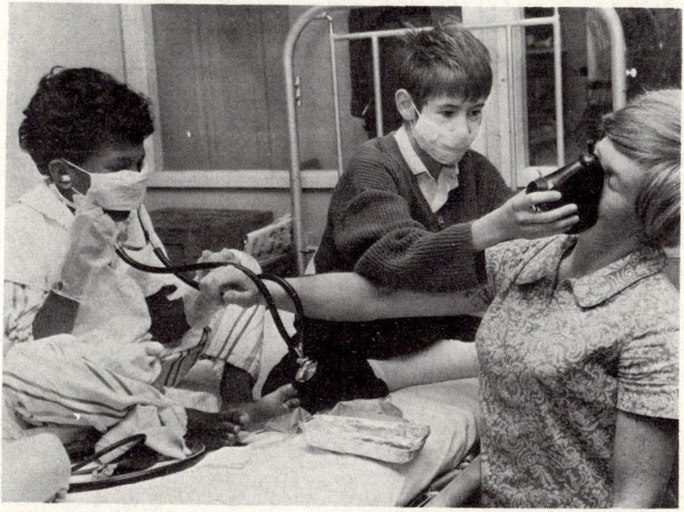

FIG. 18. Children playing at 'doctors and nurses' with their play leader as the patient, using old hospital equipment.

illness the child regresses, becoming emotionally a little younger than his normal self, only able to concentrate for short periods and he will play happily with easier toys than usual.

Often parents will ask for some guidance about suitable toys to buy as gifts. The nurse can remind them of their 'odds and ends' at home, the button box, the box of old keys, magazines, the rag bag, all of which will provide a link with home and occupational value. Other ideas that are inexpensive include, providing a special companion for the sick child with a hand puppet or rag doll, which not only provides friendship but enables the child to use the toy in dramatizing his situation. Toys that are too complicated or too involved should be avoided. Instead there should be things provided for the child to do, as well as visual stimulation, e.g. mobiles to hang on extension frames, snowstorm pictures or a felt board and scraps to make adjustable pictures. Children also need facilities for play apart from toys, for example a firm surface such as a bed table or tray, a 'play wall' for pinning pictures, 'pop star' posters or drawings up. Play containers for holding a child's precious toys may be a basket, box or bag and for some children 'play arms' are useful, such as the aids used by the elderly to pick up objects from the floor or bed. Mirrors can be used to reflect activities in the ward and elastic bands to project paper messages or pellets to companions. If the ward has a play area the child should always be taken there, providing that his condition allows it, for set periods each day. This play area should be sacrosanct and never used for treatments, medicines or medical examinations. An increasing number of children's units now have playgroups with play leaders as part of the ward team. Hospital play needs these specialists who are trained to provide suitable equipment and expertise for all ages of child confined to bed, wheelchair, or up and about, with a wide range of disabilities. The nurse needs to work closely with the play leader who should receive regular ward reports of each child's progress in order to ensure that individual needs are met. For those working in wards where there is not a play leader, the nurse should attempt to provide as much organized play as possible involving parents and volunteers. The following guide lines will provide a general framework for the nurse to use;

1. Supply materials which stimulate play and allow expression;
2. Play time should be given priority in the ward routine and should be without interruption;
3. Allow the child to play at his own pace;
4. Play for and with the child who cannot play for himself;
5. Relate play to knowledge of each child's development.

The equipment provided should include simple creative craft materials, puppets, books, building bricks, both board and card games as well as facilities for playing with sand, water, clay or dough. Children in hospital enjoy playing with ordinary household items and also hospital equipment such as stethoscopes, syringes (without needles), bandages and tubing, which allow them to act out their feelings about hospitalization. Wearing nurse's caps and face masks in bed as well as other dressing-up gear can be great fun for the child as well as being therapeutic, as an ill child who is happily occupied is likely to get well far more quickly than one who is not (see also Chapter 7).

Patient Assignment

The child should be handled by as few people as practicable. Each nurse should be allowed to become really familiar with a small number of children, rather than work all over the ward, knowing none of them intimately. She should stand by her patient when he is examined by the doctor and carry out any treatment for him herself. He will take his diet better from the nurse he knows to be his friend who has found out his favourite dish or arranges his food in a certain way. The nurse herself will get great satisfaction from 'mothering' a few children and getting to know them really well, and she will put herself out to please the child and to win his co-operation and love. A good-night kiss from his 'own' nurse can make a great difference to a homesick little child.

Nurses used to the nursing of adults often fail to realize that a few minutes spent in play or in reading to a child are as important as some complicated nursing procedure. They should never 'feel guilty' if found doing so by nursing officers or a consultant. The accompanying chart is a case in point. The child allowed to draw a picture every time he has had a drink will be willing to take extra fluids, particularly if crayons can be supplied for the purpose (Fig. 19). The gifted sick children's nurse can think of many such means of gaining the child's co-operation. Incidentally, mothers enjoy bringing a variety of drinks for their children and are grateful for suggestions of this kind from the child's special nurse.

Nurses should not be afraid of spoiling children in hospital.

Name and Age Rosemary Brown 6yrs Ward and Bed No. Charlotte Ward-3 Chart No. 5.

Date and Time	Nature of Fluid	Amount of Fluid	Urine Volume	Remarks
30.10.73 04.00 hours	Orange juice	120 ml	180 ml	
07.30 hours	Cereal, Toast and Butter			
	Milk	180 ml	N.P.U	
09.30 hours	Orange juice	240 ml	180 ml	
	Fruit			
11.00 hours	Orange juice	180 ml		
12.30 hours	Fish, potato and peas			
	Pudding refused		240 ml	
	Water	240 ml		
14.00 hours	Orange	120 ml		
15.30 hours	Tea	180 ml		
	Boiled egg			
	Bread and butter			
	Ice cream			
18.00 hours	Milk	180 ml	180 ml	
21.00 hours	Water	120 ml		
24.00 hours	Water	120 ml	120 ml	

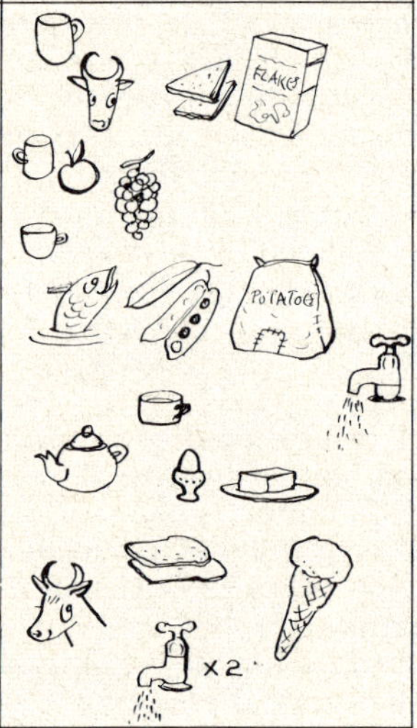

FIG. 19. Example of a chart that a child can draw himself.

It is often quite reasonable to pick up a child, to comfort and to rock him for a while. This applies especially to night time when 5 minutes comforting may be far more effective and kinder than giving the child a sedative.

Children have a way of asking very direct questions. In some it is a phase of their development, and in others it is anxiety breaking through and needing immediate reassurance. A child's questions should always be answered simply but truthfully. Children are sensitive to dishonesty or trickery. They respond far better if they are told the truth, though this can be done in a sympathetic way and encouragement given at the same time: 'this prick-injection will hurt a bit but it will not be for long, and the hurt will fade away. Hold on to Mummy's/Daddy's/ Nurse's hand.' Questions about going home should again be answered truthfully. The young child may have no conception of time and be satisfied with 'it won't be long now' while his mind can be taken off the subject by drawing his attention to a toy. The older child may be helped by making a little calendar on which he himself can tick off the days or fill in a space with a small drawing. It is surprising how much discomfort or disappointment a child can tolerate if he has confidence in his nurse and is treated with courtesy and respect by her.

Kindness and tact also achieve far more than threats and no child should ever be told that his bad behaviour might prolong his stay in hospital or make further painful treatment necessary. Adults should be careful of what they say in front of the child, since he may misinterpret what he has heard.

Some children may experience a *death in the ward.* The nurse should not be evasive or mysterious when asked about this, but give a simple straightforward answer according to the child's age. 'Michael has gone back to heaven' is often all that is needed to stop a child from brooding about the incident. But at the same time it is sometimes wise to add 'but this is not going to happen to you, you will be going back to your mum and dad'.

Emotional Reactions to Hospital

For some children a stay in hospital may actually be beneficial, prove an important stage in their social and emotional development and play a valuable part in the inevitable process of growing up.

Many children take the experience of going into hospital in their stride. Others however, may suffer disturbances and emotional trauma in varying degrees. Some of these are set out below and should serve as a warning to hospital staffs. Extra visiting, early discharge or admission of the mother should be encouraged to minimize the emotional hazards of hospitalization.

Here are some possible reactions which should be understood and treated promptly and with sympathy: Undue and persistent crying coupled with a refusal to be comforted. Regression to more immature behaviour than would be expected at the child's age, for instance bed wetting and thumb sucking. Exceptionally good behaviour or an abnormally co-operative child. The child may be very quiet and subdued and at first glance pass for a very 'good' little child, but start to cry when approached. Some children turn away from their parents when visited, others adopt aggressive or boisterous behaviour. Very young infants often fail to thrive and do not gain weight.

Older children may be very sensitive about their appearance. To talk to a patient about his physical defect, life in a wheel chair or with calipers, scarring, loss of a part, the loss or excess growth of hair, or even physiological changes of puberty, is time well spent. This need not be done formally but nurses can use any opportunity such as bath time or a few minutes when saying good night, to discuss the subject. Expressed fears are easier to cope with emotionally than suppressed ones. The patient will also be glad to know that his fears are understood and that he is not alone in his anxiety. The provision of pretty clothes suitably shaped to cover scars, wigs to cover loss of hair and other similar measures should occur readily to an understanding nurse. She might suggest to parents that they could bring such 'aids to beauty' instead of other, less useful gifts.

Giving Medicines

The medicine round in a children's ward rarely presents much difficulty as children follow each other's example and the willingness of one readily infects the others. The keynote should always be a matter-of-fact attitude on the part of the nurse giving the medicine. To approach a child with an attitude of apology and a look of disgust, coupled with elaborate promises that it will not taste bad, is likely to court disaster. The child will feel that he is, as it were, expected to dislike the taste and to make a fuss. It is far better to carry on an ordinary conversation and so take the child's mind off the subject.

Medicines for children should be camouflaged to make them palatable. This is often done in the dispensary where brightly coloured syrups of various kinds are available. Medicines are usually taken better in solution than in tablet form. Both should be placed as far back on the tongue as possible and followed by a pleasant drink or a sweet chosen by the child himself from the ward sweet tin. Sometimes it is necessary to mix a drug with a drink or some semi-solid food such as a mashed banana or jam, but even if this is done, the child should be told that the medicine is there. In these cases it is important that the food chosen is not an essential one, in case the child becomes permanently suspicious of its taste. This applies, for instance, to milk, orange juice, mince and custard. Pre-operative drugs are often bitter. If they have to be camouflaged, syrup or honey are best, as they are quickly digested and the danger of vomiting and inhalation during anaesthesia does not arise.

Some children co-operate best if they are allowed to take the medicine from a coloured spoon, through a straw or polythene tube or from a doll's tea set. The nurse should be adaptable and use her imagination to the full. The trouble taken will be richly repaid. Drugs and medicines are best given at times not closely related to meals in case the child should vomit the feed or meal with the drug.

On the occasions where there is difficulty, it is sometimes best to take the child out of his cot and sit him on the nurse's knee safely wrapped in a small blanket. She may have to shape his mouth with one hand and pour the medicine in, but it should be remembered that this method is not without danger as a screaming, struggling child may well inhale some of the medicine thus forced into his mouth. Some medicines are best given by placing the spoon at the back of the tongue and letting the medicine go down by gravity. It is as a rule, better to leave the child for a while and to return again later when his mood may have changed and he may be more co-operative. At all times, care must be taken to see that the whole dose is taken and that none is spat out or allowed to run down the chin or bib. Certain drugs are best followed by a small drink of water.

The effect of the drug given should be watched and recorded carefully and signs of intolerance reported at once. Punctuality in the giving is essential, as in many cases the efficacy depends on the concentration reached in the blood and a certain level may have to be maintained throughout the 24 hours. Children also get used to a certain routine and co-operate more readily if the medicine times follow a familiar pattern.

Dosage of drugs. Children's tolerance of drugs differs from that of adults; large dosages are often well tolerated. The dosage of drugs is often based on the child's body weight.

Accurate weight charts and the checking of weights by a fully qualified nurse are consequently important.

Resuscitation

The nurse working in a children's ward must be able to deal effectively with cardiac arrest. Not only may the heart have stopped suddenly, but breathing may also have ceased. A pulse may be absent and the pupils may be dilated.

In this situation one nurse will usually begin resuscitation of the child, while another calls for medical aid and fetches the resuscitation box or trolley. As the emergency procedure varies from hospital to hospital all nurses must acquaint themselves with the set procedure within their own hospital. As with the adult patient, success depends on team work. The aim of emergency resuscitation is the restoration of an effective circulation of oxygenated blood by means of artificial ventilation and external cardiac massage. Speed is essential to ensure survival of the brain cells which can only survive undamaged without oxygen for approximately three minutes.

Artificial Ventilation

The first essential is to establish and maintain a clear airway by hyperextending the head and pulling the chin forward, as obstruction will prevent adequate ventilation. A quick check should be made that vomitus is not present in the mouth, by placing a finger in the mouth. If the child has vomited, the vomit should be allowed to drain away by tilting the head and chest downwards.

Mouth to mouth breathing must be started if a re-breathing bag (e.g. Ambu type) is not available. The nurse using her own lungs as a positive respirator, can ventilate the patient's lungs. If the child is small enough the nurse places her mouth over both the patient's nose and mouth. In the older child she places her mouth over the patient's mouth and pinches the nose. She blows until the patient's chest is seen to expand; she then releases her mouth from the patient while expiration takes place. This procedure is repeated 16 to 18 times/minute.

External Cardiac Massage

The nurse places the heel of one hand over the lower half of the sternum, the other hand is placed on top of it. In infants this technique may be modified by placing one hand behind the infant's chest in order to give a firm base. Keeping the arms straight the nurse will depress the sternum approximately 2.5 cm (1 in) with a firm rocking movement 70 to 90 times/minute. This action compresses the heart causing blood contained within to be ejected; when pressure is released, the heart re-fills.

Ideally *external cardiac massage* and *artificial ventilation* should be combined. However, if only one nurse is available three or four good ventilations of the lungs should be performed initially, followed by one respiratory ventilation and six cardiac compressions.

Once medical aid arrives cardiac massage and ventilation will be taken over by the resuscitation team. If possible the head of the bed or cot will be removed to allow free access and a fracture board placed underneath the mattress. An intravenous infusion will also be set up to enable the following drugs to be given.

Sodium bicarbonate 8.4 per cent to counteract metabolic acidosis, Calcium gluconate 2 per cent, Adrenaline 1:10 000.

Isoprenaline (vasopressor) to sustain the blood pressure.

Effective resuscitation produces a palpable pulse in the carotid and femoral arteries. A pink colour returns to the face and spontaneous respirations and consciousness will return.

After Care

Oxygen will be administered and a mechanical respirator may be used to maintain adequate ventilation.

Pulse, respirations and blood pressure are recorded every fifteen minutes and the temperature every ½ hour. An oscilloscope may be used to monitor the electrocardiograph. To prevent inhalation of vomit, and to allow for feeding without effort for the child, a naso-oesophageal tube is passed.

Safety Measures in Hospital

Restrainers and Cot Sides

In hospital special precautions have to be taken for the child's safety. This is not only for the child's sake, but also because hospital authorities can be held responsible for any accident, and considerable compensation may have to be paid out of public funds. The use of restrainers for children at whatever time of the day or night should seldom be necessary and they should only be applied where there is no other method of managing the child while he is undergoing some form of investigation or treatment, or occasionally as a protective measure to prevent the child from injuring himself. The presence of a parent may in some cases eliminate the need for restrainers but it is very important to ensure that the parent does not leave without the staff knowing, because sometimes cot sides are inadvertently left down or the unattended child sometimes may be otherwise at risk. Restrainers should never be used routinely and should only be used as the result of a deliberate decision of the ward sister or deputy and of the consultant or member of the medical staff to whom he has delegated this responsibility. If used, restrainers should be put on with the child's co-operation as part of the process of being dressed. When put on for the first time, the mother may be asked to be present and the co-operation of both mother and child enlisted. The right approach will allay feelings of anger and frustration and will avoid psychological trauma to the young patient.

Restrainers may sometimes have to be applied when there is no other method of managing the child while undergoing some form of investigation or treatment.

Improvised restrainers must never be used (e.g. a harness made from bandages). The best restrainers consist of a close-fitting waistcoat which fastens down the back. The ties, made of webbing, should be secured to the rigid, horizontal part of the cot frame and never to the movable cot sides. The ties should be released when the child is asleep to exclude danger from strangulation and be long enough to allow changes of position.

In certain cases it is necessary to prevent children from touching their mouth or face as, for instance, after operation for cleft lip or strabismus. Simple splints can be made from wooden tongue depressors or from a piece of foam latex rolled round the arm, alternatively a roll of corrugated cardboard can be used. These restrainers are known as *elbow splints* and are applied with light, open-woven bandages. The bandage should first be carried round the child's arm, preferably over a sleeve, and then the well-padded splint is incorporated in the following

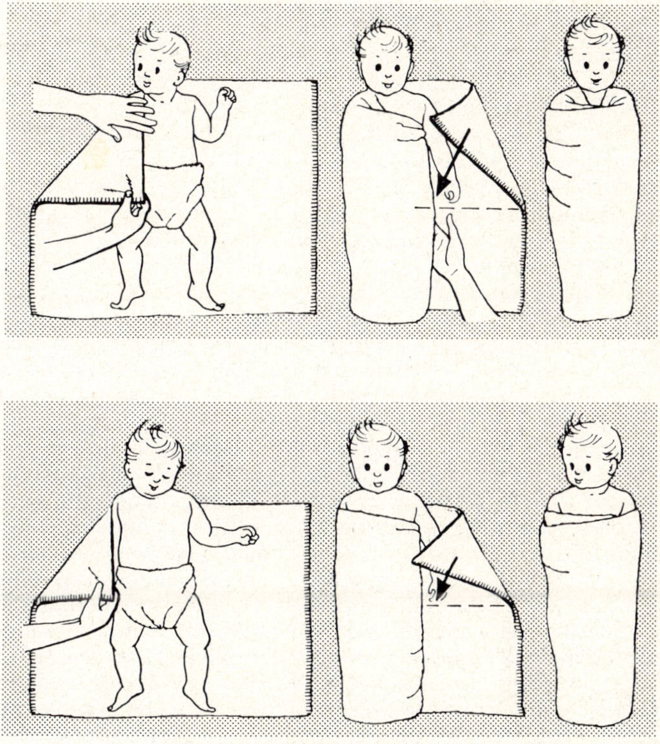

FIG. 20. Restraining the patient.

turns of the bandage. If this is not done, bandage and splint are liable to slip off like a cylinder. For *wrists and ankles* special restrainers can be made. Alternatively a crêpe bandage tied with a clove hitch may be used. Tubular gauze is another simple alternative. Infants are sometimes wrapped firmly in a blanket to avoid movement during procedures such as subdural tap or taking of venous blood (Fig. 20). Whatever restraint is used, it must be released at least at 4-hourly intervals to allow free movement under supervision.

Accidents in Hospital

Whenever possible children should be allowed to be up and about, rather than kept in bed. This places an extra burden of responsibility on the hospital staff.

The child who presents the greatest problem is the toddler. No equipment left standing about is safe from their urge for adventure. They enjoy opening and closing doors, and easily get their fingers caught. Any unguarded electrical point lends itself to investigation, and milk and other drinks are upset for the mere fun of it.

Children's wards should be as homely as possible and untidiness will never worry an understanding ward sister. But she must be able to anticipate danger and prevent accidents by wise precautions. Some of these are mentioned below but many more could be added and others need only be put into effect when circumstances warrant them.

Very young children should never be allowed out of sight, and objects which may cause accidents should be removed or suitably guarded. These include: sterilizers, radiators, lamps and light switches, thermometers, pots and bottles containing pills, lotions or medicines. All windows should have window-guards and the hot-water taps in the bathrooms should be detachable and hung out of the children's reach. Children should never be left unaccompanied in the bathroom and neither bathrooms nor lavatories should have bolts or keys. Drinking glasses and sharp feeding utensils are unsuitable for the very young and no chipped equipment must ever be allowed in a children's ward. Drinks should be just the right temperature, for a toddler will not wait to test a drink set before him but will eagerly immerse his entire face in a cup. Infants under a year should never be given a soft pillow and are usually best left without any pillows at all. If pillows have to be used they should be small, firm ones or the mattress should be raised, by placing a pillow underneath it. Hot-water bottles should never be left in the bed unless by express order and even then they should be protected by two separate flannel bags covering the entire bottle. The water is best taken from the hot-water tap rather than from a kettle. Electrical equipment should never be used unless a nurse can remain with the child for the entire time. Toys should be chosen for their safety and sharp, protruding corners or wires removed. *Mechanical toys which give off sparks are as dangerous in an oxygen tent as the striking of a match*, and watch must be kept on the type of toy given to children nursed in a tent.

Before taking a rectal temperature the bulb of the thermometer should be inspected and the nurse should keep a firm, restraining hand on the child to avoid sudden movement. When making the bed of a young child he is best lifted out or else a nurse should be on either side of the cot while the sides are down, or only one side let down at a time. A toddler can roll over with amazing rapidity and fall out on the far side. Bed trays left in position invite the child to climb on to them and make an otherwise adequate cot-side low enough for him to fall over. The vertical bars on cot-sides should be no more than 8 cm (3 in) apart. Lotion-thermometers and bath-thermometers must always be used and no reliance placed on the nurse's sense of touch. Plastic bibs should never be left on a child during sleep, as there is danger of asphyxia if the bib falls over his face. Small toys and beads are unsuitable for the under-3-year-old as they may be swallowed or inhaled. Safety pins should be used only where absolutely necessary and should always be left closed, when not in use. In many instances a piece of strapping, a tape or a stitch with needle and thread replace safety pins very satisfactorily. Finally, two nurses must always be present when injections are given, as even an apparently reliable 10-year-old may suddenly lose control of himself and move, or grasp a nurse's hand, thus breaking the needle.

Any accident should be reported at once and all details recorded. The parents should be told about it when they next visit, even if the accident was a trivial one.

Admission to Hospital

The section dealing with admission to hospital has been intentionally left to the end of this chapter. So far, an attempt has been made to describe some of the problems which hospitalization presents to both parents and children and some ways in which such difficulties can be overcome or made more easily acceptable. If these are understood a good admission routine will come almost automatically to an imaginative and sympathetic staff.

If admission is advised, the nurse should remember that, what has become so familiar to her, may be strange and frightening to mother and child. A few words about the hospital, about visiting and making enquiries, and about the ward and its staff, will give a mother comfort and will make her feel that her worries are understood. Her child will sense her confidence, and in turn will be easier to handle and happier and more content. The nurse welcoming the new arrival should act as a hostess would do in her own home. Professional bearing and a kind and understanding attitude will give confidence to the parents and this will quickly reflect itself in the child. In some hospitals it is customary for the nurse who will be looking after the patient, to come to the admission room and meet the new arrival. She should never go there wearing a mask and gown but should put them on in front of the child if his condition demands this. It is a good idea for her to take a toy for her young patient with her.

Once in the ward mother and child should be allowed to look round, meet the other patients and see the child's bed together. As she is taking the mother round, the nurse can learn something about the new patient, such as his nickname or any of his particular interests or fears. Some hospitals have a questionnaire which the nurse fills in and which gives her much interesting information (see p. 99). The nurse may here suggest to the mother of a preschool child that she may either become resident or at least arrange to be with her child for as many hours as she can spare. The ward sister will discuss these alternatives further when she talks with the mother.

Only after such a round should the nurse suggest leaving the mother to talk to the ward sister and take the child to 'find some pretty clothes'. Some hospitals arrange for the children to wear their own clothes. Where this is not possible, nurse and child can play at going to the clothes cupboard on a shopping expedition. The change to strange clothes is thus made easy and is not resented. A bath is not always necessary on admission and children rightly object when submitted to one at such an unusual time and in strange surroundings. If it is essential the mother should be allowed to be present. In a children's unit it is always wise to examine the child's head to ensure that it is clean as infestation spreads quickly to other children (see p. 402).

Since the new patient will already have had one examination in the outpatient or admission unit, the first examination by the house doctor can be delayed for a while, until the child is used to the ward. If the child is an emergency admission or a seriously ill child, the admission routine will have to be adapted accordingly, but in fundamentals the above points will still apply.

Examining the Child Patient

The physical examination of a child should include every part and system of the body. The technique adopted will have to vary according to the age of the child and the degree of co-operation to be expected. Once again, there should be an *atmosphere of leisure* and confidence and the child should be quiet and happy during the examination. A good children's physician will talk to the child first—no matter how young—for a quiet, pleasant voice can soothe even a very young baby. While doing so, he can observe many points of interest, among them the child's general attitude, e.g. whether he is relaxed or frightened. He can note the general standard of nutrition, physical care and cleanliness, the colour of the skin and the texture of the hair, and also muscle tone and general posture. Occasionally there may be a typical smell, or a certain typical facial expression may help in the diagnosis. The doctor may notice that the child's fingers are sore from sucking or that his finger nails look as if he were in the habit of biting them. The attitude towards the mother may likewise tell an important tale.

If the child is lying on the examination couch the position he adopts may be significant. He may draw up his knees to relieve abdominal colic or immobilize a limb to avoid pain on movement. His head may be thrown back and general opisthotonos be present, or he may turn away from the light on account of photophobia. He may be quiet and unresponsive or restless and anxious looking and his respirations may be characteristic of a certain disease. Some toddlers will roll or bang their heads if they have earache, or stuff their fingers in their mouths when they are teething.

All these details are of significance to an experienced paediatrician or sick children's nurse and further observations on these lines will continue after admission to the ward.

Every doctor will have his own routine in examining children but all will leave the more unpleasant or alarming procedures to the last. This applies, for instance, to inspection of the throat which few children will tolerate without protest.

Any instruments needed should be kept out of sight till the last moment and they should be warmed before placing them on the child's skin or tongue. It often pays to allow a child to handle an instrument first and to assure himself of its harmless nature before using it. Alternatively the doctor might listen to 'Teddy's chest' before he proceeds to the examination of the patient.

The doctor, or occasionally the nurse, may have to ask the mother to sign a consent form for operation. This must be carefully explained to the mother. Before doing so the child should be given a book or a toy to absorb his attention lest he overhear something that may frighten him unnecessarily. A consent form is usually required, not only for operations but also in case of an intravenous pyelogram when the injection of a dye might cause an untoward reaction.

Very young children do not understand instructions given and some little game may have to be employed to get them to do what is required. A mural on the wall or ceiling may for instance induce a child to move his eyes in the desired direction as he is told to look for a certain animal or familiar television figure. Telling him a story may absorb the child's interest and so make him relax a previously rigid abdomen and, finally, a good technique in supporting or restraining children can make a great deal of difference to the success of an examination.

Further Reading

BOWLEY, A. H. (1961) *The Psychological Care of the Child in Hospital.* Edinburgh & London: Churchill Livingstone.

CRAFT, RUTH (1976) *Play School Ideas.* London: BBC Publications.

CROSS, JOAN (1977) *The Significance of Children's Play.* London: Batsford.

D.H.S.S. (1976) *Play for Children in Hospital.* London: H.M.S.O.

GALT TOYS (1978) *Toys and Ideas When Children are Ill.* London.

GOULD, J. (ed.) (1968) *Prevention of Damaging Stress in Children*, Chapter 1. Edinburgh & London: Churchill Livingstone.

HARRISON, S. (1976) *Families in Stress.* Rcn Publications (Research Series). London.

HARVEY, S. & HALES-TOOKE, A. (1972) *Play in Hospital.* London: Faber & Faber.

HAWTHORNE, P. (1974) *Nurse I Want My Mummy.* Rcn Publications (Research Series). London.

LEAR, ROMA (1977) *Toys and Activities for Handicapped Children.* London: Heinemann Medical Books.

NOBLE, E. (1967) *Play and the Sick Child.* London: Faber & Faber.

PETRILLO, M. & SAYER, S. (1972) *Emotional Care of Hospitalized Children.* Philadelphia: Lippincott.

PLANK, E. N. (1964) *Working with Children in Hospital*, 2nd ed. London: Faber & Faber.

ROBERTSON, J. (1970) *Young Children In Hospital*, 2nd ed. London: Tavistock.

WOODWARD, J. (1978) *Has Your Child Been in Hospital?* London: National Association for the Welfare of Children in Hospital.

7

Sick children at home

WHENEVER POSSIBLE, sick children under the age of 10 should be nursed in their own homes. Chapter 6 on 'Children in Hospital' (p. 96) will have made clear the possible dangers of admitting children to hospital and separating them from their mother and their familiar surroundings. Not every child will react unhappily to the experience of hospitalization, but some few may show disturbances for life, some serious, some of a minor nature. The preschool child is the one most at risk in this respect.

Nursing the child at home, however, may tax a busy mother and housewife considerably. This chapter does not deal with special techniques of isolation, special diets or general nursing care. Where these are more complex than an average mother can be expected to manage, the doctor will call in the district nurse to advise and help. In some areas there are specialized paediatric district nurses and well-developed paediatric home nursing services (those of Birmingham, Paddington and Rotherham are well known). Where these exist, quite difficult nursing procedures and investigations can be carried out in the home. The good family doctor will also arrange for other types of relief such as Home Helps, special laundry services and help with other children in the family. In long-term illnesses Home Teachers are available.

This chapter will give a few hints on keeping the sick child happy and occupied. Few children feel ill enough to want to be quiet and inactive for any length of time. Most will want to do things, see what is going on and demand constant company. The mother's work will probably be much reduced if she brings the sick child into the living-room adjoining the kitchen, where she herself has to spend a good deal of time. Often this also means a ground-floor room with a more interesting view out of the window, a saving in heating and far less expenditure on the mother's energy with fewer journeys up and down stairs.

When the sick child is being cared for at home the mother may require advice for certain situations. The following are very basic to the nurse used to working in the well-equipped children's ward, but will prove helpful to the mother seeking guidance.

When to Seek Medical Advice

When to seek medical advice is a constant worry to parents since general practitioners are particularly busy people. It is always best to call him before 10 a.m., and the mother should be able to give a brief description of the illness. Advice should always be sought the same day for the drowsy, irritable child with a headache or earache. Also for the child with any breathing difficulty and for the child of any age with vomiting, pain and diarrhoea, when it is important that the mother should know not to give an aperient. If the child has unexplained bruising or any signs of bleeding the doctor's guidance should be sought. This also applies to the very young child under the age of 6 months, whenever he is poorly, refusing feeds or showing any other unusual signs. A child can be very ill without a raised temperature—his health should always be considered in relation to how he looks, any change of behaviour, what he complains of and the appearance of his urine and stools. When a child is ill no observation is too minor to be reported to the doctor indeed some small symptom noted by the mother will often be most helpful to the doctor in making a diagnosis. Every mother should get to know her family doctor, the health visitor as well as the district nursing sisters who are often attached to group practices in order that she can feel able to seek advice whenever worried.

Medicine Cabinets

Medicine cabinets should always be kept locked and well out of the child's reach. All tablets should be kept in child-resistant containers that are now available. All medications in current family use must be clearly labelled. Once a course of treatment is complete any medicines left over should be flushed away down the sink, unless the doctor has particularly suggested that they be retained. There are now some medicine cabinets available with in-built lights—these are more expensive but are the safest, so that when medicines have to be given at night (and often in a hurry) the labels can be clearly read.

First-Aid Boxes

All homes should maintain a first-aid box that can also be taken with the family when they go on holiday. A basic list should include:

Small pair of scissors with rounded ends;
Tweezers for removing splinters;
Safety pins;
Small stock of sterile packed dressings in assorted sizes;
Roller bandages in 1″ and 2″ (2.5 and 5.0 cm) widths;
A triangular bandage;
Small roll of cotton wool;
Small roll of adhesive tape;
Box of adhesive strip dressings;
Jar of Vaseline;
Antihistamine cream for insect bites;
Antiseptic lotion;
Protective cream for minor burns.

There is no need to spend money on toys or books. Indeed there is the obvious danger of spoiling the child who may come to expect gifts every time he is off colour. Here are a few suggestions, inexpensive, and yet perfectly capable of serving their purpose admirably.

Ages 9 to 18 Months

Magazines and comics to tear up, as well as to look at; simple toys that can be taken apart; balloons, teddy-bears or dolls with various rags to dress and undress; simple rattles made from well-sealed tins filled with pieces of wood (this will make just enough noise without deafening the family); wireless and record players if available with children's records of music and stories.

18 Months to 3 Years

Old Christmas cards and magazines; large beads to string; crayons; hollow blocks and other building bricks; a small aquarium or a budgerigar. A bird table just outside the window that can easily be seen by the patient; jigsaw puzzles or picture trays, bought or home made; conkers, daisies and other flowers to play with and examine; percussion instruments.

3 to 5 Years

Girls. Beads, conkers (through which father has made a hole); sewing cards with large, blunt needles and coloured thread; rags and bandages to dress and nurse dolls; a nurse's outfit; a doll's tea or cookery set; glove puppets (home made).

Boys. Dinkie toys, match boxes with which to build; simple construction toys; interlocking bricks.

Both sexes. Blunt, round-ended scissors; coloured paper; gummed shapes; a scribbling pad; crayons.

5 to 8 Years

Girls. Mother's button box to tidy (have a supply of matchboxes); cut-out dolls; dish-cloth yarn and thick needles for knitting dish-cloths for favourite aunts; loosely woven dish-cloths as a foundation for weaving with coloured wools and bodkin. Cotton-reels with four nails at one end for french knitting, coloured wool and a blunt knitting needle.

Boys. A book of trains and engines, old motoring and fishing magazines.

Both sexes. Tracing paper and pencils; a magnet; an old watch; a kaleidoscope; milk bottle tops to make mosaic patterns, mould or string up into 'mobiles'.

Matchboxes to build or cover in coloured paper; paints and colouring books; bits of felt or dyed lint and scissors to cut out shapes and for picture making; Plasticine; letter and number cards; toy money. Small squares of lint stuck to figures cut out of magazines, fluffy side outwards, can be made to adhere to a board covered with lint or felt.

Pipe cleaners and large beads can be made into animals and other figures. A thick notebook can be used to make into a diary (words and drawings).

8 to 12 Years

Girls. A mirror may give hours of entertainment, either together with a few ribbons, scarves and old hats for dressing up and creating hair styles or to enable the patient to 'converse' with her own image in the mirror. Scissors and thin paper for cutting out strips of people or animals and doilies by folding the paper before cutting and leaving a small piece of the contour uncut to form the link after unfolding.

Boys. Marbles; packets of inexpensive stamps, a geographical atlas and a notebook for starting a stamp collection. A mirror to play with reflections of light or sunshine; playing cards; an encyclopaedia.

A Few Points to be Remembered

Protective sheets may be necessary to prevent undue soiling of the top sheet and blankets.

Supply a good steady surface such as a tray.

Sick children tire quickly, and toys and occupations will need frequent changing.

Big or complex toys tire a child more easily than small, simple toys which can easily be changed.

A toy enjoyed today may be boring tomorrow.

Needless to say the toys given for the various age groups will please older or younger children. It is usually possible to ask friends or neighbours for the loan of books, jigsaws or other toys no longer needed by their own children (some will be only too glad to pass them on for good). The same applies to magazines, scraps of material and gramophone records.

The charm of any of these toys and occupations will fade quickly if all are left lying around all the time. Their value is greatly enhanced and their interest doubled if they are tidied away regularly to be brought out again another time.

Toys from children who have had an infectious complaint should, of course, be disinfected or destroyed in due course.

Preparing for Hospital

Sometimes the sick child at home will need to be admitted to hospital and the nurse's advice will often be sought by parents as to how their child should be prepared for this stay. Children should always be told about hospitals, doctors and nurses, from an early age, just as they are prepared for other experiences of life such as going to school. For the emergency admission it is obviously too late for detailed preparation, but the nurse will remember the child's need for comfort and security and that all questions should be answered honestly and directly without giving more detail than the child can understand. For the child on the waiting list to be admitted the time can be usefully spent in preparing for his admission. Some hospitals produce their own admission booklets which give helpful details about the ward routine and the facilities available. Often a comic or colouring section is included which helps the child to feel that this really is for him. There are also several books that can be bought, or borrowed from the local library.

Suggested Reading

ADAMSON, J. & G. (1975) *Topsy and Tim Visit the Doctor*. Glasgow: Blackie.

'ALTHEA' (1974) *Going into Hospital*. Cambridge: Dinosaur.

COCKETT, MARY (1961) *Mary Ann Goes to Hospital*. London: Methuen.

JESSEL, CAMILLA & JOLLY, H. (1972) *Paul into Hospital*. London: Methuen.

SOUTHGATE, V. & HAVENHAND, J. (1963) *The Nurse*. Loughborough: Ladybird.

WATTS, M. A. (1977) *Crocodile Medicine*. London: Andre Deutsch.

These books are suitable for children from the ages of 2 plus to 9 years. Shortly before the admission day it is helpful if the mother and child can visit the ward to be shown around and have the opportunity to talk with the sister. It is important not to place too much emphasis on the stay in hospital, but to include the preparation as part of normal family life, e.g. taking a walk past a hospital and pointing it out to the child as a place where sick children go to be made well again. It is important to the child that all questions should be answered truthfully, but in a language that they understand and is meaningful to them.

Further Reading

CHALMER, L. (Ed.) (1960) *Helping Your Child to Get Well.* London: George Allen & Unwin.

MATESSON, E. M. (1966) *Play with a Purpose for Under-Sevens.* Harmondsworth: Penguin.

8

Diseases of the respiratory system

YOUNG CHILDREN are very prone to diseases of the respiratory tract, mainly due to the small lumen of the air passages and to their poorly developed immunity to infection.

During infancy and early childhood respirations are often shallow, rapid and irregular in rhythm. At birth the baby breathes about 30 to 40 times/minute, by the end of the first year the respiratory rate at rest decreases to approximately 24 to 30 respirations/minute, by the age of two it is 20 to 24 and by the age of 5 years the respiratory rate is the same as that of an adult.

Respiration

Changes in the rate and depth of respiration occur easily in children and the cause is not always in the respiratory system. Abdominal pain may cause shallow breathing while any increase in the metabolic rate, such as fever, will send the respirations up. One can learn much from the careful observation of a child's breathing. In case of obstruction it is often important to expose the neck and chest wall and to watch for sucking in of intercostal spaces or the supra-sternal notch.

The respirations are best taken when the child is asleep.

Points to Notice

The patient's colour.

Whether the chest wall expands symmetrically on inspiration.

Whether the breathing causes restlessness or distress or is merely rapid.

Whether the child breathes through his mouth or nose, and whether the accessory muscles of respiration are being used. Posture is important. For example, children whose breathing is obstructed may throw their heads back or their arms outwards in an attempt to get more air.

Examination of the Child

It is usual for a nurse to assist the paediatrician in his examination. It is her duty to see that the patient is comfortable and well supported, and to have a small chest blanket at hand to avoid unnecessary exposure. The child who is old enough to understand should be told what is going to happen and it is usually well worth while to allow a few moments in which to gain his confidence. He might be allowed to handle the stethoscope or to listen to his own or his Teddy's chest. The stethoscope should always be warmed as the touch of the cold object will frighten the child and cause him to protest.

The paediatrician will first watch the child's breathing for depth, regularity, complete and symmetrical expansion of the chest wall, any undue wasting and any drawing in of the intercostal spaces. He will note whether the respirations are abdominal or thoracic, and determine the position of the apex beat. By now the child will have gained confidence and only then will the physician use his stethoscope.

Special point. When using the stethoscope on the back of a young child it is often a good plan for the doctor to hold the patient in his arms for he will know from experience that, as so often when dealing with sick children, orthodox methods are not always the most suitable ones.

X-Ray Examination

It is often difficult to obtain good radiographs of young children, but it will help a great deal if someone with whom the patient is familiar can accompany him to the department. With a little forethought, it is often possible to arrange for the patient's mother to be present and to assist. It is well to remember the fear a child may feel when confronted with a dark, unknown room or with the enormous structure of the X-ray apparatus. The X-ray plates and the table should be covered with a soft, warm material or protesting screams may well make the procedure both difficult and unsuccessful.

Position may be a problem in babies and toddlers, particularly when they are feeble and limp. Further problems arise if the child is crying. Nor can the child be expected to hold his breath during exposure. Often therefore more than one picture has to be taken and both lateral and posterio-anterior pictures are required.

Special Investigations

Bronchoscopy

Bronchoscopy may be done for various reasons. At times it may be performed in order to suck out pus or viscous secretions; at other times to determine and if possible remove the cause of collapse of a lobe of the lung as for instance a foreign body or a tuberculous gland. Occasionally some tissue is removed for biopsy.

The procedure is the same as for adults, but children are usually given an anaesthetic and preparation is done accordingly. In addition the throat may be made insensitive by means of a cocaine or Decicain spray. Bronchoscopy is not entirely without danger. The small air passages may go into spasm during the bronchoscopy and cause asphyxia. A drink, given before a good swallowing reflex has returned and the effect of the local anaesthetic has worn off, may have serious consequences. Approximately 4 hours should elapse between spraying the throat and giving the first drink, and the nurse has a special responsibility in this respect. A test drink of 7 ml (0.25 fl oz) of plain water should always be given.

Bronchography

In preparing the patient for bronchography postural drainage should be carried out at night and by a physiotherapist or nurse immediately before the child goes to the X-ray department, in order to empty the bronchial tree of as much stagnant pus or mucus as possible.

Bronchograms are done in the X-ray department or operating theatre under a general anaesthetic. Good premedication will ensure that the child is fast asleep before being moved from the familiar surroundings of the ward. Before taking the radiograph, a radio-opaque substance, usually iodized oil, is introduced into the main bronchus. This is either done by passing a fine catheter over the back of the tongue into the trachea or by inserting a needle through the cricoid membrane into the trachea. The radio-opaque substance, e.g. Dionosil with sulphanilamide powder is then injected by means of a syringe and allowed to outline the bronchial tree. According to the positioning of the patient the radiograph will show the bronchial tree in the selected lobes of the lung. Irregular filling will be proof of abnormalities which were suspected on clinical grounds and from straight X-ray.

On return to the ward, postural drainage is started almost at once. Thus, the danger of the iodized oil, pus or secretions spilling into the healthy parts of the lung is reduced. Frequently the patient may complain of a sore throat after a bronchogram and there may be a productive cough for some days.

Dionosil with sulphanilamide powder, or any other oily substance used for bronchograms, may set up sensitivity reactions due to its iodine content, and it is important to carry out a simple sensitivity test the previous day. A consent form must be signed previously by the child's parents.

Chest Aspiration

The requirements for chest aspiration are similar to those needed for adults.

The procedure is not really a painful one but it is very uncomfortable and may prove alarming to a young child. He should be told as much about what is going to happen as he is likely to understand, and a sedative should always be given.

The patient is made comfortable lying over a pillow, or sitting up and resting on a bed table and pillow. He should be kept warm and, if he is awake, the nurse should distract his attention by reading to, or playing with him while the aspiration is carried out. Warning of any injection should be given immediately before the prick and care taken not to let the child see anything of the preparations. Occasionally it is useful for the nurse to have the patient on her lap and to comfort and restrain him in this position.

A warm, sweet drink at the end will often help to settle a somewhat agitated patient and may induce a restful sleep.

Steam Tents

Various types of steam tents are in use, but the aim should always be to achieve maximum benefit from the warmed air while allowing for a clear view of the child, as well as for free circulation of moistened air within the tent.

The usual precautions are taken, such as not directing the steam towards the patient's face, but in addition children should wear a loose safety bodice and some sisters like them to wear cotton mittens as well. The spout of the kettle may be protected by bandages as an extra safety measure. A steam kettle may also be a danger to other children running around in an open ward and suitable precautions should be taken to avoid accidents.

Whenever possible, a special nurse or the child's mother should stay with the patient while steam therapy is in progress. Alternative methods of humidifying air are steam cubicles and Croupaire, a cool-vapour humidifier, or a Humidaire tent. As soon as the acute stage of the illness is over, plenty of occupation will help to keep the child at rest and this will also help to avoid accidents.

Oxygen Therapy

It may be dangerous to give oxygen in excessive amounts, or in too high a concentration (see p. 85). Therefore when oxygen is used for the sick child *the amount to be given* per minute should be ascertained from the doctor and mentioned on any report. An accurate flowmeter is needed. To count the flow by means of a *Woulfe's bottle* is rarely satisfactory, and it should be realized that a speed at which individual bubbles can be counted, only delivers 500 ml of moistened oxygen per minute. The usual precautions when giving oxygen apply. With children the danger from striking a match and smoking does not exist, but explosions can also be caused by sparks given off from mechanical toys and visitors need to be warned about this.

Children soon show signs that they lack oxygen by being

restless and looking anxious. The respirations become rapid and gasping, and the lips and extremities cyanosed.

Methods of Giving Oxygen

Not all methods used for giving oxygen to adults are suitable for children. In newly-born infants oxygen given in an endotracheal tube or oxygen via an *incubator* are the most commonly used. Later there are various models of oxygen tents for use at different ages.

Patients having a tracheostomy may have to be given oxygen. In these cases humidified oxygen will be delivered directly into the tracheostomy tube by means of a polythene catheter, or a specially designed Perspex collar and fittings.

Acute Bronchitis

Upper respiratory tract infections are very common in childhood, and may occur in the prodromal period of measles or pertussis. They may be mild or severe. When the inflammation spreads down into the bronchial tree, the patient suffers from bronchitis.

Acute bronchitis most frequently attacks children from overcrowded homes who are ill-nourished and debilitated. It is a common complication of measles or influenza, and children suffering from fibrocystic disease of the pancreas, mongolism or congenital heart defects are particularly prone to this and other chest infections. Allergic bronchitis, a familial condition, may also occur. In young children the illness remains a serious one.

Signs and Symptoms. The child suffering from acute bronchitis looks and feels ill. His cheeks are flushed and his skin and mouth are dry due to a fever of 39.4° to 40.6°C (103° to 105°F) or more. Respiratory difficulties make him restless and irritable. The accessory muscles of respiration come into play and the alae nasi may be working. The respiratory rate is increased and the respirations may be shallow due to pleural pain. A cough, harsh and dry at first but later productive, is present throughout the 24 hours and is both an early and an exhausting feature of the illness.

In young children the sputum is swallowed and this may at times lead to gastric irritation and vomiting. Occasionally the mucous secretions form a plug in one of the bronchial tubes causing collapse of a lobe or segment of the lung.

Specific Treatment. Oxygen therapy may be of use, provided the atmosphere is kept moist during the early, dry stage of the illness. Steam may be used to warm and moisten the atmosphere of the room but the high concentration achieved by putting up a steam tent is not as a rule suitable for patients with acute bronchitis.

Drugs. Appropriate drugs, such as penicillin, sulphonamides and antibiotics are given to combat the infection. Antispasmodic drugs are used in selected cases. Cough mixtures and expectorants are rarely of value for children, particularly if the patient is very young.

Complications. Collapse of one or more sections of the lung, anaemia, tuberculosis and general debility may follow the acute stages of the illness, while in young babies diarrhoea and vomiting are frequently associated with it.

Nursing Care. Children suffering from acute bronchitis should be barrier-nursed in a warm, well-ventilated room for the first few days until a communicable disease has been ruled out. Several pillows arranged to give maximum support are usually needed, but the child should be allowed to adopt any position he or she finds comfortable. Alternatively the foot end of the bed may be raised and all pillows removed to promote drainage by gravity. Unless the patient does so himself, the position should be changed frequently so as to move the secretions and to avoid the formation of mucous plugs. When secretions are profuse and the patient too weak to cough them up, the use of a sucker and occasionally even of bronchoscopy may become essential. Clothing should be light and warm.

For the relief of coughing, warm drinks should be given and often warm milk and honey are enjoyed and very effective.

Fluids should be given freely, but sore throat, tracheitis and cough may cause the patient to be reluctant and difficult. For bottle-fed babies the feeds are best given diluted during the acute phase and spoon feeding may prove less exhausting than sucking. The feeds should be small and frequent so as to avoid distension of the stomach and resulting pressure on the diaphragm.

Temperature, pulse and respirations are taken 4-hourly and any changes reported at once. The pulse volume should be watched with special care. Intake and output charts should be kept well up to date as intake may be small. As the illness is as a rule an acute one, and of short duration, mouth toilet, treatment of pressure areas and the care of the bowels present few problems.

Young infants may show signs of intolerance to certain antibiotics, such as Achromycin (tetracycline). A preparation of vitamin B is given at the same time to try and prevent diarrhoea and thrush. If diarrhoea should develop it can often be improved by adding Arobon or arrowroot to the bottle-feeds (for the treatment of thrush see p. 242).

Bronchiectasis

Bronchiectasis is a dilatation of the bronchi and bronchioles, resulting from the blockage of a bronchus, and may occur as a result of repeated chest infections, pertussis or measles. One or several sections of the lung may be involved. Additionally, a swallowed foreign body that has 'gone the wrong way', e.g. a peanut, resulting in bronchial obstruction will lead to bronchiectasis. It is inadvisable to give peanuts to young children in view of this danger.

Children so affected are pale, undernourished, underdeveloped and generally suffer from poor health. They usually have chronic upper respiratory tract infections and frequently the mother gives a history of several attacks of otitis media, sinusitis and chronic cough. In its severest form which fortunately is now being seen far less than some years ago, clubbing of fingers may be present. The teeth may be carious and the tongue coated. Halitosis is common and these children usually breathe through their mouths on account of the chronic nasal obstruction which is present. Hearing is frequently impaired. The chest wall may be deformed, there is shortness of breath and often a low-grade fever. Sputum is profuse, greenish, purulent and very offensive in advanced cases. The younger children are inclined to swallow the sputum, which causes gastric irritation and loss of appetite. Interrupted schooling, the result of frequent admissions to hospital, adds to the impression of dullness so often seen in these children.

Straight radiographs and bronchograms are done to confirm the clinical diagnosis. The sputum is sent for culture and for tests to determine the sensitivity to various drugs of any organisms present. White blood counts, blood sedimentation rate, Mantoux test, and sinus X-ray are performed. Antrum washout may be necessary for the frequently associated sinus infection, and dental treatment should be given when indicated.

Medical Treatment

In mild cases, or in those in which the disease is scattered through several lobes of the lung, postural drainage and physiotherapy remain the treatment of choice. In cases in which the

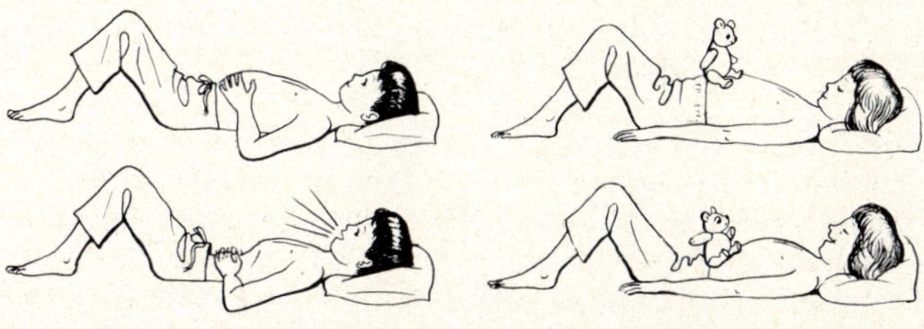

FIG. 21. Breathing exercises can be made to be fun.

diseased areas are well defined, lobectomy gives very good results.

In either case, the patient should have intensive physiotherapy and should be taught breathing exercises to develop his chest (Fig. 21) and the correct position to encourage drainage at night.

Postural Drainage of the Lungs. When the internal passages of the body become inflamed, the membranes lining them produce mucus or phlegm. If the phlegm gets too thick or too much, it may hinder recovery by blocking the passages. Usually phlegm is brought up and spat out, though in children it is often swallowed and does very little harm. If the phlegm is very thick, it cannot come up so easily and may stagnate. Postural drainage is done to remedy this.

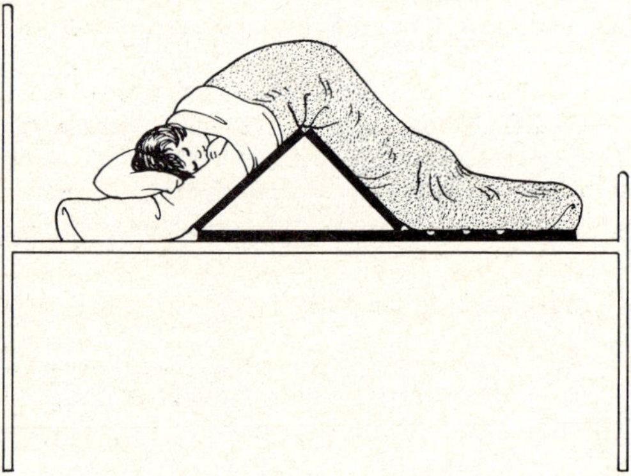

FIG. 22. If a child tips over with hips above the head, it helps the phlegm to run out of the chest.

From the physiotherapist, nurses and parents can learn to understand the positions which allow for maximum drainage of the affected lobe. The child should be allowed up and should have plenty of fresh air and exercise to improve the general tone as well as the finicky appetite. Activities such as hospital school or occupational therapy improve morale, and nurses should treat these children with sympathy and kindness, remembering the tedious nature of the treatment and the repeated admissions to hospital. Morning and evening temperatures are taken and observations are made on the nature of the respirations and the type and persistence of cough. The sputum must be accurately measured and its appearance noted. The child should be encouraged to expectorate, particularly on waking in the morning, and a warm drink given first thing may help him to do so. A teaspoonful of compound mixture of

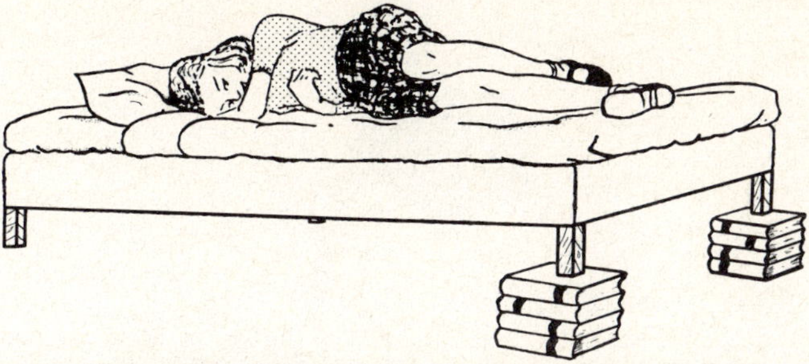

FIG. 23. Postural drainage. To clear the middle lobe you lie on your left side; to clear the left you lie on your right side.

sodium chloride in hot water, sipped slowly and given three times a day before meals is also helpful. Disinfectants should never be placed in a sputum mug in a children's ward but chlorophyll tablets added to the sputum will combat offensive smells.

Inhalations and nose drops may help to loosen secretions. When giving inhalations the nurse must remain with her patient throughout the treatment to ensure his safety and to see that the treatment is efficient. She should encourage both coughing and

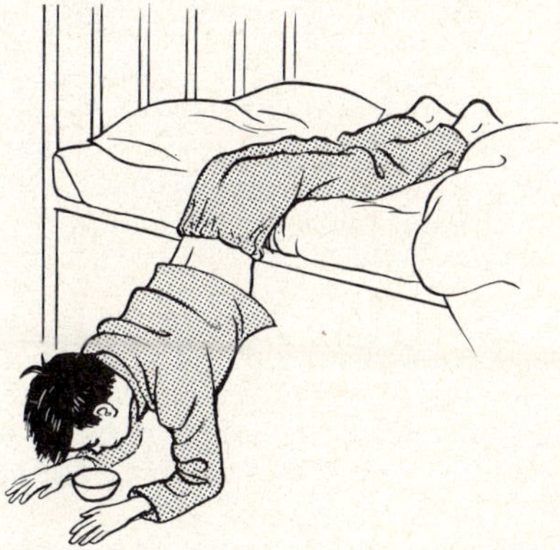

FIG. 24. Postural drainage for bronchiectasis.

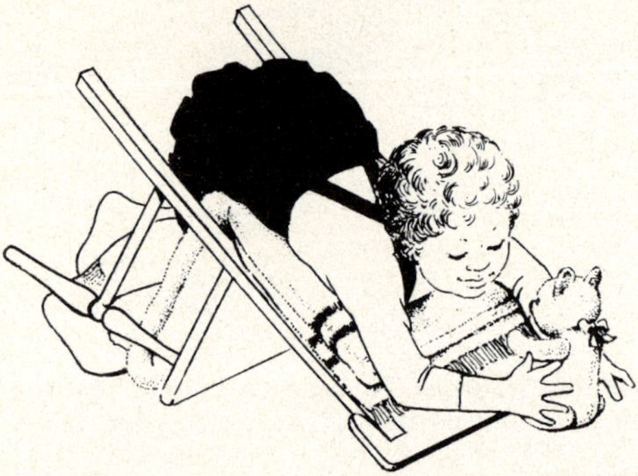

FIG. 25. A position for draining the right and lower left lobes.

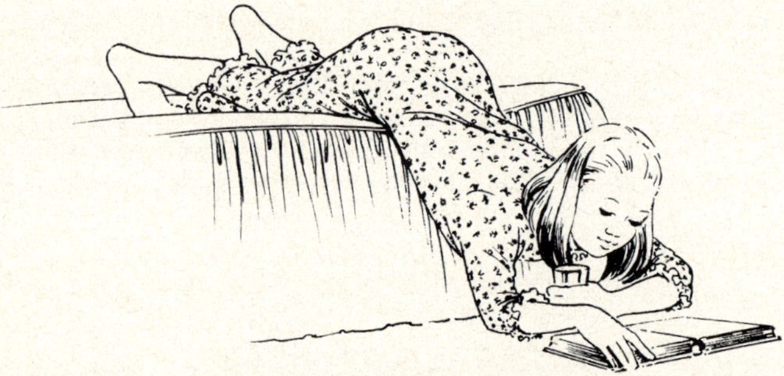

FIG. 26. Postural drainage. Keep this position for 10 minutes 3 times a day following a hot drink.

expectoration. Paper handkerchiefs should be provided and the child taught to clear his nose thoroughly on waking and frequently during the course of the day. It often helps to allow the child to hang his head downwards over the edge of the bed for a moment or two before blowing his nose in order to drain his sinuses.

Nose drops are sometimes useful for clearing the phlegm before postural drainage is attempted. Put five drops in each

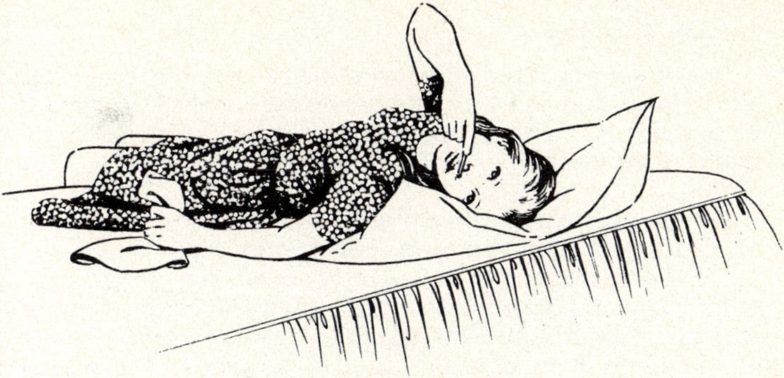

FIG. 27. Putting in nose drops.

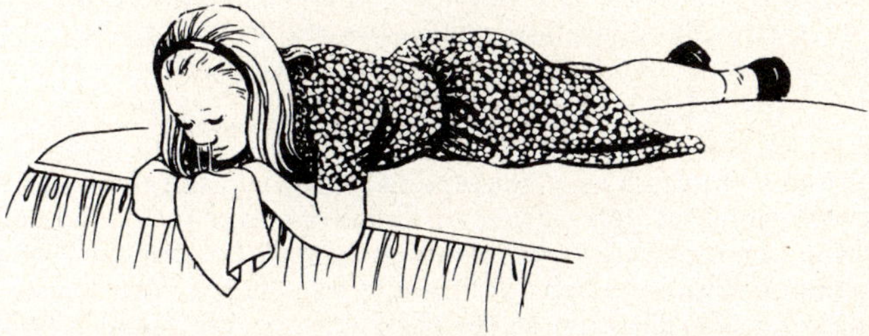

FIG. 28. After waiting half a minute, allow the nose drops and phlegm to run out.

nostril, keep the child still for half a minute then ask him to turn over and let the fluid run out of his nose (Figs 27 and 28). A hot drink and postural drainage should then follow (Fig. 26).

The diet should be nutritious and the addition of protein often helps to build up general strength.

The medical social worker and school medical officer can arrange for the child's admission to an open-air school where regular medical supervision, additional rest periods and physiotherapy are available during school hours.

Surgical Treatment

In cases in which the disease process has become irreversible and in those cases in which the changes are confined to one lobe or one side of the lung, segmental resection, or operative removal of the diseased lung or lobe may be considered.

Pre-Operative Preparation. Pre-operative preparation aims at eliminating all septic foci, and carious teeth, septic tonsils and infected ears should receive attention. Fresh-air therapy, antibiotics, postural drainage and intensive physiotherapy coupled with attempts at improving the patient's health generally, are all important if the operation is to be successful. The general management of all cases of thoracic surgery are similar and details can be found in Chapter 10.

The improvement in the child's condition is often dramatic, once the septic organ has been removed. The physical handicap following lobectomy is minimal. The child is allowed up 2 or 3 days after the operation and in the majority of cases a full, active existence can be resumed within 6 weeks.

Lobar Pneumonia

Various organisms may be responsible for causing the lungs to become infected and setting up inflammation. In lobar pneumonia one or several lobes of the lung may be affected. Lobar pneumonia rarely affects young infants. The patients are as a rule otherwise healthy, active children who are taken ill with great suddenness. They appear very ill with little warning though occasionally an attack of vomiting or a convulsion may herald the illness.

Signs and Symptoms. The temperature rises rapidly to 39.4°C (103°F) or more and may continue to swing at a high level for several days. The face is flushed, the child is bright-eyed and anxious-looking. The alae nasi may be working. The cough is painful and the child appears to suppress it in order to reduce the pain which may radiate into the abdomen, so that at first it is not always easy to exclude acute appendicitis. The child may hold himself so stiffly as to resemble a case of meningitis and the pain in the region of the kidneys may suggest pyelitis. The breathing is shallow, rapid and inverted, that is to say, a pause occurs between inspiration and expiration instead of normally after expiration. As a rule the rise in the respiration rate is much greater than the rise in the pulse rate. Even at an early stage the skin feels hot and dry and herpes frequently develops around the lips. As the cough becomes productive, the patient brings up sputum, which the younger children are likely to swallow rather than expectorate. Older children should be given a sputum carton and observations of the sputum may show it to be rust-coloured and frothy.

As the illness progresses the patient may become drowsy and if response to treatment is delayed, delirium may set in. Sometimes oxygen needs to be given and the congestive stage is quickly followed by formation of exudate which soon becomes absorbed. This is called resolution. The white cell and polymorph counts are high and the urine may contain albumin. Typical changes in the affected lobe show up on radiographs.

Drugs. With modern drug therapy lobar pneumonia is as a rule an illness of short duration. The infection responds well to sulphonamides, Orbenin (a penicillin derivative), broad spectrum antibiotics or a combination of any two of these.

Recovery is as a rule complete, though sudden collapse, herpes, pleurisy and occasionally convulsions may complicate the illness.

Nursing Care. The patient is best nursed sitting up, supported by firm pillows but otherwise allowed to find the position which gives him greatest ease in breathing and maximum comfort. Alternatively the special harness used in cardiac failure, a special chair, or the 'Baby Sitta' made by Ekco, may be used.

The colour of the child's face should be watched and pallor or cyanosis reported. The mouth must be treated carefully and the lips should be kept supple with petroleum jelly. Herpes, if present, is best treated with dusting powder.

The nasal passages should be kept clear, using pledgets of cotton wool if necessary.

On account of the high fever, the urinary output will be low and the urine concentrated, and special care should be given to the buttocks of incontinent children. Constipation is

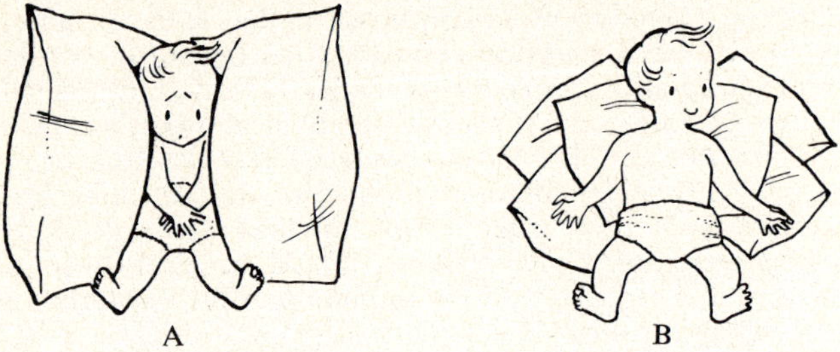

FIG. 29. Correct use of pillows in upper respiratory tract infections. (A) *Wrong*: Young children should never be given large, soft pillows as there is a danger of suffocation and overheating. (B) *Right*: The pillows are arranged to allow air to circulate, important in cases with pyrexia, and to allow for full expansion of the chest on inspiration.

common but opinions vary as to whether or not this should be treated. It will help both these conditions if copious fluids are given.

The bedclothes should be cradled and an electric fan can be used to assist in bringing down the temperature. Cool sponging of hands and face may do the same and also induce rest and sleep. The room should be of even temperature, but well ventilated.

Four-hourly temperature and fluid charts are kept up and during the acute stage observations should be recorded frequently and fully. Glucose drinks and diluted milk feeds are suitable in the early stage of the illness but when improvement sets in a normal diet can soon be adopted.

Bronchopneumonia

In contrast to lobar pneumonia, bronchopneumonia most commonly affects babies and children who are already weak and debilitated and this is one of the reasons why it is by far the more severe of the two illnesses. It often affects very young infants and is a fairly common complication of whooping cough, measles, severe burns and fibrocystic disease of the pancreas.

Signs and Symptoms. Occasionally the onset is acute but more often there is a history of an apparently harmless cold for 2 or 3 days. Then cough and fever develop and the child soon appears to be severely ill. Convulsions are common at the onset.

The respirations become rapid and distressed and are often of the inverted type with an expiratory grunt. The accessory muscles of respiration are brought into action, and the child may throw his arms above his head in an attempt to increase the air entry. His colour is often ashen grey or cyanosed, and the eyes are dull in contrast to the hectic flush and the bright eyes seen in lobar pneumonia.

Prostration is marked and becomes aggravated by the exhausting nature of the attending cough. The temperature is raised, though less so than in lobar pneumonia, and both respiratory and pulse rate are so high that they are at times uncountable.

The radiograph shows a mottled appearance with small, widely scattered areas of consolidation over both lungs.

Treatment. Treatment is similar to that for lobar pneumonia but in addition to sulphonamides or antibiotics, digitalis preparations may have to be given if there is evidence of cardiac failure. Oxygen therapy is given and occasionally the oxygen in the tent is moistened with a fine water or Alevaire spray by means of an atomizer connected to a cylinder of compressed air. As oxygen must be given in constant concentration nursing care and medical examinations necessitating the opening of the tent, should be reduced to a minimum and carried out with speed and efficiency.

Complications. In spite of modern therapy bronchopneumonia continues to be a serious illness. As large areas of the lung are congested, pulmonary circulation is restricted causing considerable strain on the infant's heart. One or more lung segments may collapse, later leading to bronchiectasis. Other complications include convulsions, diarrhoea and vomiting, and pleurisy.

Nursing Care. Most of the nursing points applicable to lobar pneumonia are the same for bronchopneumonia. It is, however, important that all necessary medical examinations, treatment and nursing attention be so co-ordinated as to make any disturbance of the patient as infrequent and brief as is compatible with efficiency. The acutely ill child usually resents being touched and every movement or struggle sets off a new bout of coughing. Long periods of rest and sleep are an essential to recovery. If the child is being nursed in an oxygen tent only a minimum of clothing is needed. In the later stages fresh air is good for the child provided he is kept warm and well covered. During the acute stage glucose fluids or milk and Bengers are very suitable foods. Tube feeding is often less exhausting than sucking and care should be taken not to embarrass respirations further by giving large feeds which distend the stomach. Warm, diluted honey is readily digested and is soothing to the cough.

Convalescence. Following discharge the child may not be quite ready to return to school. If possible the parents should be encouraged to take a family holiday, and, during that time, every attempt should be made to achieve an increase in weight and to build up general health and resistance. Medical supervision should continue until the doctor is satisfied that the lungs are once more fully expanded.

Pleurisy

When the pleura become inflamed, as may happen as a complication of pneumonia, the condition is known as pleurisy.

As the inflammation spreads from the lungs, the two layers of pleura rub against each other and cause severe pain. The child restricts both breathing and coughing to a minimum on account of the pain, and this causes both rapid and shallow respirations. He may also lean towards the affected side in an attempt to splint and immobilize it. Sometimes the pain is referred to the iliac fossa and may cause the doctor to suspect acute appendicitis. As an effusion forms, the inflamed surfaces are separated and the pain subsides.

A Mantoux test (see p. 422) and a radiograph of the chest must be taken to exclude tuberculosis and, if an effusion is present, some fluid should be sent for examination and culture.

Treatment. Treatment of the underlying cause is often all that is required. In mild cases the effusion is absorbed spontaneously but when it causes respiratory distress or displaces the heart and mediastinum, chest aspiration must be performed. In either case fibrous adhesions form and often show up on routine radiographs throughout the patient's life. Apart from this, recovery can be complete but a good follow-up and prolonged convalescence are desirable.

Thoracic Empyema

Sometimes thoracic empyema (pus in the thoracic cavity) occurs as a complication of pneumonia and occasionally when a pleural effusion fails to absorb, an empyema may develop. The infecting organism is as a rule the staphyloccocus. Pus in the pleural cavity is a serious condition, especially in the very young.

Signs and Symptoms. The patient with empyema looks toxic, his colour is grey and he is apathetic. His appetite is poor and he is often anaemic. The tongue is coated and the temperature may swing at a high level.

Medical Treatment. Daily aspirations of the pleural cavity and instillation into the cavity of an appropriate antibiotic are carried out. In addition the antibiotic will also be given orally or by injection.

Nursing care aims mainly at relieving symptoms and building up the child's strength and weight. A good general nursing routine is obviously called for as the illness may be a long and tedious one. The diet should be nourishing and appetizing, iron and extra vitamins may be prescribed. The nurse should always remember the alarming and uncomfortable nature of repeated chest aspirations (see p. 134) and do all in her power to make the procedure a more tolerable one. Plenty of occupation and frequent visiting will also help to keep the patient happy and at rest.

Occasionally empyema does not respond to the above treatment and surgical drainage becomes necessary.

Surgical Drainage. Surgical drainage of empyema may be done either through a wide-bore tube into a dressing (open drainage) or, if the pus is sufficiently thin, by means of closed drainage through a narrow-bore catheter connected to an underwater seal. In order to insert the narrow drainage tube it may be sufficient to introduce the catheter by means of a trochar and cannula. If a wider tube is used for the drainage of thick pus, rib resection is necessary and the empyema cavity is widely opened. In that case the dressings are changed at least twice a day at first and the tube may be removed and reinserted on alternate days. In either case intensive physiotherapy is important to achieve full expansion of the underlying lung and obliterate the empyema cavity. The nurse should encourage her patient to cough effectively and may play games with him which encourage deep breathing and lung expansion. As soon as the condition permits and the temperature has settled, the patient is allowed to get up as this will encourage deep breathing and good posture.

Drugs. Hand in hand with drainage, the empyema is treated by antibiotics, given orally, by injection or into the empyema cavity by instillation through the drainage tube.

General Treatment. Fresh air, a high-calorie diet, adequate vitamins and iron to correct the anaemia which is usually present are all important adjuncts to surgery. Whatever the treatment adopted, the young patient is likely to be frightened by the various procedures and the drainage tubes and sympathetic handling by his nurses will be needed to reassure him and to restore his confidence.

Asthma

Asthma is a respiratory disorder which presents as bronchial spasms, expiratory difficulty, wheezing and a feeling of suffocation. Asthmatic children are very frequently seen in paediatric departments and, during the course of an attack, may present an alarming and pathetic picture. The first attack may occur as early as the first year of life, and occurs more often in boys than girls. Infantile eczema may be replaced by asthma in the older child.

Signs and Symptoms. The following is a typical picture of an acute attack of asthma; after several hours of peaceful sleep the child awakes suddenly with a feeling of suffocation and in great terror. By the time the parents are roused he looks grey or cyanosed, his pyjamas are damp with perspiration, the breathing is laboured and wheezing, and expiration appears to be more difficult than inspiration. The accessory muscles of respiration are working. If the temperature is taken it is found to be only slightly raised or even normal, while the rise in the pulse rate is in keeping with the impression of an acute emergency. The respiratory rate is increased. At other times the attack may start during the day and would sometimes seem to be associated with over-excitement or frustration. In young babies the early signs of the disease may be noisy, harsh breathing and a cough. These attacks are usually diagnosed as teething or acute bronchitis and, though they may clear in one to two weeks, will gradually change to wheezing or obvious asthma. The *duration* of an attack may vary from a quarter of an hour to several hours and the patient may be shocked and exhausted by the time the attack subsides.

Examination. On examination, chronically asthmatic children appear pale, underweight and undersized. Their posture is often poor. A slight expiratory wheeze can be heard, as there is a constant, mild degree of bronchial spasm. In the majority of cases the patient is alert and intelligent, but at the same time highly strung and nervy. On closer acquaintance he may be found to be rather anxious, insecure and aggressive in his relationship to others. Very often the parents are over-protective and managing, or there seems to be emotional trouble or discord in the home. It is interesting to note that in many cases children known as established asthmatics never have an attack while in hospital or away at school.

Investigations. Investigations include X-ray of chest, bacteriological examination of sputum, blood sedimentation rate, sensitivity tests, and inspection of teeth and tonsils. The possibility that psychological factors may bring on attacks must always be borne in mind.

Treatment. Disodium cromoglygate (Intal) or Intal Co is effective in preventing asthmatic attacks when inhaled through a Spinhaler. Various anti-spasmodic drugs in common use include aminophylline given by mouth, intramuscular or intravenous injection, or as a suppository, pethidine, ephedrine and antihistamine drugs. Occasionally antispasmodic drugs are given in the form of a spray or via an oxygen tent. A sedative of the barbiturate group is often ordered at the same time. In addition to these drugs the following are now coming into common use, although they are frequently reserved for severe or resistant cases: isoprenaline (10-mg tablet dissolved under the tongue), by inhalation as a 1 per cent hand spray, or through an aerosol propellant and steroids. Dosage of the last two drugs is usually high at the start and gradually reduced to the smallest dose which will control the asthma. Cortisone therapy is not without danger and is reserved for status asthmaticus. After the attack has subsided, attempts are made to determine the factor which produced it.

Common Causes of Asthma. An attack of asthma in the sensitive child may be precipitated by various factors:

Allergic factors. Allergies are thought to be inherited as other members of the family are commonly found to suffer from hay fever, eczema or migraine. In asthma, the allergic factor is most usually inhaled and can usually be traced to the environment. Sensitivity to the house mite, found in dust around the home, is the most important of this group and explains why these children commonly develop their attacks at nights as the house mite finds an ideal dwelling in bedding and mattresses. The house mite lives on shed human skin and prefers humid, warm and dark living conditions. If the child's attacks are noticed to be seasonal, pollen is most likely to be the causative factor. Occasionally, sensitivity to pets occurs and it may be necessary for the pet to be taken care of elsewhere. This is a difficult family decision, but much unnecessary illness can be avoided for the child, and this should always be explained to him.

Emotional factors can often be observed in the child's relationship with his parents. Very commonly the child is described as being quiet and introspective and is often of above average intelligence.

Infection may trigger an attack in a child and this is usually of viral origin.

General Management. In the general management of asthma, known precipitating factors must be avoided. All pillows and quilts should be Terylene and the mattress should be enclosed in a dust-proof cover. Other beds in the house should be treated in the same way. The mattresses and the house should be vacuumed once a week with the windows open preferably when the child is out at school. Over-enthusiastic vacuuming more frequently should be avoided as this only stirs up the dust. Bedroom blinds rather than curtains should be used, and upholstered furniture avoided. The bedroom should be kept warm, dry and well ventilated.

Care should be taken to explain to the parents the nature of asthma, and that the treatment is aimed at reducing the number of attacks. It is important that the parents should not treat the child as an invalid, but encourage him to participate in all school activities. Psychotherapy may be required for the asthmatic child who is emotionally disturbed. Although the majority of children improve as they grow older physiotherapy will be needed throughout childhood in order to prevent the development of a 'pigeon chest' which in itself leads to repeated chest infections in later life. Breathing and postural exercises can be taught to the child and his parents, in order that they can be carried out regularly in the home.

Nursing Care. By and large, nursing care is symptomatic and consists of carrying out the doctor's orders, and reassuring the patient and his parents. The patient may get relief from sitting up well supported. Dunlopillows and cotton blankets should be used. Fresh air is often helpful and the room should be evenly warm but not stuffy, nor should the atmosphere be too dry. As soon as the condition permits, the child should be offered occupation and diversion. Though the attitude should be sympathetic, a degree of firmness is often essential.

Status Asthmaticus

When one attack of acute, spasmodic asthma virtually runs into the next attack, the patient is said to suffer from status asthmaticus.

Treatment and management initially are similar to that in ordinary attacks but, as this state may persist for many hours, exhaustion may be extreme. Relaxation and rest must be achieved by any means available, and this may tax the nurse's ingenuity severely. As so much energy is expended on the act of breathing it is difficult to get the child to take sufficient fluids. Sponging the face and hands, changing and turning the pillows and gentle massage of the patient's scalp with a hair brush can be very soothing. Quiet reassurance by speaking to the child may do much to calm his fears, and hot drinks, given in small amounts as often as possible, help as much as drugs, in getting the patient off to sleep.

The child may develop respiratory acidosis, and require intravenous therapy to correct the pH balance and prevent dehydration. Unfortunately, death can no longer be regarded as rare in this condition, and the use of a respirator giving intermittent positive pressure may be life saving.

N.B. One of the reasons for the present increase in deaths of these children whilst in status asthmaticus, is due to the intensive usage of anti-spasmodics before admission to hospital. It is important that an accurate history of the drugs received by the child is known on admission to avoid giving a lethal dose. The greatest danger comes from aminophylline which is very toxic in high doses, and should not be repeated if there is no response to the initial full dose. Severe asthma may persist throughout life, but mild cases may have cleared by the age of 15 years.

Acute Spasmodic Bronchitis

An acute spasmodic bronchitis attack may follow a common

cold, and bronchial spasm, cyanosis, pyrexia and a troublesome cough may continue for several days. The same drugs as those used for spasmodic asthma are usually effective and the nursing treatment too is the same. Any infected focus should be cleared up as soon as the patient's condition permits.

Further Reading

HUME, K. M. (1970) *Asthma: A Guide for Patients.* London: Health Horizon.

9

Diseases of the ear, nose and throat

EAR, NOSE and throat conditions are very common in childhood, and may account for much minor illness and frequent admissions to hospital or visits to the out-patient clinic. Repeated attacks of catarrh, otitis media, obstructed breathing and sinusitis may contribute to poor general development and diminish mental alertness; loss of schooling may affect the child psychologically as well as educationally.

For children prone to ear, nose and throat infections and congestion there are some simple measures which are well worth trying in an attempt at improving the tendency to recurrent infections. Among these are simple but thorough education in nose blowing and encouragement at breathing through the nose. Occasionally simple practices such as allowing the child to sleep with the head lower than the rest of the body may encourage drainage and parents should be made to realize that plenty of fresh air, particularly during the day, is as a rule more beneficial than keeping the child indoors for fear of his catching cold.

The Common Cold

Owing to an infant's small air passages, *a cold in infancy can be a serious illness*. Nurses must always remember this and avoid going near babies when they themselves have a cold; they should realize that a day off duty may prove a greater degree of conscientiousness than being on duty while they are a source of danger. The importance of meticulous care in hand washing and attention to every detail of hygiene is evident. Taps should always be manipulated with the elbows, and the hands thoroughly dried. A liberal supply of suitable towels and a hand cream are usually provided to prevent the hands from getting sore or chapped from frequent washing. Fingernails must be kept short and neither rings nor watches must be worn on duty. Masks and gowns, if used, should be put on and taken off as described in Chapter 3 (p. 46). If a nurse herself has to use a handkerchief, this must be done away from the baby's cot and should be followed by hand-washing and a change of mask.

Very young babies breathe wholly through the nose and find mouth-breathing difficult. Nasal obstruction may therefore interfere considerably with feeding as sucking is made almost impossible.

Complications which may arise from a common cold in infancy include otitis media, pneumonia and gastro-enteritis.

Laryngoscopy

When a doctor wants to inspect the larynx, trachea or the vocal cords, or if he wishes to remove secretions such as blood, mucus or vomit by suction, laryngoscopy is performed. With very young infants laryngoscopy can often be done without an anaesthetic; with older children, except in dire emergency, a general anaesthetic is given.

Before being placed on the table the child is securely wrapped in a blanket leaving the neck and upper chest exposed. Laryngoscopy may have to be performed in the neonatal period and for some of the conditions described below.

Choanal Atresia

Choanal atresia is a congenital abnormality in which the openings at the back of the nose are blocked by plates of tissue. Since the newborn infant has not yet adapted himself to breathing through the mouth, the condition has to be corrected as an urgent surgical measure or the baby will die. As the baby struggles to breathe the lips can be seen to move as in a flutter, a typical sign of this condition. An oral airway is introduced and the obstructing plates pierced by means of a probe. If the condition is unilateral treatment can be delayed until the baby is stronger and the structures involved less minute. In this case babies should always lie on the affected side to ensure an adequate airway.

Congenital Laryngeal Stridor

Congenital laryngeal stridor is not a dangerous condition and children usually outgrow it by the age of 1 year or 18 months. Parents, however, are concerned about the noise the child makes on inspiration and about the sucking in of the intercostal spaces. The condition is best observed when the child is crying or when asleep. Congenital abnormalities, such as laryngeal web or papilloma must be excluded as both are dangerous forms of respiratory obstruction, but in the majority of cases the parents can be reassured and told that no treatment is needed although it may take several months for the condition to disappear.

Croup

Laryngitis stridulosa, or croup, is an acute laryngeal spasm causing the patient to struggle for breath in a sudden attack of dyspnoea. The condition affects children of 3 to 5 years who are of a nervous disposition. The stridor usually occurs in connection with a cold. In a typical case the child awakens in the middle of the night, apparently struggling for air, sweating profusely and in a state of acute anxiety. The attack may last as long as an hour and is followed by normal sleep. Often the child has no recollection of the episode on waking in the morning. While the attacks are very frightening to the parents, they can be reassured about their harmless nature. A warm drink and a sedative may be helpful, and late, heavy meals should be avoided.

Laryngotracheitis

Laryngotracheitis, inflammation of the larynx and trachea, is probably caused by a virus, although *Haemophilus influenzae*, haemolytic streptococci and staphylococci are often isolated but are thought to be secondary bacterial invaders. Children most commonly affected are aged between 6 months to 2 years.

The chief manifestations of the disease are respiratory obstruction and inspiratory stridor caused by inflammation and congestion of the respiratory tract. The whole of the larynx and trachea is coated with thick, viscous secretions so that the air passages are narrowed. Adequate oxygen exchange becomes impossible and this leads to serious respiratory difficulties and general exhaustion.

Although pyrexia is occasionally absent, the temperature is usually 39.4° to 40°C (103° to 104°F). The child looks anxious, grey and collapsed, the pulse rate is rapid and the volume poor. An almost incessant cough adds to the exhaustion and leads to extreme restlessness. Respirations rise to 60 or more per minute as the child struggles for air, and the intercostal spaces and supraclavicular region are drawn in and the stridor increases.

Treatment. Treatment is required urgently. A *steam tent* is invaluable as the moisture prevents the secretions from drying up, but care must be taken not to overheat an already feverish patient. A *Croupaire tent* may be beneficial provided that the atmosphere is kept moist by means of a vaporizer with Alevaire, a non-toxic detergent which helps to liquefy tenacious sticky secretions. Occasionally an *emergency tracheostomy* may have to be performed as a life-saving measure, and fine judgement and careful observation are needed when caring for these patients as sudden deterioration is common. All necessary equipment for tracheostomy should be at hand, including an *electric sucker* for the extraction of the viscid mucus.

Drugs. A course of intramuscular benzyl-penicillin and gentamycin is commenced pending the bacteriological results of nose and throat swabs taken on admission. In exceptionally severe infections steroids may be given. Sedatives may be tried but are rarely of much value in the acute stages. If an aerosol is used the margins of the eyelids frequently become inflamed, but this is of little importance since the inflammation clears as soon as treatment is stopped.

Nursing Care. To procure rest should be one of the prime concerns of the nurse. Well-positioned pillows, frequently turned, loose, comfortable clothing (sometimes nothing beyond a napkin if the child is being nursed in a tent), sponging of hands and face, frequent, small sips of water or a glucose drink and even soothing stroking of the head may help to induce rest and so to preserve the strength of these children. The giving of oral fluids may be difficult, but small quantities should be offered if the child is able to take them.

Tracheostomy

Tracheostomy has to be performed whenever the lumen of the larynx has been so narrowed by disease as to make adequate air entry impossible. The trachea is opened by a surgical incision and held open either by dilators or by insertion of a tracheostomy tube. This may happen for several reasons, including:

Congenital abnormalities such as papilloma, laryngeal web or cysts;
Trauma, e.g. oedema following intubation or scalding;
Infections such as diphtheria or laryngotracheitis;
Paralysis, e.g. in anterior poliomyelitis.

Signs of obstruction

Distressed respirations, wheezing inspiratory stridor.
Restlessness.
An anxious expression.
Sucking in of the intercostal spaces, the diaphragm, neck muscle, sternal notch and the lower end of the sternum.
An increasing pulse and respiratory rate.
Cyanosis in most, but not all, cases.

With the above signs in mind it should normally be possible to appreciate the impending need for this life-saving procedure and only rarely is an unprepared tracheostomy required. Occasionally a bronchoscopy is done before the tracheostomy and sometimes an endotracheal tube is also passed.

When tracheostomy is to be performed the position of the patient is very important. He should be placed on his back with a firm pad under his shoulders so as to achieve full extension of head and neck (Fig. 30). Spine and neck must be absolutely straight in order to have the trachea in midline and unless a

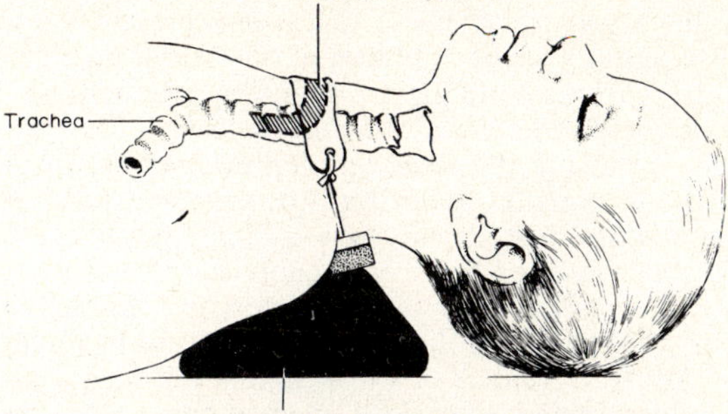

FIG. 30. Tracheostomy. Note position of pad extending the neck.

general anaesthetic is given he should be wrapped in a draw-sheet or thin blanket with the arms securely fixed to make any struggling impossible. One nurse should control the child's body and another assistant steady the head.

At the conclusion of the operation the tube is fastened securely round the neck by means of tapes and the inner tube inserted. The tape should always be tied with the neck flexed, as in this position the neck is narrowest. If this is not done, the tube may slip out of place when the head is brought forward. It is wise to use coloured tape or to colour white tape with ink, in order to avoid any confusion with the tapes of the child's bib or nightgown and, for the same reason, to tie the tapes at the side of the neck; a small pad of polyurethane foam will prevent the ribbon cutting into the skin. Improvement in the patient's condition is dramatic. Cyanosis is instantly relieved, breathing becomes normal and quiet and if he is conscious, the patient relaxes and falls into a deep, restful sleep.

Nursing Care. The patient is received back into a warm room and the air should be humidified. Barrier precautions may be carried out if indicated by the primary disease.

The patient's position should be a restful one and as a rule it is best to have him sitting up, well supported by pillows except in the case of diphtheria, when the heart may be affected by toxins. Care must be taken to keep the chin off the opening of the tube, and this is of special importance with young infants as they have very short necks. This may present a problem, which is one of the responsibilities of the special nurse who will have to be with the child all the time. She may achieve this by placing pillows in such a way that the the baby's head falls back slightly, so exposing the neck, or even by holding up the chin herself. It is equally important to prevent clothing from covering the opening of the tube and no fluffy clothing or blankets must be used for these children.

It must be remembered that speech is impossible, that the patient is often seriously ill and that he may be frightened and nervous. Wrist restrainers or elbow splints will be necessary for young children and for delirious or unco-operative older ones. While with the patient the nurse must keep a careful watch on his general condition, his colour, the quality of his pulse and the ease of his respirations. Any bleeding from the wound must be reported. It may happen that the tube slips out of the trachea while still remaining in the tissues. A deterioration in the patient's colour, respiratory distress and restlessness are all indications this may have happened (Fig. 31). If there is any doubt, a tiny wisp of cotton wool held in front of the lumen of the tube will show if air is blowing in and out. No time must be lost in sending for help if the tube has actually slipped. If it cannot be made to slip back into the trachea the tapes may have to be cut, the tube removed and the tracheal dilators used to make an airway. Occasionally air may leak into the tissues around the tube, causing surgical emphysema. As long as the tube is in the trachea and as long as it is kept well cleaned, the patient's breathing should be inaudible. An electric suction pump may be used to keep the tube free from secretions. Some surgeons allow a few millilitres of 0.9 per cent saline solution to be instilled into the tube to help clear it. The electric sucker must be ready to suck the tube out at once, if this is done. Disposable gloves may be worn during this procedure. Mucolytic agents to loosen viscid mucus may be used. Acetylcysteine, used with a nebulizer attached to an oxygen or compressed air cylinder, is one of these.

The nursing equipment needed by the bedside is the same for children and adults. Nurses should, however, remember that

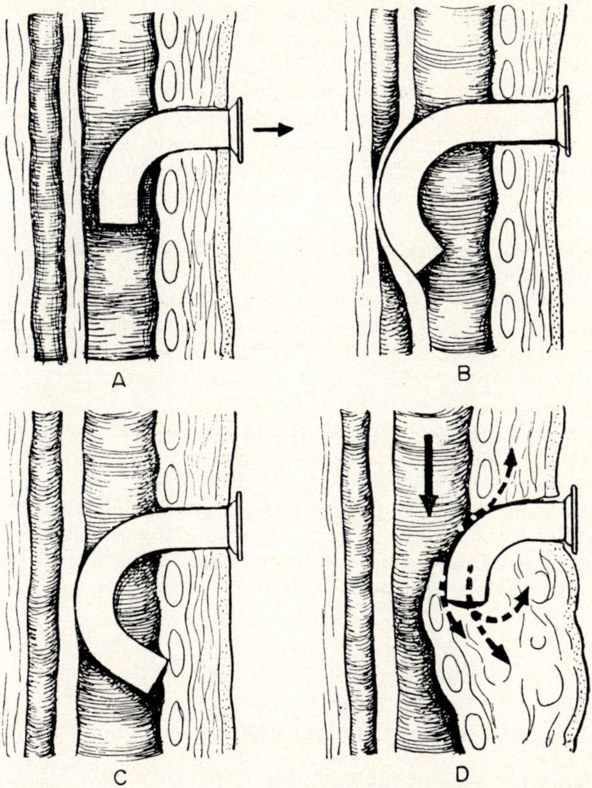

FIG. 31. Dangers of badly positioned or accidentally displaced tracheostomy tubes. (A) Tube of correct dimension comfortably in place. (B) Too long a tube. The child will have dysphagia. (C) Too long and too curved a tube. Ulceration of the interior tracheal wall may occur from pressure. There will be a continual cough. (D) Disaster. Too short a tube has been inserted. It has been loosely tied in. The tube has slipped. Air enters through the narrowed larynx and the wound. The result may be asphyxia, surgical emphysema and possibly tension pneumothorax.

they must be familiar with the type of tracheostomy tube in use. It is particularly important to be absolutely certain about the number of parts which make up a particular pattern and to understand their maintenance.

A tracheostomy does not interfere with feeding and the child should be given fluids and a light diet as soon as his condition permits, but extra care is needed to avoid any fluid from dribbling down the chin and into the tube. In paralytic conditions, however, feeding by naso-oesophageal tube may be necessary.

Tracheostomy performed in cases of acute illness, as in laryngotracheitis, can often be allowed to close after only a few days after plugging the tube for experimental periods. In cases of congenital abnormalities or neoplasm it may have to be permanent. Parents and children then have to learn how to manage the tube. The patient may be able to lead a fairly normal life.

After having had a tracheostomy for several days, children are rather apprehensive when the tube is to be removed. It is often helpful to give a sedative before attempting to do so. Occasionally the tube can be best removed while the child is drinking some favourite drink, as at this time normal rhythm between swallowing and breathing is easily established before the young patient is aware of what has been done.

Catarrhal Children

Children are very prone to upper respiratory tract infections, partly due to the close relationship of the organs concerned, partly because they have not acquired the necessary immunity against these infections. A great deal of schooling is missed in the first school years due to absence caused by coughs, colds, earache, throat infections and wheezy chests. Enlarged tonsils and adenoids are sometimes blamed for these periods of sickness, but it seems likely that they are not the cause but the effect and that they play a useful part in developing immunity.

Tonsillitis

Throat infections, such as tonsillitis, most frequently caused by the haemolytic streptococcus, are very common in children. The patient is often severely ill and this applies particularly to children under school age.

As children are not always capable of describing pain accurately, they may complain of abdominal pain. In addition, vomiting may be present and it is thus not easy to exclude acute appendicitis. As the neck is frequently held stiffly the condition may at first be mistaken for meningitis. Often mesenteric adenitis develops simultaneously causing general rigidity and confusing diagnosis still further.

The child is generally ill and fractious. The face is flushed, the temperature perhaps as high as 39.4°C (103°F) and headache may cause him to turn away from the light. Saliva may dribble from the mouth or alternatively the lips are parched and cracked.

When any other conditions have been excluded, a throat swab is taken to determine the causative organism and its sensitivity to drugs. Penicillin, given by injection, is the drug most commonly used.

Nursing Care. Patients suffering from tonsillitis should be barrier nursed for at least 24 hours after commencing treatment. If there is a high temperature the bed clothes should be light and supported by a bed cradle. An electric fan, well out of reach of the patient, may be used, and tepid sponging may be carried out with the doctor's permission. Mouth toilet, including mouth washes with a mild antiseptic such as glycothymoline or with saline, will help to keep the mouth clean.

Aspirin gargles may relieve the pain and are often given about 20 minutes before meals to make swallowing easier. As the child is likely to refuse solid food in the early stages of the illness, he should be encouraged to take frequent drinks of cool, bland fluids. Ice cream is soothing and is often taken eagerly when other foods are refused. Later, extra nourishment in the form of milk and eggs should be given.

If the child is treated with modern drugs improvement is as a rule rapid and he may be ready for discharge in 4 or 5 days. On the other hand, the infection may spread to the middle ear and the cervical glands. Convulsions occur fairly frequently but are rarely of a serious nature, and the parents may be reassured about this.

Special Points. If nursed in an open ward, these children should never be placed next to others suffering from acute rheumatism, nephritis or congenital heart disease, as streptococcal infections are serious in patients suffering from these conditions.

Retropharyngeal Abscess

Retropharyngeal abscess occurs fairly frequently in young debilitated children. The abscess forms in a lymph gland in the pharynx and is situated underneath the mucous membrane between the post-pharyngeal wall and the cervical vertebrae. As it protrudes into the back of the throat it causes a swelling (which is always central), pain and difficulty in swallowing and breathing. The child is ill and toxic with a high temperature, flushed cheeks and sunken eyes. Fluids are obstinately refused and the child moves around restlessly in an attempt to find a position which allows for easier breathing. The head is held stiffly as every movement causes pain.

The illness is extremely acute and progresses with great rapidity. The abscess may burst spontaneously but although this may be followed by relief and general improvement there is a danger of inhalation of pus and subsequent lung infection. As a rule operation is therefore preferred. If time permits the child is prepared in the usual way in the ward and placed on the operating table with the head below the level of the body, or in the same position as for tonsillectomy. Occasionally the situation is a very urgent one and the opening has to be done without anaesthetic. In this case the child is wrapped in a blanket and restrained by an assistant. With the child's head well down a mouth gag is inserted and a pair of closed sinus forceps or a guarded scalpel used to puncture the abscess. Immediately this is done, the child is turned on his side with the head well below the level of the shoulders and the pus is removed by means of an electric sucker, and mouth and throat are thoroughly cleared with gauze swabs. A specimen of pus is sent to the laboratory for sensitivity tests.

Improvement is usually rapid and may be hastened by giving an appropriate antibiotic, abundant fluids, a light, high-calorie diet, vitamins and iron.

Quinsy or Peritonsillar Abscess

Quinsy is much rarer in childhood than retropharyngeal abscess. The abscess often follows tonsillitis and forms in one of the crypts of the tonsils. The swelling is therefore always a one-sided one. Pain is severe and prevents the patient from opening his mouth (trismus) and from swallowing. The illness may continue for a week or two and the difficulty of swallowing, taking nourishment and finding rest may seriously affect an already debilitated patient.

Treatment. Treatment may be conservative or surgical. In the first instance hot gargles, warm compresses to the neck, Disprin-swallows, antibiotics and careful mouth toilet are given. Surgical treatment follows the same lines as those for retropharyngeal abscess. In either case removal of the diseased tonsils should be considered at a later date and treatment given for any dental caries or oral sepsis.

Tonsillectomy and Adenoidectomy

Operation for the removal of tonsils and adenoids is among the most common surgical procedures in a children's unit. Some nurses feel that they are here dealing with an undramatic and uninteresting routine job, but if they are made to realize how often the removal of diseased tonsils and hypertrophied adenoids improves the child's general health and how other illnesses such as recurrent tonsillitis, otitis media, sinusitis and even bronchiectasis and general development can be improved, they will realize the importance of this type of surgery and will find it of real interest.

Ideally, patients for tonsillectomy should be admitted the day before operation in order to allow them to get used to the ward and the nurses and to be fully examined. They should be told simply what is about to happen and expectations about parties, ice cream and the like, which some parents still promise, should be tactfully but firmly dispelled.

Temperature, pulse and respirations are taken and recorded 4-hourly but as most of these children are mouth breathers, it is usually best to take the temperature in the axilla. Any fever and any other observations, such as coughs or purulent nasal discharge, are reported. Routine urine testing is carried out. A glucose drink is given 2 to 4 hours before the anaesthetic. The teeth should be cleaned as part of the immediate pre-operative preparation. Premedication should include a sedative which will cause amnesia but at the same time is sufficiently light to allow for a rapid return of the cough reflex following operation. The hair of little girls should be kept out of the way with narrow ribbon and the operation gown should be left unbuttoned as the anaesthetist will want to slip it well off the shoulders when the patient is placed on the theatre table. In some units pyjama trousers only are worn by both girls and boys.

The operation differs in no way from that done in adults and on return to the ward the usual 'tonsillectomy position' is adopted, i.e. the child lies on his side with the upper leg bent and the upper arm flexed in front of the head with the body leaning forward (Fig. 32). A pillow in the back will assist in

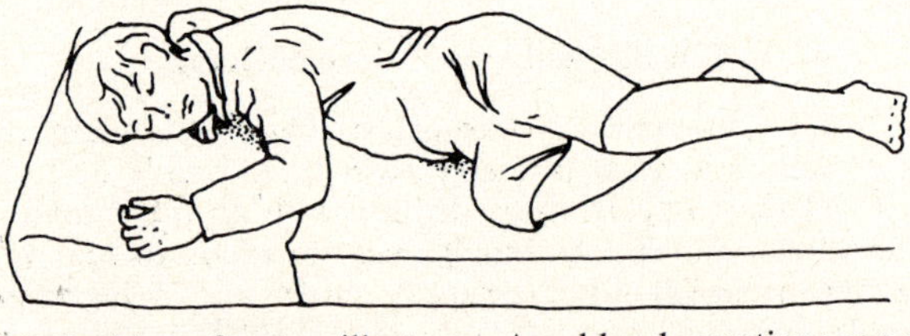

FIG. 32. Position after tonsillectomy. Any blood secretions can easily drain out of the mouth and inhalation is thus prevented.

maintaining this position which will ensure that any blood trickles out of the mouth rather than down the throat. In that way the danger of inhaling blood is greatly reduced and any abnormal bleeding can easily be observed. The neck should remain exposed as regular swallowing movement of the neck muscles may be the first sign that there is some bleeding and that the child is swallowing blood. Some surgeons return the patient to the ward with tongue clips still holding the tongue safely forward, others ensure that the cough reflex is fully recovered before the patient leaves the theatre and that the level of consciousness is such that there is no danger of obstruction from the tongue falling back. Cold sponging of the face will hasten the return to consciousness and refresh the patient as he comes round from the anaesthetic. In some wards one prophylactic dose of procaine penicillin is given by intramuscular injection immediately after return from the theatre. The pulse is recorded very frequently for the first 24 hours, and some surgeons prefer the temperature not to be taken orally for the first three days.

Post-Operative Bleeding. Restlessness and noisy, moist respirations are early indications of bleeding. If this goes unnoticed, the pulse rate may rise and the pulse volume become weaker. These signs and any vomit should be reported at once and vomit, if any, kept for inspection by an experienced nurse. Stale blood in the vomit is of little importance as it probably dates back to the time of operation, but any signs of fresh blood should be viewed with suspicion, and vigilance should be increased. If there is any bleeding, the mouth and naso-pharynx are carefully swabbed and cleared of blood and the patient raised to the upright position, well supported by pillows and an injection of Nepenthe, previously ordered in case of any complication, given. In the majority of cases this is all that is needed. Sometimes however a clot on the tonsils or adenoid bed is the cause of the trouble and has to be removed with a sterile swab and forceps. Serious haemorrhage necessitates a return to the theatre and ligaturing of the bleeding point. Blood loss can quickly prove serious and may have to be made good by blood transfusion or, in less serious cases, by iron therapy.

The younger the patient, the less severe are pain and general malaise. Fluids should be given as soon as the effect of the anaesthetic has worn off. Oedema and stiffness of the throat, associated with pain, can be greatly reduced by encouraging the child to swallow early. Cool drinks of fruit juice and ice cream are suitable but milk is inclined to coat the tonsil-bed and is best omitted for the first 24 hours. Children under the age of 8 years are usually ready for a light breakfast the morning after operation. Disprin 0.3 g crushed and dissolved in a little water can be given 20 minutes before meals and this reduces the pain and so encourages eating and drinking. A cheerful, matter-of-fact attitude by the nurses contributes considerably to an early recovery of these children.

Post-operatively these patients often complain of earache and of a stiff neck. In most cases neither of these conditions is serious and the referred pain causing the earache, and the stiff neck caused by the position on the theatre table can be relieved by the application of warmth.

Breathing through the nose should be taught as soon as the post-operative oedema has subsided and the child told that the doctor will be looking forward to seeing how well he can do it on his next visit. Since modern antibiotics have become available the fear of infection and secondary haemorrhage is much reduced and it is, therefore, unjustifiable to forbid visiting. The presence of the mother up to the time the premedication has taken effect and a short visit of mutual reassurance soon after the operation can be beneficial to both mother and child and may be the best means to ensure that there are no psychological after effects.

Deafness

Deafness in childhood may be temporary or permanent. Permanent deafness may be congenital nerve deafness caused, e.g. by an attack of rubella in the mother, during the first 12 weeks of pregnancy. Cerebral palsy sufferers often also have an associated nerve deafness.

Among the acquired causes are repeated attacks of otitis media and perforation of the ear drum with subsequent scarring and adhesions or radical mastoidectomy. Transitory deafness may be caused by an accumulation of wax, a foreign body in the meatus, meatal boils and blocking of the Eustachian tube due to a cold, sinusitis or adenoids.

Total deafness is rare. Once any doubt about a child's hearing has arisen, no time must be lost in seeking expert advice—a 'wait and see' attitude may prejudice the entire future of the child. Tests to assess the degree of deafness can now be carried out on very young babies at special audiology centres staffed by specialists in the diagnosis of deafness in children. Once the deafness has been confirmed a training and stimulation programme can be planned with the child's parents who will have a great part to play in developing any potential of hearing, speech and intelligence. They should therefore be encouraged to participate in the training from the start. The 1944 Education Act provides for education from the age of 2 years. Deaf children should be allowed to mix with hearing ones in nurseries and by attending special classes within ordinary schools. The problem of placing a child in a residential home for the deaf at an early age must be carefully considered as separation from the family may add to the heavy handicap these children have to bear.

Otitis Media

Otitis media is inflammation of the middle ear. In young children the structures of the ear, nose and throat are particularly closely related to one another, and their smallness easily accounts for frequent congestion and blocking and for the spread of infection from one to the other. Otitis media is common as a secondary infection following a common cold, tonsilitis, infections of the mouth, infectious fevers and carious teeth. In babies the short, straight and rather wide Eustachian tube may even become blocked by vomitus, and special care should be taken with babies suffering from any kind of vomiting.

Signs and Symptoms. The onset of otitis media may be insidious and the first signs may be that the young child rolls his head on the pillow, pulls his ear and is abnormally irritable. Pain soon becomes severe, the temperature rises as high as 39.4° (103°F) and the patient resents being touched. He looks toxic, and diarrhoea, vomiting and convulsions are common. On examination the blood vessels of the ear drum are found to be dilated and congested, the cone of light normally reflected from it is absent, and the usual mobility of the drum is lost. The ear drum may be bulging and opaque owing to the pus which fills the cavity of the middle ear.

Treatment. Treatment may be conservative, i.e. by means of drugs such as ampicillin given systemically in fairly large dosage. The application of local heat may be soothing. At night several pillows should be used, as pain is more severe when the patient lies down flat. Disprin or some other analgesic should be given, as it is senseless to allow the child to suffer pain, and the loss of sleep which goes hand in hand with it can only prejudice the course of the illness. Sometimes sleep can be induced by such simple measures as a hot drink and a 'cuddle' from a sympathetic nurse. One per cent ephedrine nasal drops, which have the effect of shrinking the mucosa of the nose and Eustachian tube, may be ordered to promote drainage, and older children can be given inhalations with the same purpose in mind.

Myringotomy. If there is no response to conservative treatment of middle ear infection, and if the presence of pus is suspected in the middle ear, the tympanic membrane may be incised to allow the pus to escape. This procedure is called myringotomy, but is seldom required nowadays. It is done as it is better to have a clean surgical incision which later heals by first intention than a spontaneous perforation with ragged edges which will result in scarring and adhesions of the ear drum. As soon as the tympanic membrane is perforated and pus released, pain subsides and the general condition of the patient improves.

Myringotomy is an exquisitely painful operation and for that reason should always be done under a light general anaesthetic, even though it takes only a matter of moments to perform.

Nursing care following myringotomy. On return from the theatre the patient is placed on the affected side to encourage drainage. The auditory meatus may have been loosely packed with a ribbon gauze wick to aid drainage of pus by capillary action and a light pad and bandage applied. These should be inspected and changed as soon as they have become saturated with discharge. Routine ear mopping (and in some cases syringing) is ordered, and started 12 hours after operation.

The procedure is a sterile one and is repeated as often as the need arises. The pain is as a rule relieved by the myringotomy, and analgesic drugs are rarely necessary. The patient may be allowed up the next day, as running around promotes drainage and means a happier patient. The course of ampicillin will probably be continued. The diet should be a full, well-balanced one. Aural toilet is carried out as often as is necessary until the drainage has completely dried up and the ear drum has healed. In favourable cases there is little or no impairment of hearing.

Grommet Tubes. An alternative method of draining the middle ear is by sucking out the fluid via the myringotomy. If this does not appear to be sufficient, tiny drainage tubes called Grommet tubes are placed in the ear for further drainage. The tubes have small flanges at each end and they act as aerators as well as as drains. They are left in situ until the Eustachian tubes, blocked by catarrh, have cleared.

Otorrhoea

Serous or purulent discharge from the ear may be either acute or chronic. In either case treatment will consist of three main factors:

Treatment by drugs such as sulphonamides, penicillin and other antibiotics.
Regular, thorough aural toilet by syringing or mopping.
Building up the patient's general health.

Ear Mopping. Ear mopping carried out by an efficient, experienced nurse, should be painless. All the same the preparation involved may frighten the young patient, and it is well worth gaining the child's confidence before starting the actual procedure. Once he has learned that there is nothing to fear, even the youngest child will prove co-operative, and it is only the quiet patient, who needs little if any restraint, who makes thorough, gentle aural toilet possible.

Position. Infants and toddlers are best allowed to lie on their side either on their cot or on the nurse's knee. The nurse's one forearm can rest lightly on the child's head, the other on the body, thus giving light restraint and acting as an indication to the patient that he is required to keep still. Older children may be asked to stand between the nurse's legs as she sits, with the head on one of the mopper's knees (the left knee for the right ear and vice versa). Unco-operative patients and young babies may have to be restrained, as in Fig. 33.

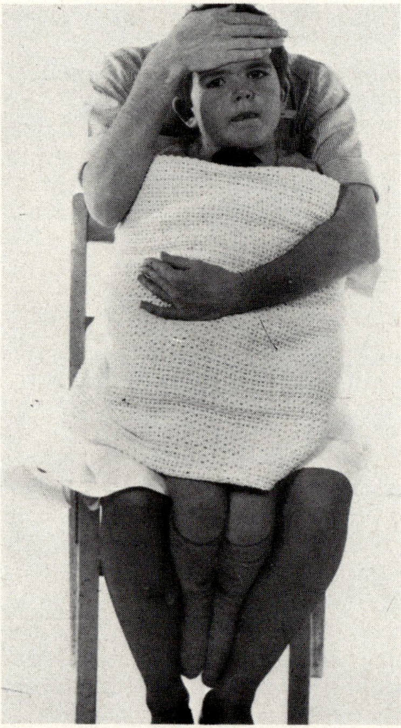

FIG. 33. This comfortable and secure method of holding a child for examination of the mouth and throat is also used for gastric lavage. If the head is turned to one side, this position can also be used for examination of the ear.

Method. Whichever method is adopted the nurse should hold the wool carrier so lightly that she can easily let go as soon as the child moves his head. No harm is likely to come to the child who momentarily has a wool carrier sticking out of his ear, whereas a movement of the head with the operator clinging to the rigid stick may easily damage, and even perforate the ear drum, or at the least, is likely to cause pain. Alternatively the nurse can rest her hand on the patient's head so that they move together and so avoid trauma. Once the child has lost confidence the repeated aural toilet will also mean a repeated struggle.

Ear mopping is essentially the same in children as in adults. The auditory meatus in young children is, however, of different anatomical shape and in order to straighten it sufficiently to reach the bottom of the meatus when mopping, the pinna should be gently pulled in a backward direction up to the age of approximately 18 months, but in older patients in a backward and upward direction.

In some wards a graph record is kept of the number of mops used and the time intervals between treatments. The type of discharge, whether serous, purulent or blood-stained, its nature, whether ropy or watery and whether odourless or offensive, should all be reported.

The delicate skin of children easily becomes excoriated by aural discharge. The area around the ear should be gently washed with cotton wool and saline, and zinc ointment or lanolin applied. As in the case of any open wound (and a discharging ear means a perforated drum, i.e. an open wound), it is important to keep all hair well out of the way. In little girls this can be achieved by wearing an Alice-band, hair grips or even a hair net. Any short, stray hair can be controlled by applying a little petroleum jelly to keep it away from the aural orifice. Babies and toddlers may have to have their arms restrained in order to prevent spread of infection. In all cases pillow slips should be changed whenever they become soiled.

Syringing Discharging Ears. In some units the doctor may order 4-hourly or twice daily syringing for a discharging ear. In young children this is best done with a sterilized rat-tail rubber bulb-syringe, in older children a sterilized Higginson's syringe with a special attachment is sometimes used. In either case the greatest care should be taken to use lotion at the correct temperature [37.8°C (100°F) in the jug] and to direct the stream on to the wall of the meatus and never on to the ear drum. The meatus should be straightened as described above. Careful drying of the meatus following the syringing is essential and the toilet is completed as described in the preceding paragraph. Note that ear syringing must never be undertaken except on doctor's orders. *N.B.* Whatever the type of otitis media, it is important that treatment is continued until the normal mobility of the tympanic membrane returns. Hearing should always be checked before the child is discharged from medical care.

Disease of the Mastoid Bone

Mastoiditis may be an immediate complication of otitis media or the sequel to long standing, badly drained infection of the middle ear. The organism is as a rule the streptococcus or staphylococcus but occasionally the mastoid infection is caused by the tubercle bacillus or *Escherichia* (*Bacterium*) *coli.* Chronic mastoiditis is associated with poor general health and aural discharge; at operation, granulations of the middle ear and necrosis of the mastoid bone are found. Neglected mastoid disease may lead to meningitis, brain abscess and lateral sinus thrombosis.

Acute Mastoiditis

With the advent of antibiotics acute mastoiditis is now very rare. When it does occur the child appears a picture of misery, looking toxic and febrile. The mastoid process is acutely tender and swollen, causing the pinna of the ear to be pushed forwards. Often there is a history of otitis media or upper respiratory tract infection. Most cases respond to the correct antibiotic therapy, surgery is rarely required.

Myringoplasty

Occasionally a long-standing perforation of the ear drum is closed by skin graft. The necessary skin is taken from the upper arm, inner aspect of the thigh, a vein or from the ear. Working with the help of a microscope throughout the operation, the surgeon cleans the ear carefully and removes the upper skin of the tympanic membrane before applying the graft. The graft is kept in position by tiny plastic or nylon sponges, packed tightly into the auditory meatus and left undisturbed for at least 10 days. The operation is a very delicate one and only about half the cases are entirely successful. If the graft has taken discharges cease and the danger that infection might enter the middle ear is eliminated. Hearing is restored to a useful level.

Cleft Lip and Cleft Palate

Approximately one baby in every thousand is born with a cleft lip or cleft palate so that most nurses are likely to meet this abnormality in the course of their paediatric experience. Cleft lip and cleft palate are often hereditary and are caused by a failure of development in the first 3 months of pregnancy. Many degrees of severity of this deformity occur and either condition

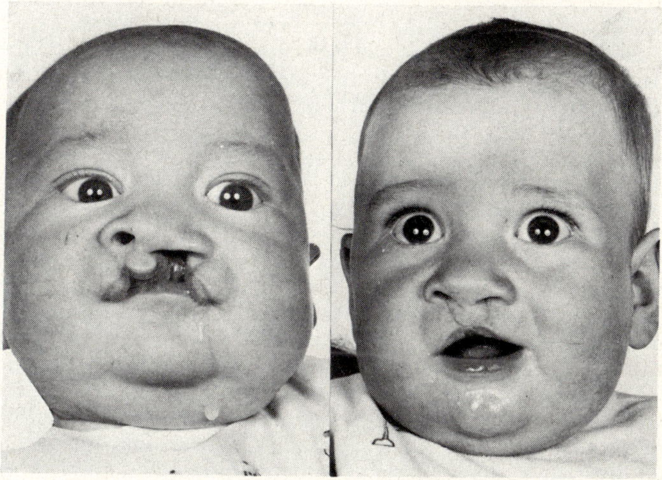

FIG. 34. Baby with severe cleft lip and palate (*left*). The same baby after successful repair of the cleft lip (*right*). Note the gross deformity of the nose and the clearly-defined pre maxilla.

can be present without the other. The cleft may be unilateral or bilateral, it may merely be a small notch in the upper lip, and it can be incomplete or extend deep into the nostrils. If the cleft is centrally placed the deformity is known as hare lip. Cleft palate may involve only the uvula or be a small hole in the soft or hard palate, but more often the cleft extends through both hard palate and soft palate. The cleft may be narrow or wide and may include the alveolar margin and if associated with a bad cleft lip causes an ugly protrusion of the premaxilla bone. In the majority of cases cleft lip is associated with an asymmetry and flattening of the nose.

Cleft Lip

General points. A mother who has a baby with a cleft lip is likely to be deeply distressed at the time of the birth. This can be greatly relieved if the midwife can show the mother some photographs of similar babies before and after surgical repair (Fig. 34). Some paediatric surgeons repair a cleft lip within the first few days of life before the mother takes the baby home. At the same time the closure of the cleft may help to push back the protruding premaxilla and later produce a better dental arch and a more regular development of the teeth. A small prosthesis achieves the same thing. More usually, however, the operation is postponed until the baby is well established, that is to say when he is 3 months old and weighs about 5.5 kg (12 lb).

Cleft lip without cleft of the palate often does not interfere with sucking and in many cases breast feeding can be carried out successfully. Alternatively special nipple shields and teats are available and only severe cases of cleft lip and cleft palate need to be spoon-fed from birth. Even then the breasts should be expressed and the milk given to the infant as long as lactation can be maintained. When the cleft is complete feeding may be very difficult as regurgitation through the nose causes the baby to cough and sneeze. When spoon feeding, the milk should be allowed to run on to the back of the tongue or into the cheek, as this reduces regurgitation through the nose and checks irritation. Upper respiratory tract infections, inhalation pneumonia and otitis media are common.

Babies with cleft palates tend to swallow much air during

feeding and special care must be taken when 'bringing up the wind'. A little boiled water is often given after feeds to clean the mouth and prevent crusts of milk from forming around the edges of the cleft.

Repair of Cleft Lip. The baby is usually admitted to a cubicle several days before the operation. The surgeon may wish to have a photograph taken for record purposes and nose and throat swabs are sent for culture as it is important that the baby should be free from infection. The haemoglobin level should be 80 per cent (14–16 g/dl). Spoon feeding is started and the baby should be nursed by as few nurses as possible, so that both baby and nurse can get used to each other. Ideally the mother is admitted with her baby and can be allowed to look after him herself most of the time. For spoon-feeding, a special spoon with the sides bent in to form a trough is often useful and great care must be taken not to injure the mucous membrane of the mouth. After feeds the chin should be well dried to avoid the skin getting sore from dribbling while being fed. Systemic penicillin is sometimes ordered to help reduce the risk of infection. Feeds are discontinued 4 to 6 hours before operation but a drink of 90 ml (3 fl oz) of dextrose 5 per cent may be allowed 2 hours before the child goes to the theatre. The child will be prepared for theatre in the usual way. Atropine 0.3 mg by hypodermic injection will be given ½ hour before surgery.

Post-operatively the baby is received into a warmed cot protected from draughts. While unconscious he is nursed on his side and the foot-end of the bed may be raised to help with the drainage of any saliva and blood, although bleeding is not likely to occur. A stimulant tray, oxygen and an electric sucker with sterilized suction catheters should be by the cot side. The sucker is used only if other means of evacuating secretions or blood prove ineffective, as the suture line can easily be damaged. It is of particular importance to watch the infant's colour and to ensure an adequate air-way as the closure of the cleft and the oedema arising from the local anaesthetic and surgical manoeuvre may obstruct much of the airway to which the infant has been accustomed. When a general anaesthetic has been given, via an endotracheal tube, laryngotracheal oedema is a common complication which may require treatment by steam therapy.

On the bedside locker, a sterile tray is kept for the toilet of the suture line and nostrils. This should be changed every time it has been used. It should contain fine dressing forceps, swabs, sterile saline and, if desired by the surgeon, some antiseptic lotion such as an aqueous solution of acriflavine 1:1000, or Roccal 1:160. Sometimes liquid paraffin or Polyfax ointment, a mild antiseptic, which keeps the scar soft, may be applied. While the infant is still unconscious elbow splints are applied and in addition it may later be necessary to secure the splinted arms to the cot frame. The splints are removed at least twice daily and the child allowed to exercise his arms. As soon as the baby has regained consciousness, he is sat up well supported by firm pillows to facilitate breathing and avoid chest complications. As it is vital that all tension on the stitches should be reduced to a minimum everything possible should be done to stop the baby from crying. Picking him up and nursing him will not spoil the infant but is mere common sense at such a time. Occasionally a Logan's bow is applied to relieve tension. Feeding can usually be resumed about 2 hours after return to the ward. As the infant has had atropine he is as a rule particularly thirsty and liable to cry for that reason. The first feed given is plain boiled water or sterile dextrose 5 per cent. If this is well tolerated, the next feed can be half-strength milk and this can be rapidly increased to the feed the baby has been used to before operation.

Local care includes careful mouth toilet. If a nasal plug is in position, this is changed as soon and as often as it becomes soaked until it can be omitted according to the surgeon's instructions, probably after 48 hours. The lip is cleaned and any crusts gently removed. Hydrogen peroxide in a 1:8 solution may help to loosen any crusts of blood. If a Logan's bow is used, the skin should be watched for reaction to the strapping.

The catgut sutures used on the mucosa of the lip are not removed, as they gradually become absorbed, but the fine silk sutures should be removed on the sixth and seventh days respectively. Skilled restraint of the baby during this procedure is essential if scarring is to be prevented. Special care should be taken not to overlook the fine stitches which often continue well up into the floor of the nose.

In uncomplicated cases the infant may be ready for discharge once the sutures have been removed. Breast-feeding and sucking from a teat can be started again as soon as the stitches have been removed, provided that an associated cleft palate does not make this impossible.

Cleft Palate

Repair of Cleft Palate. The usual age for repair of cleft palate is 12 to 24 months, that is to say before the child begins to talk, so that any bad habits of speech may be prevented from developing. Children with cleft palates are often late in commencing to talk. Long before this however, orthodontic treatment may have been started with the intention of moulding the maxilla into a well-shaped arch and to stimulate growth of the under-developed maxilla.

As in the case of babies admitted for repair of cleft lip, these children are brought to hospital a few days prior to operation for thorough assessment and to allow them to get used to the unfamiliar people and surroundings. Elbow splints are applied for short periods so that the child may gradually become used to them. Nose and throat swabs are sent for culture and sensitivity tests and blood is taken to ensure that the haemoglobin is no lower than 80 per cent. As post-operative blood transfusion is occasionally necessary, the blood is also grouped.

Feeding and pre-operative care differ little from that for any other operation, and the immediate post-operative care is similar to that described under the heading of cleft lip. The danger of an obstructed airway is, however, even greater. Careful watch has to be kept for excessive oozing of blood from the suture line. If vomiting occurs, stale blood may be seen. The immediate post-operative considerations and nursing observations are, for obvious reasons, very similar to those necessary for patients who have had a tonsillectomy (see p. 169). Sometimes ribbon gauze packs soaked in Whitehead's varnish are used to relieve tension either side of the suture line. Although they are as a rule kept in position by the normal pressure of the tongue, the mouth should be inspected from time to time to see if they are still in position, as the child may try to dislodge them with his tongue. In this case his attention should be distracted and a sedative given. Elbow splints are used continuously until healing has taken place.

For the first 10 days all food should be liquid or semi-solid and meals should be followed by a drink of plain water to wash down any remains of food. The diet should be rich in vitamins, protein and iron.

Drugs. Sedatives should not be withheld for the 2 or 3 days, as crying and fretfulness may prejudice the good result of the operation. Iron in the form of Colliron is often given and vitamin C in the form of ascorbic acid or fresh fruit juices will enhance healing. Orange juice is inclined to sting on the raw wound edges and for that reason is best discontinued for the time being. Catgut is used for suturing and as this dissolves, removal is not necessary. Some surgeons favour silk sutures. These can be 'sucked out' by the patient and will disappear within about 10 days. Even though the child's arms are effectively splinted, the toys chosen to occupy and amuse him should be of a kind which cannot be put into the mouth, as this would easily cause damage to the suture lines and might introduce infection. It is important that neither boiled, hard sweets, nor toffees should be given and this should be explained to the mother.

Speech Therapy. Speech therapy is of great importance in promoting early, normal speech. As soon as the post-operative oedema has subsided the nurse can start to play games, such as blowing bubbles and practising the consonants K and T in order to encourage normal articulation. On discharge the child is referred to a speech therapist for assessment, and in some cases the mother can be taught exercises which can be practised at home until such time as the child is old enough to benefit from organized speech therapy. The best results are obtained where there is good team work between surgeon, nurse, speech therapist and orthodontic surgeon.

Points of Interest. Cleft palate occurs in 1 in 1000 babies. Mental handicap is ten times more frequent in children with cleft lip or palate than in others.

Grades of deformity:

Lip only: 25 per cent Palate only: 25 per cent
Complete: 50 per cent

Two males are affected to every female, and the deformity occurs in a proportion of two left clefts to every right.

Pierre Robin Syndrome

Sometimes babies are seen who have a series of abnormalities referred to as Pierre Robin Syndrome.

These babies have a small, receding mandible (retrognathia) and a widely cleft palate as well as an abnormally small mouth (microstoma). The tongue seems to have insufficient anchorage so that it slips down the back of the throat (glossoptosis). It follows that the tongue obstructs the airway when the baby lies on his back; normal feeding is impossible.

The nursing care of these babies is all-important. The nurse must build up pillows or wedges of polyurethane which make it possible to nurse the baby face down so that the tongue falls forward by gravity. Sometimes a wooden frame or plaster cast can be constructed; tube feeding is usually necessary until the baby weighs about 2 kg (4 lb), but a plate made of acrylic resin may help to occlude the cleft palate during feeding. Sucking should be encouraged, as this strengthens the tongue and develops the mandible. Furthermore peristalsis starts in the mouth, so that sucking aids digestion.

The surgeon may stitch the tongue to the mandible and cause adhesions to form—Douglas operation, or he may transfix the tongue with wire to prevent it from slipping back. As the baby grows bigger the difficulties resolve themselves sufficiently so as no longer to endanger the child's breathing and life.

Complications including aspiration pneumonia and cyanotic attacks which, if severe, lead to brain damage.

Further Reading

BOWLEY, A. H. & GARDNER, L. (1972) *The Handicapped Child*, Edinburgh & London: Churchill Livingstone.

BOYLES KORKIS, F. (1968) *Ear, Nose and Throat Nursing*, 2nd ed. Edinburgh & London: Churchill Livingstone.

WHETNALL, E. & FRY, D. B. (1970) *Learning to Hear*. London: Heinemann.

10

The cardiovascular system

THE RELATIONSHIP between temperature, pulse and respirations in children is of great importance and should therefore always be reported together.

The Pulse

Owing to the small size of the structures involved, even simple procedures such as taking the pulse or the blood pressure and obtaining a sample of venous blood may present special difficulties in children; the younger the child, the more difficult it may be to feel and count the pulse beat over the radial artery at the wrist as he may resent being touched and may struggle or cry; also, overlying fat may make it hard to feel the pulse and may alter the volume and make assessment difficult. It is often a good plan to try to take the pulse while the patient is sleeping and this is often best done over the temporal artery immediately in front of the ear or in the case of infants over the fontanelle. The pulse should be taken and counted for 1 min. Changes in the rate, volume or rhythm should be reported at once. In certain diseases, for instance in some types of congenital heart disease, the pulse can be plainly seen at the side of the neck, in others it is not palpable in the groin, as it is in normal children. The pulse rate alters as the child grows older and during exercise, excitement or disease. An increased pulse rate (tachycardia) may be associated with pyrexia, the administration of certain drugs and following haemorrhage. An abnormally slow pulse (bradycardia) may be due to raised intercranial pressure or hydrocephalus. Infection and febrile conditions in infancy are not, however, necessarily accompanied by a rapid pulse as with adults, a fact which must be borne in mind when assessing a child's condition.

The sleeping pulse. When metabolism is at its lowest during sleep the pulse rate normally drops to approximately 10 beats per minute below the waking pulse rate. Overactivity of the heart, as it occurs in certain diseases, may cause both sleeping and waking pulse rates to be raised and at the same time the beat may be irregular. In certain diseases such as rheumatic carditis, there may be little or no difference between the sleeping and waking pulse and both may be significantly raised. A special record of the sleeping pulse is usually kept in these cases. It is of course important to avoid rousing the child when the pulse is taken. The temporal pulse is often the site of choice.

The apex beat. In some diseases not every beat of the heart is transmitted to the radial pulse and it is important to record the difference by counting not only the peripheral pulse but also the apex beat. In children the apex beat is usually found just below the left nipple and can be heard with the help of a stethoscope. A difference between the apex beat and the radial pulse is known as pulse deficit.

Sinus arrhythmia is often noticed in children and, when present, does not necessarily imply disease. The pulse rate is accelerated during inspiration and slowed during expiration.

Extrasystole or premature contraction may be present in the healthy child but occurs more commonly when the heart is diseased. The extrasystole can be heard with a stethoscope or may be felt in a peripheral pulse. It is rhythmic and is sometimes likened to an 'echo' of the real beat. This 'echo' may take the place of the next beat and so cause a beat to be missed. Another abnormal pulse is known as *heart block*. In this condition there is failure in the conduction of nerve impulses from the atrium to the ventricle through the atrioventricular node. In consequence, although the atria may be beating rapidly, the ventricles and consequently the pulse rate may be slowed to below 50 beats/minute or with partial heart block be irregular in rhythm. It is rare to find this abnormality in children.

Atrial fibrillation is caused by rapid and ineffective auricular contractions. The pulse is irregular in rhythm and volume as not all contractions of the heart are sufficiently powerful to be felt as a pulse. The atrial contraction may occur as a flutter as often as 250 times per minute while the ventricle contracts after every third or fourth contraction. Heart block is often associated with atrial fibrillation. The condition usually indicates cardiac damage following rheumatic heart disease.

Ventricular fibrillation deprives the circulation of blood and is fatal. Electric defibrillators and cardiac massage may succeed in restoring normal contractions and so save life.

Taking the Blood Pressure

In infants and young children it is difficult to estimate the blood pressure with accuracy. Special narrow cuffs may have to be used but they should be narrower than two-thirds of the length of the child's upper arm. Variations may be considerable even in healthy children, but average systolic readings are likely to be 60 to 80 mmHg and the diastolic pressure 50 to 60 mmHg in the first year and 100 to 110/80 (systolic/diastolic) at 10 years of age, while at rest.

Daily blood pressure readings may be required in certain heart diseases, diseases of the kidney, when increased intracranial pressure is suspected and in the case of patients on steroid therapy. A nurse who experiences difficulties should always seek help and advice, as the paediatrician will rely on the accuracy of the charting notwithstanding the difficult nature of the procedure. Children are sometimes frightened by the apparatus, and it may be wise to 'reassure' them by taking the teddy bear's blood pressure first and letting them handle the rubber bulb, making the mercury rise and fall themselves.

Cyanosis

Lack of oxygen in the circulation causes cyanosis more readily in young children than in adults. Central cyanosis is always a serious sign. It should be relieved without delay by the administration of oxygen. It may be particularly marked in respiratory abnormalities of the newly born, congenital heart lesions and in obstructed breathing. Occasionally young children have breath-holding attacks which cause cyanosis. These attacks are often due to behaviour disturbances.

Types of Heart Disease in Childhood

There are two main types of heart disease in childhood:

1. Congenital malformations of the heart or great blood vessels;
2. Inflammatory lesions in the heart, causing carditis.

Both these will interfere with the action of the heart and lead to heart failure, in an attempt by the heart muscle to compensate for the extra strain placed upon it, thereby becoming weakened and failing to push the necessary amount of blood to the body.

Heart failure in childhood is usually acute. Chronic heart failure develops gradually.

Heart Failure

Instant recognition and treatment of developing heart failure in the infant is necessary in order to preserve life. The young baby may collapse in a matter of hours or days, while the older child or adolescent may take weeks before his condition becomes serious.

The Most Common Causes of Heart Failure Are:

1. Congenital heart disease;
2. Carditis;
3. Pulmonary conditions;
4. The anaemias.

The infant in heart failure may be sweating, cyanosed or grey and pale with marked respiratory difficulty. Tachycardia is present or respirations are rapid and the airway quickly becomes blocked by thick viscid secretions. Because of difficulty in breathing, the infant is often restless and irritable and throws back his head to improve air intake. A persistent cough is common and sub-costal recession will be observed on inspiration. Feeds are taken slowly and are rarely finished. Vomiting is a common feature. Despite refusal of feeds, weight gain is noticed but this is due to retention of fluid which may produce oedema. Abdominal distension may be marked.

Nursing Care. Babies in heart failure need rest above all. They should be nursed in an oxygen tent (Fig. 35), extra humidity can

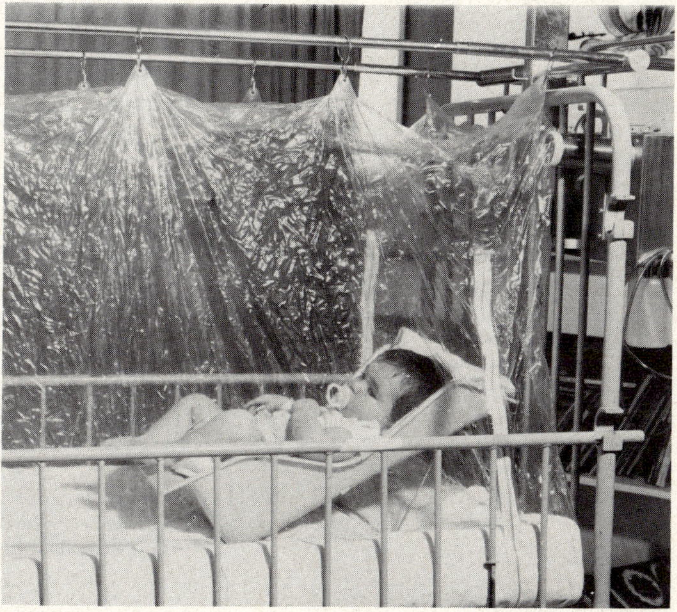

FIG. 35. Young infant nursed in the Vickers 58 Oxymist Tent providing an oxygen concentration of 60 per cent.

be added via a humidifier or nebulizer. An older child might tolerate a face mask. The child is best nursed in the upright position in order to prevent the abdominal organs pressing on the diaphragm and therefore will allow greater lung expansion. Sometimes a special frame is used in order to maintain this position. Heat is easily lost and a rectal temperature of 36° to 36.6°C (97° to 98°F) should be maintained. The clothing if any, should be light enough not to restrict breathing by its weight.

A daily blanket bath should be given, with careful attention to pressure areas. Reduced peripheral circulation coupled with comparative immobility make these children very prone to pressure sores which are difficult to heal once they have occurred. Mittens and socks may be worn to keep the extremities warm and more comfortable. The mouth will require frequent toilet hygiene in order to prevent mouth ulcers and dental caries. Breathing exercises are given by the physiotherapist. They will often be done by playing games such as blowing cotton wool balls across the table or making soap bubbles. Nurses can assist by interesting children in play activities which are at the same time breathing exercises (Fig. 21).

Tracheostomy (see p. 160) often relieves the respiratory difficulties and make it easier to suck out the viscid secretions. It also serves to reduce the 'dead space' in the trachea. Secretions may be further loosened by instilling $\frac{1}{2}$ to 1 ml of normal saline into the tube prior to suction with a fine catheter (Nos. 3 to 5 Jacques) well down the tube.

Constipation is often a troublesome feature associated with the anorexia. In order to prevent further strain on the heart during defecation regular aperients should be given in order to ensure soft motions. A flatus tube should be passed whenever the child becomes distended with 'wind' in order to prevent further impairment of respiration.

A daily weight record must be kept in order to detect any incipient collection of fluid and also to assess the patient's general growth. A fluid balance chart must be maintained.

Feeding. Children in heart failure and therefore lacking in oxygen, need a high-calorie intake for metabolism, also a high-protein diet in order to meet tissue needs for growth and repair.

Infants. Ordinary milk feeds of 150 to 175 ml/kg body weight /24 hours are suitable for these babies. The total amount should be given in small, frequent feeds. In order to avoid the undue exertion of sucking, the baby should be fed via a fine naso-gastric tube which will not occlude the airway. Portex tube PP 30 or PP 50 is suitable. Care should be taken when passing these tubes as they can easily slip into the lungs. The nurse should always test that the tube is in the stomach before each feed by syringing 0.5 ml of air in and listening for the 'plop' in the stomach with a stethoscope. A 2-ml syringe fitted on to the tube by means of a disposable needle should be used for administering the feed slowly. This type of tube can be left down in the stomach for long periods without causing trauma to the mucosa lining the upper alimentary tract.

If the sodium intake of feeds needs to be reduced due to the presence of oedema *SMA* milk may be used. *Breast milk* is also relatively low in sodium but these babies are unable to suck well at the breast and mother's milk supply often disappears on learning that her baby has heart failure. Unfortunately expressed breast milk is hard to come by and very expensive.

The milk *Edosol* a very low sodium milk should be avoided as the infant can quickly enter a state of sodium crisis as the milk contains insufficient sodium to meet basic needs, this milk is also low in calories and other minerals.

A weaning diet may be offered when the baby is strong enough to take food from a spoon.

Older Children. In order to tempt the appetite the diet should be carefully prepared and appetizingly served in small amounts and at frequent intervals. Mother should be consulted by the nurse to ensure that the child's favourite foods are given and dislikes avoided. No added salt should be given, but it is important to remember to give fruit juices and vitamins. The calorie content of the diet can be increased by giving ice cream and high-calorie milk shakes.

Drugs. *Digoxin*, this acts as a tonic to the heart muscle enabling it to work with greater effect without increasing its oxygen consumption.

Initial digitalizing dose in 24 hours:

0.1 mg/kg body weight;
First dose half the total;
Second dose a quarter of the total;
Third dose a quarter of the total.

Maintenance dose:

0.02 mg/kg body weight/24 hour.

The pulse or apex beat should be taken before this drug is administered as undue slowing of the heart beat may occur. Other early toxic symptoms to observe are vomiting, anorexia and irregular or coupling of the heart beat.

Lasix (frusemide) is a quick-acting diuretic which is given in order to stimulate kidney function and therefore the excretion of water and salts from the body.

Dose per 24 hour
Intramuscularly—½ mg/kg body weight.
Orally—2 mg/kg body weight.

The side effects of this drug include rapid fluid loss leading to dehydration. Potassium levels in the blood should be frequently assessed and extra potassium given.

Aldactone (spironolactone) a longer-acting diuretic is occasionally given in divided doses combined with Lasix in patients with severe heart failure.

Morphine is commonly given in order to sedate the patient and reduce the metabolism. This drug also reduces the respiratory rate.

Dose
0.2 mg/kg body weight every 6 hours as necessary.

Choral hydrate is also a useful sedative for the restless anxious older child in order to ensure that he is able to rest.

Antibiotics are often prescribed prophylactically as the risk of infection is high in these children.

Children in heart failure tend to be irritable and tire easily, feeling great frustration at not being able to do all the things that their friends are able to do.

While doing everything for the patient, the nurse should encourage him to make small efforts to help himself such as cleaning his teeth, but at the same time she should watch to see how each small effort affects her patient.

The nurse should learn to choose suitable toys and educational games which do not require too much energy. Parents and the 'play leader' can do much to help keep the child occupied with interesting activities and games.

The welfare and well-being of the parents may have a great effect on the patient's general condition. The mother's anxiety is easily conveyed unconsciously to the child, and will increase his restlessness. Free visiting should be encouraged and financial help given towards fares if necessary. If possible, the patient's mother should have a room with her child where she can stay and be resident. Parents must be well informed about their child's condition by the doctor, and the nurse should be available to listen and to support the parents through this difficult illness. A medical social worker should be available to help with particular problems as they arise.

Congenital Heart Disease

Congenital heart disease can be divided as follows:

Acyanotic	*Cyanotic*
Patent ductus arteriosus	Fallot's tetralogy
Coarctation of the aorta	Transposition of the great vessels
Ventricular septal defect	
Atrial septal defect	
Aortic stenosis	
Mitral stenosis	

Patent Ductus Arteriosus

The ductus arteriosus is necessary to the fetal circulation, failure to close after birth causes oxygenated blood from the aorta which is under pressure as it leaves the ventricle, to be pumped back into the pulmonary artery where the blood is under low pressure. The flow of blood from the aorta into the pulmonary artery may reach great volumes and the cardiac output is increased. It is not clear why the ductus arteriosus should fail to close in some children although research has shown it to be commonly associated with hypoxia during and after birth. Statistics show that more girls than boys are affected; ratio of 2:1.

Growth is often stunted although otherwise there may be no

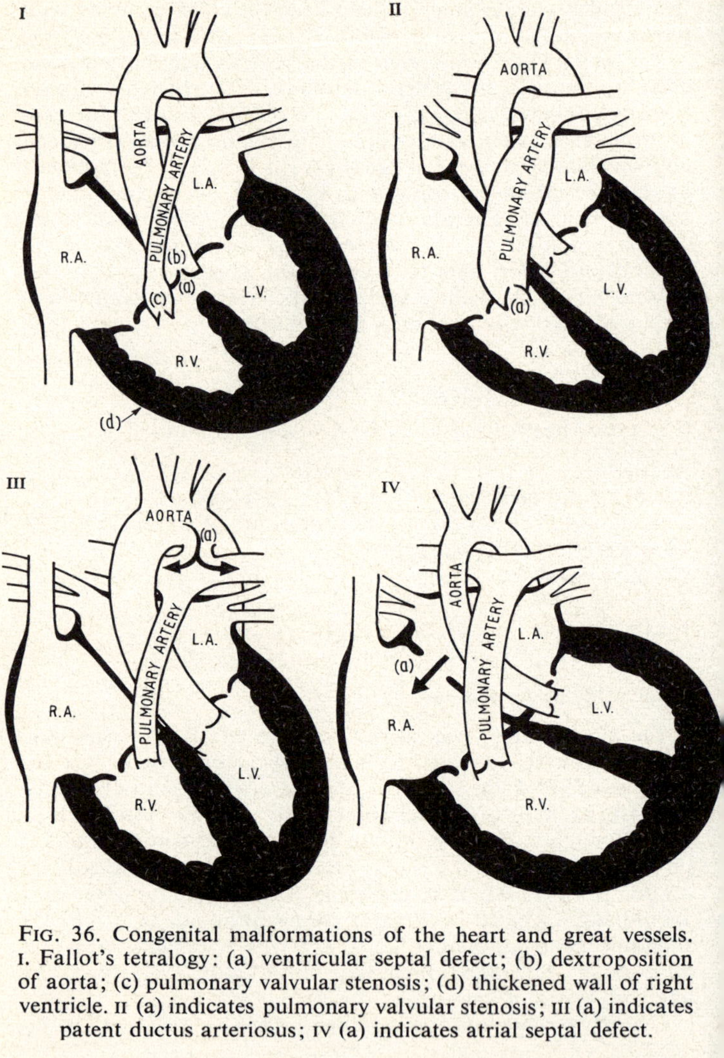

FIG. 36. Congenital malformations of the heart and great vessels. I. Fallot's tetralogy: (a) ventricular septal defect; (b) dextroposition of aorta; (c) pulmonary valvular stenosis; (d) thickened wall of right ventricle. II (a) indicates pulmonary valvular stenosis; III (a) indicates patent ductus arteriosus; IV (a) indicates atrial septal defect.

other symptoms. Diagnosis may not be made until the child is 3 or 4 years old, when a heart murmur may be heard on routine medical examination by a doctor. Ligation of the patent ductus is best carried out as soon as the diagnosis is made. The operation is carried out through a left thoracotomy, the heart is not entered. Following successful surgery the patient can expect to lead a normal life.

Coarctation of the Aorta

Coarctation means narrowing; in this case narrowing occurs along the course of the aortic arch. The blood supply to the distal part of the aorta is thus reduced, whilst pressure is high in that part of the aorta and the arteries supplied by it which lie between the left ventricle of the heart and the narrowing, the proximal part. The systolic blood pressure in the arm is high, the myocardium hypertrophies in an attempt to increase cardiac output, subsidiary or collateral vessels develop. Pulsation in these vessels can be felt on the chest and back, but the femoral pulse is feeble or absent.

Operation consists of resecting the coarcted area with direct anastomosis. The age that this is performed depends a great deal upon the condition of the individual child and the surgeon, but the surgical correction is recommended before adult life.

In successful cases the prognosis is good. The circulation becomes normal, the blood pressure falls to ordinary levels and the patient is able to lead an active unrestricted life.

Ventricular Septal Defect

Septal defects between the right and left ventricle vary in size. Small defects (maladie de Roger) are characterized by loud systolic heart murmurs, but the child is often completely asymptomatic and the prognosis is good. No treatment is indicated. It has been reported that some defects close spontaneously.

With large septal defects the situation is different. Due to the higher pressure in the left ventricle, a shunting of blood occurs from the left to right ventricle during systole. This increases the work load of the right ventricle and hypertrophy occurs.

Symptoms may be severe, with marked feeding difficulty, frequent upper respiratory infections and dyspnoea. Growth is impaired. Urgent treatment is required. Operative repair is carried out with the aid of a heart–lung machine. The defect may be repaired by direct closure or with a specially prepared patch, sutured in position. With surgery the prognosis is favourable but the outcome depends upon the amount of resistance which has developed in the pulmonary vascular bed.

Atrial Septal Defects

An atrial septal defect is an abnormal opening in the atrial septum resulting in shunting of blood from the left to right atrium. This produces an increase in the right ventricular output and resultant pulmonary engorgement. The diagnosis is suspected by the presence of a soft blowing systolic murmur in the area of the pulmonary artery that may be found at a routine medical examination.

The child usually appears slight, noticed to tire easily with poor exercise tolerance. Susceptibility to pneumonia and rheumatic fever is increased. Operative repair is possible both by closed and 'open-heart' surgery. Since the prognosis for most of these children is good, the risks of operative repair have to be carefully considered for each individual child.

Aortic Stenosis

When a thickening of the aortic semilunar valves occurs it is spoken of as aortic stenosis. The narrowing restricts circulation and causes a lowering of blood pressure in the peripheral arteries; hypertrophy of the left ventricle develops as the heart attempts to overcome the obstruction. Valvotomy is carried out by opening the heart and operating under direct vision.

Mitral Stenosis

Mitral stenosis may be congenital or acquired. In the latter instance it is associated with rheumatic heart disease. The mitral valve becomes narrowed causing dyspnoea on exertion, repeated respiratory tract infections and failure to thrive. Surgery is indicated and involves the use of a heart–lung or cardiac by-pass machine as the heart is opened for direct vision during surgery.

Cyanotic Heart Lesions

Fallot's Tetralogy

The tetralogy of Fallot varies in severity but is characterized by the combination of four defects:

1. Pulmonary stenosis;
2. Ventricular septal defect;
3. Over-riding aorta;
4. Hypertrophy of the right ventricle.

As a result some of the right ventricular output goes to the aorta. Cyanosis in varying degrees occurs, which is most marked on exertion. It is the most common defect causing cyanosis in patients surviving beyond 2 years of age.

Attacks of paroxysmal dyspnoea may occur in children with Fallot's tetralogy especially before the age of 2 years. The child becomes distressed with deep cyanosis and air hunger which may be followed by loss of consciousness and convulsions. The child should be placed in the knee–chest position to increase cardiac efficiency and oxygen should be given if available. Older children learn amazingly well to adapt their activities, so that during play he takes frequent rest pauses and adopts the characteristic squatting position.

Correction of this anomaly is a major procedure in which the cardiac by-pass machine is used. The best age for such surgery depends upon the individual patient but is usually between the years of 2 and 15. Temporizing operations have been developed in order to assist the very severely affected younger child:

Waterston's operation—anastomosis of the side of the pulmonary artery directly to the side of the ascending aorta.

Blalock–Taussig operation—anastomosis of either subclavian artery to the pulmonary artery.

The aim of these shunting operations is to increase the pulmonary blood flow by creating an artificial ductus arteriosus. This results in improvement of the child's general condition so that when older, he is able to tolerate the major surgery necessary for this anomaly.

Transposition of the Great Vessels

In this anomaly the aorta arises from the right ventricle instead of the left ventricle and the pulmonary artery from the left ventricle. Unless surgical treatment can be given, death usually takes place within a few weeks. A palliative procedure has been developed. *Rashkind balloon atrial septostomy* which creates an atrial septal defect sufficient to maintain similar right and left atrial pressures. This procedure is carried out under a local anaesthetic at cardiac catheterization, before the age of 2 months whilst the septum is reasonably supple. A surgical septostomy through a thoracotomy is performed in the older infant and child—Blalock–Hanlon operation.

Complete correction of the transposition is not possible at this present stage of cardiac surgery. However the Mustard Procedure has been devised to bring about an internal redirection of blood flow in order that de-oxygenated blood will flow into the pulmonary artery. This major surgery is carried out with the use of the cardiac by-pass machine usually after the age of 6 months. The change of colour in the child is most dramatic. He often feels for the first time that he can play without having to sit down at the slightest exertion.

Surgery of the Heart and Great Vessels

In the course of the last 30 years many abnormalities of the heart and great vessels have become amenable to surgery assisted by new methods of anaesthesia, hypothermia, extra-corporeal circulation, pace makers and other advances. Under ideal conditions cardiac surgery can now be accepted in the same way as other types of surgery. Heart and great vessels can be regarded as specialized muscular tubes rather than inaccessible structures.

Pre-Operative Care

Ideally children are admitted 3 to 4 days before operation to allow time for exploration of their new surroundings and to make friends with the ward team and other children in the ward. The parents, prior to admission, should be offered resident accommodation, especially those with a young child or with one who is very homesick, and those far from home. Parents should be given detailed explanation and guidance by the doctor as to the details of the operation and the attendant risks before the consent form is signed. The ward sister or staff nurse should listen to the parents' fears and anxieties and help them to understand their role as part of the team aiding the recovery of their child. Co-operation of the parents is the greatest asset in helping the child through this difficult time.

Many of the children admitted for elective surgery look well and appear most active, they often find it difficult to understand why they need an operation. Explanation appropriate to the age of child should be given by his nurse some time on the day before operation. The child and his parents should be shown the room where he will wake up. The equipment to be used

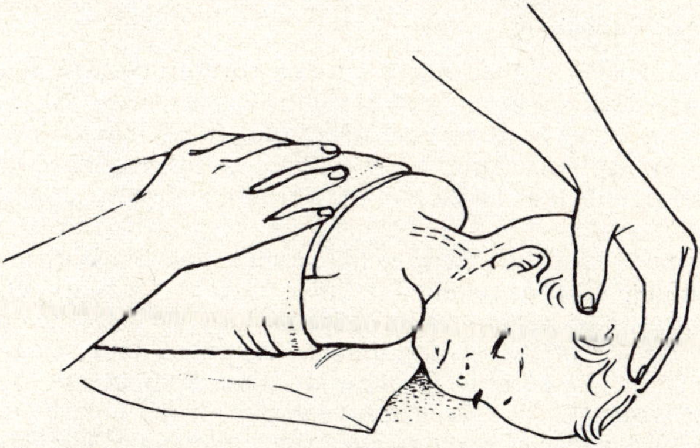

FIG. 37. Method of restraining and positioning an infant for venepuncture. Owing to the small size of the veins, either the external or the internal jugular vein are often used when a blood sample is required.

should be explained, oxygen tents can be called space ships and the monitors special TV sets.

Investigations carried out before surgery include the taking of blood for cross matching, bleeding and clotting times, haemoglobin and electrolyte estimation. Electrocardiograms and radiographs are taken. The doctor will carry out a thorough phsyical examination. The nurse will collect and test a specimen of urine. Height and weight will be recorded, also blood pressure, temperature pulse and respiration rates. If there is any suspicion of infection the operation is postponed.

The physiotherapist will teach the child breathing exercises in order that he can do this effectively post-operatively, the nurse should be present to aid and encourage as she will often have to carry out these exercises in the absence of a physiotherapist. A mild sedative may be ordered in order to ensure a good night's sleep.

The immediate pre-operative preparation is the same as with any other surgery. When the premedication is given the child is encouraged to empty his bladder. The parents or the nurse should then stay quietly at the bedside until he goes to theatre.

Cardiac Surgery

The detail of cardiac surgery varies according to the technique of individual surgeons and sometimes unexpected decisions have to be made at time of operation. In all cases however thoracotomy is performed and sometimes this may have to be bilateral to include division of the sternum and resection of one or more ribs.

Using special anaesthetic techniques it is possible to inflate or deflate the lungs as required in order to reach the heart. When the surgeon wishes to operate inside the heart he is able to do so with the aid of the heart–lung machine which takes over the circulation temporarily in order to allow clear access to the heart structure. The heart–lung machine works in two ways; by ensuring adequate ventilation of the lungs and by circulation of the blood around the body, by-passing the heart. Blood loss is carefully measured (all swabs used are weighed before and after use) and replaced by blood transfusion.

Drugs used during surgery may include intrapericardial

procaine to reduce the irritating effect of the handling of the heart to the minimum, injection of potassium citrate to stop the heart temporarily. Hypotensive agents to control the bleeding from enlarged collateral vessels in the chest.

Post-Operative Care

Following cardiac surgery the child is nursed flat, with a wooden board placed beneath the mattress for resuscitation purposes if the need should arise. The bed is made up with clean linen and warmed with an electric pad that is later removed when the patient is placed on to the bed. Usually the prepared bed, complete with oxygen tent and attached cylinder, carriers for drainage bottles and clamps is taken to the theatre for reception of the child.

In the recovery area all equipment required is prepared,

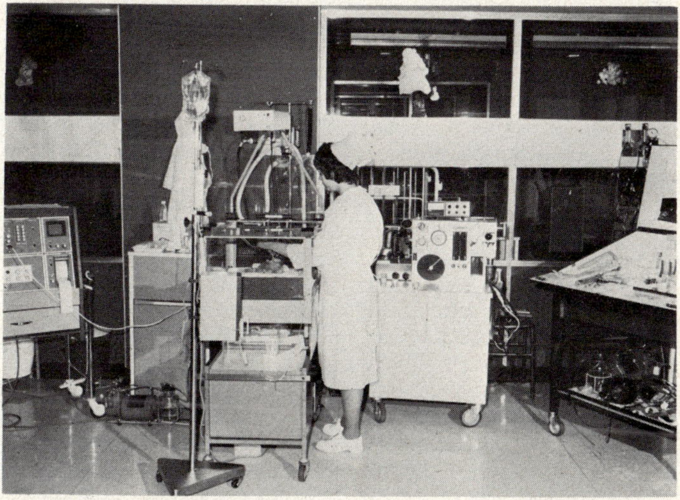

FIG. 38. This photograph illustrates the complexity of equipment and technology required in post-operative care of children following major cardio-thoracic surgery. Specialized nursing skills are called for during this demanding post-operative period.

e.g. monitoring equipment for recording apex beat, blood pressure and temperature should be checked and switched on ready for use. Suction pumps, e.g. Roberts, should be plugged in and ready for immediate attachment to the drainage bottles. Electrodes should be prepared and ready.

All that is necessary for general nursing care should be at the bedside, including a mouth tray, also a tray for naso-gastric aspiration. Splints and strapping ready for limb immobilization should be within easy reach. Charts should be prepared for recording vital signs, fluid and blood balance.

During the first post-operative 24 hours a special nurse should be always at the child's bedside, closely observing and recording details of the child's condition. Temperature, apex beat and respirations need recording $\frac{1}{4}$-hourly together with blood pressure (from the monitor) and central venous pressures (if required). Fluid balance must be maintained. The in situ urinary catheter should be released hourly and the amount measured and recorded, also the naso-gastric aspirate. Blood loss into drainage bottles should be measured $\frac{1}{2}$-hourly and according to the amount present, blood will be replaced according to the doctors' instructions through the intravenous infusion. In order to ensure that the measurement of this drainage is accurate, tubes must be checked $\frac{1}{4}$-hourly to prevent kinking and 'milked' to avoid clogging of the tube lumen. Following some operations the child may be attached to a ventilator.

When the child is fully rousable post-operative sedation, e.g. Pethidine or Omnopon may be given for pain. Nursing routine should be established to minimize fuss and disturbance to the child, procedures as far as possible should be combined to fit in with 2-hourly turning or 3-hourly mouth care. The parents should be brought in with a nurse to see and comfort their child and their questions answered. As soon as possible a member of the surgical team should explain to the parents details of the operation.

Throughout this important recovery phase the nurse should be calm and unhurried taking care to comfort and talk to the child during any procedures. Any complications that arise are most likely to do so within the first 24 hours. The nurse should be most observant and understand the significance of any change reporting these promptly and quickly.

After 24 hours the lungs are usually fully expanded and following X-ray confirmation the intercostal drains may be removed and if all is well the child sat up with two or three pillows. Deep breathing and coughing exercises continue, whilst the nurse supports the chest and abdomen to make it easier. If fluid balance is maintained and kidney function good the urinary catheter is taken out. It is usual to send a specimen of urine to the laboratory for culture and sensitivity to ensure that infection is not present. Mouth care should continue 3-hourly and as the lips often become sore, petroleum jelly may be applied.

During the second to third day oral feeding may be commenced with clear fluids in small amounts, if absorbed the nasogastric tube can be removed. The intravenous infusion is usually left a little longer until all oral feeds are absorbed and tolerated. If an atrial line is still in position this is now removed if good progress continues. The child may be sat out of bed for a short time whilst bed linen is being changed. Ambulation is gradually increased and more occupation given to the child in the form of games, jigsaws and puzzles. If the bowels are not opened with the introduction of a light diet, a glycerine suppository should be given. After a week dressings should be taken down and if necessary sutures removed.

If the recovery period continues uneventfully the child is discharged home about the tenth day post-operatively. Parents should be advised as to the best routine to follow at home for the needs of their child. The child initially should be encouraged to rest in the afternoons, gradually doing more and more. After relief of a serious cardiac disability babies often find themselves enjoying their feeds for the first time. They are inclined to take them greedily, demanding more than is offered. The temptation to overfeed must be resisted to avoid overdistension and pressure on the diaphragm.

A follow-up appointment for all patients to visit out-patients is given usually 4 to 6 weeks after discharge. It is most rewarding for the nurse to see her patients when they come back looking very well, able to play more games with their friends and also most noticeable a relief of tension and anxiety in the family.

Complications of Cardio-Thoracic Surgery

Complications of cardio-thoracic surgery may be:

1. Pneumothorax (spontaneous filling of the pleural space with air);
2. Haemothorax (filling of the pleural space with blood);
3. Cardiac arrythmias;
4. Horner's syndrome—damage to the sympathetic cervical chain which may be irreversible, resulting in ptosis and pupil dilatation on the affected side;
5. Posture deformities, counteracted with physiotherapy and encouragement to the child;
6. Cerebral thrombosis;
7. Post-operative euphoria and confusion, temporary, lasting a few days, treated with Valium;
8. Irreversible shock—death.

Mechanical Artificial Ventilation

Increasingly artificial ventilation is required in paediatric care for a variety of conditions, e.g. following major cardiac surgery or as part of the treatment of respiratory failure. There are many different makes of ventilator available, but the majority now in use are intermittent positive-pressure machines. Which ventilator to use is not a choice that the nurse has to make, but she needs to recognize the principles involved in the use of these machines and should make herself familiar with the type of ventilator in use for any patient in her care.

There are basically 2 types of ventilator using intermittent positive pressure—flow generators and pressure generators. The aim of artificial ventilation is to maintain gas exchange in the lungs. When a ventilator is used, the intrathoracic pressure changes are reversed. The ventilator does this by driving an air/oxygen mixture through the connecting airway into the lungs. The alveolar pressure rises above the atmospheric pressure which interferes with the return of the blood to the heart. During expiration the chest wall returns to its resting position, the alveolar pressure falls and blood returns to the heart. Amongst the complications of using ventilators is rupture of the lungs due to high pressure in the alveoli and pneumothorax.

Nursing Management of a Child on a Ventilator

As the child is attached to the ventilator by means of a tracheal tube, the airway must be kept clear of secretions. Aspiration should be carried out whenever the child is turned (at least 2-hourly), whenever the nurse can hear the rattle of secretions in the trachea and more often if the patient's condition indicates the need. Tracheal aspiration requires a swift and gentle aseptic technique. It is a good rule to follow that the whole procedure should only take as long as the nurse can hold her own breath (see p. 160). The tube must be kept firmly in position and the tapes securing it should be checked at regular intervals. The ventilator tubing itself is heavy and will need to be supported, if it is not to pull on the tracheal tube. Frequent observations should be recorded showing the rate of ventilation, flow rate of inspiratory gases, inspiratory—expiratory ratio, tidal volume, pressure attained on the manometer of the ventilator and the patient's colour. Records should also be kept of the patient's pulse, blood pressure and temperature. All these are best kept on a graph chart in order that any change can readily be seen. All children nursed on ventilators require humidification of the inspired gases, water is usually used, although some paediatricians prefer saline.

When the patient's condition has improved to allow for normal respiration to be re-established, weaning from the ventilator may take some time. All respiratory depressant drugs must be discontinued and time allowed for their elimination. The easiest method of weaning from the ventilator is to allow the child to breathe spontaneously for short periods, which can gradually be increased, providing the child does not get too tired or anxious. A great deal of encouragement and reassurance will be needed. The same method can be used for young infants. An alternative method for older children only, is to adjust the trigger mechanism, thus encouraging the child to greater effort in establishing the onset of inspiration. This method is only possible with a few ventilators.

The child on a ventilator requires constant nursing support, and should never be left unobserved. Even if the child appears unconscious he should be spoken to in a kindly reassuring manner, as hearing is often the first sense to return. The nurse should never feel self-conscious about this, and it will be particularly comforting to the parents.

For the child attached to a ventilator for a long time, life must go on. A nursing routine should be devised which meets his needs for stimulation and comfort, thus minimizing the stress of this situation. The presence of the tube will interfere with speech, and it is a good idea to have a writing board or slate always available for use, even for the child who cannot yet communicate by writing, as a great deal can be conveyed with simple line drawings.

Hypothermia

The ability of certain organs of the body to remain undamaged if deprived of oxygen at normal temperature is known to vary and it is known that the brain tissues are the first to suffer, the maximum period of deprivation for the brain being 4 minutes without causing irreparable damage. By cooling the body to temperatures as low as 12° to 15°C (53° to 60°F) the metabolism is slowed down and therefore the oxygen requirements reduced. Operations involving a temporary interruption of circulation can therefore be undertaken while the patient is in a state comparable to that of a hibernating animal.

Cooling of the body can be achieved by the use of ice packs, by immersion in cooled water or by allowing the blood to flow through a cannula and tubing from the superior vena cava to a refrigerating circuit and pumping it back into the circulation via the inferior vena cava.

At this low body temperature the heart can be opened and the operation performed under direct vision.

The return to normal temperature must be very gradual and has to be carefully controlled. To this end an oesophageal temperature (by means of an electrode) is taken every 10 to 15 minutes. A rise of more than 0.2°C in this time is a signal to slow further active warming-up procedures.

Intercostal Drainage

Following intrathoracic surgery one or two tubes are stitched into position to allow fluid and air to escape from the pleural space. The drainage tube connects to a drainage bottle either containing a measured amount of water or suitable disinfectant or in some cases a 'Redivac' sealed bottle. This forms an air-tight seal.

Expansion of the chest on inspiration increases the intra-pleural vacuum and as fluid and air drains out the lungs re-expand. Drainage must be carefully measured, and fluctuations in the tube noted. The tubes should be 'milked' at frequent intervals to prevent blockage of the tube lumen.

When the lungs are fully expanded drainage ceases; following X-ray confirmation of this, the tube is removed under aseptic conditions carefully sealing the tube entry point with sterile vaseline on a gauze dressing to prevent air entry.

The tube leading to the drainage bottle must be clipped off securely when changing the bottle and it must never be raised above the level of the patient or air and fluid may be sucked back into the pleural space.

Special Diagnostic Procedures

Angiography

Radio-opaque dye is injected into the venous circulation. Serial radiographs or cine-recording follows the passage of the dye through the heart outlining abnormal shunts or any obstruction. This procedure is commonly combined with cardiac catheterization.

Cardiac Catheterization

Under deep sedation an opaque catheter is inserted by way of a vein commonly one of the femoral veins, into the superior vena cava, the right atrium, right ventricle and pulmonary artery. Pressures and oxygen saturations are measured repeatedly during the procedure revealing a great deal of information about the function of the heart. The use of serial radiographs and/or cine-recording enables the doctor to follow the progress of the catheter.

Catheterization of the left side of the heart in the absence of any shunt is much more difficult and must be performed either through the aorta or by perforation of the atrial septum within the heart as in Rashkind's procedure.

Cardiac catheterization is not without risk. This procedure should be carried out in specialist paediatric centres. After the procedure the child should be carefully observed for blood loss from the site of the venous incision and resultant shock. Nursing care is aimed at keeping the child quiet and rested. Oxygen and humidity being given if necessary. Providing all observations are satisfactory the child may be up and about in 24 to 48 hr. The wound should be kept dry and the sutures removed about the seventh day.

Haematocrit

The haematocrit or packed cell volume becomes elevated with cyanosis and is accompanied by an increased viscosity of the blood. This increased viscosity heightens the patient's susceptibility to cerebral thrombosis.

Inflammatory Heart Diseases

Although endocarditis, myocarditis and pericarditis are separate entities, any one of them is bound to affect all parts of the heart as the various structures are intimately connected.

Inflammation may be caused by toxins reaching the heart as in pneumonia, influenza, general septicaemia and especially diphtheria and the result may be heart failure. Alternatively the heart may be affected by bacterial invasion, e.g. bacterial endocarditis. Inflammatory heart disease is one of the possible complications of rheumatic fever and chorea. Permanent cardiac damage may result.

Bacterial Endocarditis

Bacterial endocarditis is an acute or more commonly a subacute infection of the endocardium and this condition often follows, throat, dental or middle ear infections caused by the *Streptococcus viridans*. Bacterial endocarditis usually arises as a complication of congenital or rheumatic heart disease. It is rare in childhood.

The symptoms are similar to those of rheumatic carditis but the child is extremely toxic. He looks seriously ill, the eyes are sunken and surrounded by deep shadows and though he seems weary he tosses about restlessly. Pulse and respiration rates are increased and the temperature may rise to 40°C (104°F) or more. The skin becomes dry, the urinary output is diminished, the tongue is furred, the lips dry and inclined to crack. Petechial spots may appear on the skin.

Nursing Care. The child will be nursed in a similar manner as that described for a child with cardiac failure.

Drug therapy is directed towards overcoming the infections by giving large doses of the appropriate antibiotic usually one of the penicillins. In very severe cases this may be given intravenously. Steroids are prescribed because of their anti-inflammatory effect and to minimize the production of scar tissue.

Recovery may be complete but the illness and period of convalescence may extend over many months. A careful follow-up by the paediatrician must be maintained over several years.

Complications

1. Embolism as a result of breakdown from the septic valves;
2. Permanent damage to the valves requiring operation at a later date.

Further Reading

RENDLE-SHORT, J. & GRAY, C. P. (1967) *A Synopsis of Children's Diseases*, 4th ed. Bristol: John Wright & Sons.

ROBERTS, K. D. & EDWARDS, J. M. (1976) *Paediatric Intensive Care*, 2nd ed. Oxford: Blackwell Scientific.

VENABLES, A. W. (1964) *Essentials of Paediatric Cardiology*. Springfield, Illinois: Charles C. Thomas.

11

Rheumatic and collagen diseases

ALL THE DISEASES described in this chapter are thought to be due to a hypersensitivity or an autoimmunity reaction. In persons affected by any of these conditions, the normal immune reaction is replaced by an abnormal sensitivity to infection or a definite destructive reaction within the body. In addition to the conditions described in this chapter, the following diseases are sometimes included in this broad group;

Anaphylactoid purpura (see p. 222);
Idiopathic and symptomatic thrombocytopenic purpuras (see p. 235);
Nephritis, nephrosis (see pp. 335 and 338);
Ulcerative colitis.

Acute Rheumatic Fever and Rheumatic Carditis

In acute rheumatic fever there is commonly a history of a sore throat or tonsillitis 2 or 3 weeks before the onset of symptoms.

Streptococcus pyogenes is usually the causative organism, but this is not always present on culture when a throat swab is taken. The infection may have been overcome although the streptococcal toxin has set up an autoimmune reaction in the body.

The child suffering from acute rheumatism often has a moderate pyrexia of about 37.2° to 37.8°C (99° to 100°F), but it may be much higher. The pulse rate is raised and toxic signs such as headache, vomiting, furred tongue, sweating and constipation are likely to be present. The child may complain of severe pain in the knee, elbow, ankle and wrist joints. These severe pains may affect one joint one day and others the next and although there may be redness, heat and swelling there is no permanent damage to the joints. In long-standing cases anaemia may develop and there is danger of permanent cardiac damage. The latter fact makes good medical care and careful nursing all-important. A constant watch has to be kept for early signs of carditis (see p. 208).

Occasionally a faint, slightly pink rash appears on the trunk and this may recur intermittently for several months (erythema marginatum). On examination rheumatic nodules are sometimes found over the elbows, shins, knuckles, knees, occiput and spine. These nodules are better felt than seen, but when the skin over them is stretched they show up clearly as raised, white areas. They may appear in crops for many weeks and may go only after some considerable time. These nodules are usually a sign that the illness is taking a serious course and they are rarely found unless the heart has become affected.

Treatment

Little treatment can be given apart from adequate drug therapy and careful nursing care and rest.

Drug Therapy. Salicylates are the specific drugs for the treatment of acute rheumatic conditions. Usually at least 0.6 g four times a day are given in the form of Disprin or Solprin. Relief from pain may be very rapid. Signs of intolerance or overdose, which used to be very common when sodium salicylate was used, are now unusual but if they occur they should be reported at once. They include nausea, tinnitus, vomiting, deafness, albuminuria, a discrete erythematous rash, sighing respirations and purpura. Prophylactic drug therapy against recurrent streptococcal infections is sometimes prescribed and usually carried on for a period of at least 5 years or until the child leaves school, whichever is the longer. During that time the patient may be ordered penicillin by mouth or one of the sulphonamide group of drugs. Steroids are valuable in severe cases or where there are signs of cardiac involvement, since the early use of these drugs has been found to prevent or minimize permanent cardiac damage. If there is any cardiac incompetence due to carditis, digoxin may be ordered. Phenylbutazone may be given in certain selected cases for the relief of severe pain.

Unfortunately this drug occasionally produces agranulocytosis, therefore all patients receiving this treatment should at frequent intervals have white cell counts.

Nursing Care. Children suffering from acute rheumatism should be nursed in a warm, well-ventilated, pleasant room. If admitted to a ward they should be given a bed in a quiet corner where there is little danger of other children or passers-by knocking into their beds, as at first pain is severe and even slight vibration, caused by someone passing or holding on to the bed while talking to the patient, may cause the child to cry out in agony Complete rest is enforced, that is to say he is not allowed to do anything for himself. The nurse will have to explain this if the child is old enough and capable of co-operation. He will be washed and, unless a very light patient, two nurses will be required for giving a bed pan which he is asked to use in a lying-down position. In many cases the child will have to be fed, but some paediatricians feel that, provided the patient is well supported by pillows, he may be allowed to feed himself as this may improve the appetite and is often less strain than being fed. When pain is present the use of small pillows or pads of cotton wool to support the affected limb may give comfort. A soft, firm mattress should be used and the weight of the bedclothes taken by a bed cradle. But no definite rule can be laid down and the nursing routine will largely depend on the history, the severity of the illness, whether the heart is involved and the patient's response to treatment. It is, however, always best to be too careful in view of the serious consequences a neglect of the illness may have.

The *diet* should be light and nutritious as the illness is a long and debilitating one and no trouble should be spared in tempting the child with dishes he enjoys.

Drinking in the recumbent position can be a serious problem. A feeding cup may be used and the nurse can play a suitable game with her patient while teaching him how to drink from it. Polythene tubing is more suitable than a straw to assist with drinking, as it bends easily. Owing to its transparency, the fluid can be seen going up and down the tube, a fact which amuses children and makes drinking a pleasure. Nowadays coloured straws which can be bent and moulded have become available.

A story told or read while feeding a child is permissible if this means a contented patient who takes his food willingly.

As exertion should be reduced to a minimum, it is useful to let the child wear an open-back gown in the acute stages as this makes dressing and undressing easy and also prevents him from lying on wrinkles and creases. The nurse can use her nursing skill and imagination in many ways to relieve pain and boredom and to make the irksome rest and the difficulties of taking food in the recumbent position as bearable as possible. Some ways of relieving pain and preventing painful movement are mentioned above. In the relief of boredom a good paediatric staff will co-operate in setting some time aside during which the nurse can read to the child or sit down beside him to talk to him or draw for him. A book-rest may be supplied to make reading possible without exertion or light toys or comics may be provided. It may be possible to move the bed near a window and let the child watch the happenings in the street by means of a spy mirror fixed to the bed. Extra visiting helps to allay boredom and a radio or television set by the bedside is often greatly appreciated and may give hours of restful entertainment.

Rheumatic carditis most commonly follows an attack of acute rheumatism often preceded by a sore throat, but may occasionally arise without any evidence of previous infection. Endocarditis with some involvement of the myocardium is the most common manifestation and the pathology is similar to that of endocarditis in the adult. The lesions resulting from the inflammatory process are scarring and growth of vegetations around the cardiac valves; the most commonly affected one being the mitral valve. Over a period of years, mitral stenosis accompanied by aortic regurgitation and enlargement of the left ventricle develops. In the young adult this damage leads to dyspnoea, congestion of the lungs, oedema and generalized cardiac crippling.

The child who has an attack of acute rheumatism fails to improve and remains tired, irritable and unhappy. His appetite is poor, his sleep restless, his colour grey or dusky, his skin feels clammy and the face looks pinched and the nose pointed. The pulse rate is rapid and the sleeping pulse rate may rise to approximate the waking pulse. Irregularities of volume and rhythm may occur. A mild pyrexia of 37.2° to 37.8°C

(99° to 100°F) is common. The child frequently suffers from dyspnoea.

On examination heart murmurs can be heard and the erythrocyte sedimentation rate may be raised from 10 mm to 60 or 80 mm/hour. The urinary output is often diminished and oedema may develop due to heart failure.

Complications. Complications arising from rheumatic carditis may become apparent during the attack or occur later, and are due to permanent damage to the heart and its valves. They include heart failure, mitral stenosis, aortic valve incompetence and pericarditis. All these are likely to make the patient into a permanent invalid and to shorten life. No trouble or expenditure of time is therefore too much to give when nursing those children and a very great responsibility rests upon the nurse in this respect.

A child with rheumatic carditis will be in bed for a number of weeks or months and passive exercises, particularly to the limbs, are sometimes given to help to maintain muscle tone and prevent foot drop, without causing the patient any exertion. The position in the bed will depend on the wishes of the physician and on the degree of dyspnoea present. A semi-recumbent position with two or three pillows giving adequate support to the trunk, neck and head, is often considered more satisfactory than the recumbent position with only a small pillow for the head, as it may be difficult to keep a child quiet and content with most of his outlook confined to watching the ceiling. If one pillow only is allowed, raising the head end of the bed on blocks overcomes some of the difficulty. It is sometimes considered wise to nurse these children in a cubicle or side ward to ensure better rest and quiet. This needs to be considered carefully, however, as many children will lie still more readily when they can watch what is going on around them, provided a long night's rest and a good sleep at midday can be guaranteed. The blanket bed, so commonly used at one time, is now not considered necessary but a small flannelette blanket next to the patient may give comfort and extra warmth. A daily blanket bath should be given, particularly if perspiration is profuse. Oral toilet and regular attention to all pressure areas are important in a patient who will be ill for some time and who as a rule has to lie still, is on a very light diet and is probably thin and in indifferent general health.

Charts and Observations. Four-hourly recordings of temperature, pulse and respirations will be made and the sleeping pulse taken and recorded 4-hourly throughout the night. The nurse should note particularly the quality and rhythm of the pulse rate and report any irregularities without delay, as they may be the earliest signs of cardiac involvement. The nurse's intelligent observations and careful recording can be of great value to the doctor in charge. A fluid balance chart is kept up and the urinary output watched conscientiously. An imbalance in the intake and output may be an early sign of cardiac failure. The child's weight is checked weekly, provided special scales which enable even older children to be weighed lying down, are available for the purpose.

The *erythrocyte sedimentation rate* is taken weekly and together with sleeping pulse recordings will give a good indication as to the patient's progress. Guided by these and a lessening in the abnormal heart sounds, a gradual increase in exercise is allowed, though the child may need to remain at rest for several weeks or even months. If symptoms persist and the heart lesion fails to improve, transfer to a long-stay hospital and special schooling may have to be arranged.

Chorea (Sydenham's Chorea, 'St Vitus' Dance')

Chorea is sometimes described as rheumatism of the brain. Attacks may be so mild as almost to escape notice or of extreme severity. In its severest form, chorea is now rarely seen, but the seriousness of the attack cannot be overestimated even if it is a mild one. In this chapter a severe case and its nursing care is described and the intelligent nurse will modify the nursing treatment according to her patient. The characteristic features of the disease are the involuntary, unco-ordinated and purposeless movements.

Signs and Symptoms. The onset is often insidious but emotional factors do appear to play a part in starting the disease.

Anxieties over schoolwork, sudden frights or bereavement are among these emotional causes. Parents and teachers may merely complain that the child has become fidgety, that he is dropping things at school and that his handwriting is deteriorating. The usually bright pupil becomes inattentive and giggles and grimaces during lessons. As time goes on the movements become more marked and emotional disturbances develop. The child laughs and cries without any apparent reason. Examination of the patient includes some simple but almost diagnostic tests. The child who is asked to put out his tongue does so, but moves it in and out, unable to keep it still. Asked to unbutton his coat he is unable to do so on account of irregular, unco-ordinated movements and when asked to hold out his hands in front of him he shoots them forward like a gun. Hyperflexion of the wrists and hyperextension of the metacarpophalangeal joints causes a 'dinner fork' deformity of the hands. Speech is jerky and difficult to understand and in the severest form may be altogether impossible. During the medical examination the child is sometimes asked to count rapidly, a task he finds himself unable to perform. He finds writing and drawing extremely difficult and it is often interesting to give the patient a weekly drawing task in which improvements in the co-ordinated movements can be seen when the successive drawings are compared. The child has a friendly smile which may seem very attractive, but it is exaggerated in relation to the circumstances and to his emotional state. He easily bursts into tears and has emotional upsets and temper tantrums.

Eating and drinking are difficult as the patient is constantly moving and throwing himself about. The difficulty of getting the child to take sufficient nourishment, together with the constant movements, leads to wasting and this coupled with the rubbing of occiput, elbows and heels on the bedclothes presents a serious nursing problem if bedsores are to be prevented. An interesting feature is the fact that movements cease during sleep.

Nursing Care. The child is best nursed in a separate room or quiet part of the ward. Cot-sides should be used to prevent him falling out of bed and in severe cases these need to be padded to prevent injury. The head bars of the bed should be protected by tying a pillow in position. The child may be nursed by lying on a sheepskin to prevent friction sores. As movements are so uncoordinated, there is a real danger of suffocation and loose, soft pillows must never be used. Sudden noises or lights should be avoided and all excitement kept from the patient. All sources of danger such as buttons, pins, long fingernails and sharp or even hard eating utensils must be eliminated. The mouth should be given special attention as the child frequently bites his tongue, lips or cheeks and ulceration easily occurs. The corners of the mouth should be protected against the constant dribble of saliva by lanolin or petroleum jelly. Feeding presents many difficulties. The child will move his head around continuously and it is often almost impossible to 'aim' at the mouth. Inhalation of food, drink and saliva is a real danger and not easy to prevent. Plastic spoons and polythene tubing are useful but at times it becomes necessary to resort to tube feeding. The diet should have a high-calorie value and should require little mastication.

The giving of bed pans may also present difficulties. As the patient cannot keep still on the bed pan, abrasions must be prevented from the start by padding the hard edges or by using rubber bed pans. The temperature must be taken in the groin or axilla to prevent accidents.

Every attempt should be made to ensure as much rest and sleep as possible by good nursing attention. Warm sponging may not only keep the skin healthy but may help to induce sleep. Toys should be of a simple, soft type and should have no hard bits or parts which could come off and be swallowed. Hairslides should be replaced by ribbon.

The temperature, pulse and respirations are recorded every 4 hours and observations on the pulse and the recording of the sleeping pulse are of particular importance. Whenever possible a weekly weight chart is kept, as well as a note on the patient's emotional behaviour, movements and general condition. A weekly sample of his writing or drawing performance can be filed for comparison (Fig. 39).

Treatment. Apart from careful nursing, every effort should be made to reduce exertion and excitement to a minimum. The nurse should spare the time to sit by the child and read and

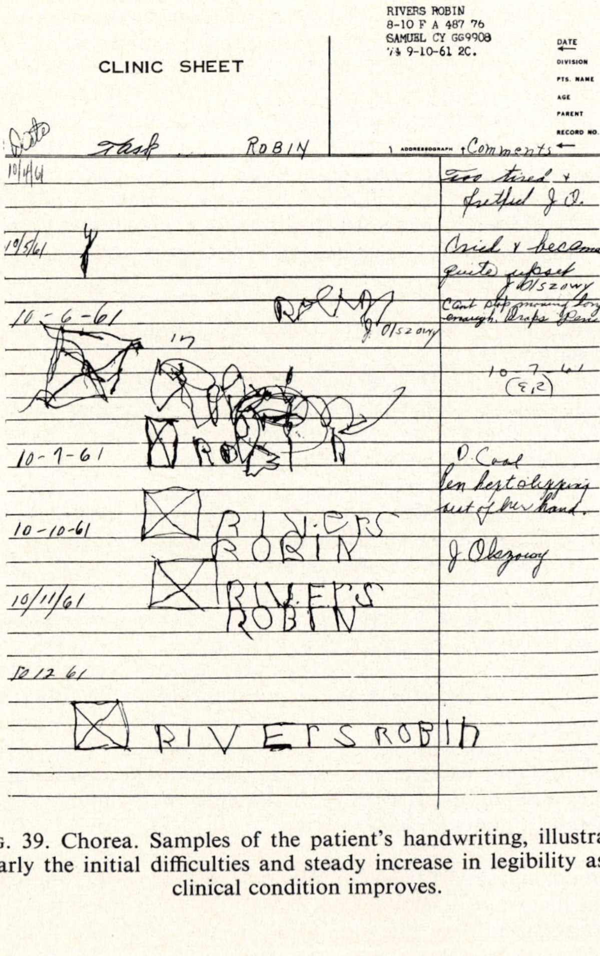

RIVERS ROBIN
8-10 F A 487 76
SAMUEL CY GG9908
7¼ 9-10-61 2C.

DATE
DIVISION
PTS. NAME
AGE
PARENT
RECORD NO.

CLINIC SHEET

ADDRESSOGRAPH

Date	Task	ROBIN	Comments
10/4/61			Too tired + fretful J.O.
10/5/61			Cried + became quite upset J Olszowy
10-6-61	ROBIN	J. Olszowy	Can't stop moving long enough. Drops pen.
			10-7-61 (E,C)
10-7-61	ROBIN		O. Cook Pen kept slipping out of her hand.
10-10-61	RIVERS ROBIN		J. Olszowy
10/11/61	RIVERS ROBIN		
10 12 61	RIVERS ROBIN		

FIG. 39. Chorea. Samples of the patient's handwriting, illustrating clearly the initial difficulties and steady increase in legibility as the clinical condition improves.

talk to him and extra visiting by the mother will help to keep him happy and occupied. There is little medical treatment apart from sedatives. Some physicians prescribe a course of penicillin or sulphonamides prophylactically over a period of years. Erythrocyte sedimentation rate and cardiography give a useful guide to progress.

Complete recovery may be expected after several weeks but there is a strong tendency to recurrence and the danger of cardiac involvement is considerable.

Rheumatoid Arthritis (Still's Disease)

Still's disease (Fig. 40) is an inflammatory condition of the joints, similar to the more common, crippling condition known

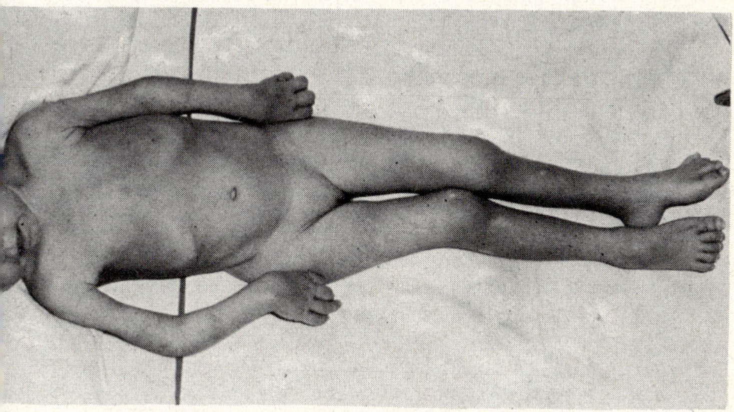

FIG. 40. Still's disease. Note deformities of joints.

as rheumatoid arthritis in adults. Although not common in childhood, Still's disease is of interest to the paediatric nurse because of the characteristic manifestations and the careful nursing called for in this disease.

Still's disease most commonly starts between the age of 18 months and 6 years and the earlier the onset the less favourable the prognosis. The cause remains unknown.

Signs and Symptoms. The first manifestation of the disease may be a single swollen joint (often the knee). A carefully taken history may reveal recurrent complaints of a stiff neck or stiffness in other joints. Occasionally the onset is acute and may easily be mistaken for acute rheumatic fever. The child is feverish and complains of general malaise. Pain and swelling of the joints may be both acute and severe. More often, however, the disease develops gradually. The usually bright child becomes listless, miserable and pale. Loss of appetite soon causes him to lose weight and he fails to make general progress. He has a high, swinging temperature, the skin is moist and clammy and the blood sedimentation rate is raised (50 to 100 mm in one hour) and the Rose Waaler test may be positive. The haemoglobin level falls and there may be a mild degree of tachycardia. On examination, subcutaneous nodules may be found although more rarely than in rheumatic fever. As the illness progresses the joints become painful and swollen and the overlying skin looks white and shiny, though at the same time it may be hot to the touch. Periarticular swelling and wasting gradually cause the fingers to take on a spindle-shaped appearance.

As a rule the fingers, wrists, elbows and knees, feet and cervical spine are affected most and the swellings and deformity occur symmetrically. Despite marked swellings in the acute stages, the joints are not always permanently damaged, though fibrous ankylosis is very often the cause of extensive crippling and may necessitate corrective orthopaedic surgery. Osteoporosis may be considerable and may be the cause of pathological fractures. Occasionally a fine erythematous rash appears and may not fade for many weeks. Both the peripheral lymphatic glands and the spleen may be enlarged. Pericarditis is an occasional complication.

Treatment. In the acute stage this aims at resting both the patient and the affected part, and splints are applied to avoid deformity. The child should be nursed in a well-ventilated room and the bed should be protected from any jarring movement. Whenever possible he should be carried on to a balcony or into the garden but draughts and cold should be avoided. The bedclothes should be light and bed cradles should be used. Sand bags, small pillows and foot rests and light plaster of Paris splints help to make the patient more comfortable and may prevent deformities. Even in the acute stages physiotherapy should ensure movement throughout the whole range at least once daily. Movement may be made easier by heat therapy prior to physiotherapy and this can be achieved by the use of radiant heat, wax baths or infra-red ray treatment, but it should be remembered that the child must not be left even for a short time during such treatment.

The diet should be attractive and nutritious and should contain adequate amounts of vitamins. Fresh fruit is wholesome and may help to prevent constipation. Poor general health and immobility make careful attention to all pressure areas important. Children with Still's disease are inclined to become over-anxious and introspective, and schooling and adequate occupation should be provided to keep up the child's morale and interest. At the same time occupational therapy will help to keep the affected joints moving.

Drug Therapy. Salicylates which abolish pain and fever in acute rheumatism are also effective in Still's disease. The possibility of salicylate intestinal bleeding must be kept in mind. but Disprin and other analgesic drugs may relieve pain. Iron is given to combat anaemia and occasionally a small blood transfusion may help to build up the child's health generally, as well as raising the haemoglobin level. Steroids are used with some success, but the side effects which occur, and the need to keep up the steroid therapy, limit their usefulness. If only one or two joints are affected, intra-articular hydrocortisone may be of value. However, if this treatment is used for weight-bearing joints, caution must be observed lest the relief of symptoms leads to excessive use of the joint thus causing further damage.

Prognosis. Inadequate or late treatment may lead to complications which include general ill health, retarded growth, deformities and blindness from iridocyclitis. About half the children suffering from Still's disease and treated within a year of onset, may be expected to have no residual joint lesions 5 years later, the disease may, in others burn itself out over a period of 1 to 2 years.

Other Collagen Diseases

Sometimes a hypersensitivity or autoimmune reaction affects the connective tissue, and in that case one of five rare diseases, grouped together as collagen diseases, may occur. These diseases are briefly described below. They may have a poor prognosis in spite of treatment with steroids and death is often caused by renal failure. The serum proteins are abnormal and the erythrocyte sedimentation rate is raised.

Henoch-Schönlein's Syndrome (Anaphylactoid Purpura)

Henoch-Schönlein's purpura, which is one of the collagen diseases, is seen fairly commonly in childhood, but rarely before the age of 3 years. The small purpuric haemorrhages seen on the skin are at first of a purple colour but later they turn a dusky red and still later brown, until they gradually disappear. A faint urticarial rash is usually present. The areas most commonly involved are the legs, the back of the elbows and arms, the lumbar region and buttocks. Any pressure, such as sitting on a bed pan, may cause localized purpuric spots. If the haemorrhages involve the intestinal tract, there may be severe abdominal pain of a colicky nature which may last for several hours. This may be followed by the passage of bright blood or a melaena stool. The child may be shocked and occasionally an intussusception may complicate the picture. For that reason there is a certain danger in giving drugs such as pethidine to relieve pain, as this may mask symptoms which should urgently be recognized. The Henoch-Schönlein syndrome may also involve the large joints causing pain and swelling although there is no actual haemorrhage into the joint itself. As different joints become involved, pain flits from one site to another but it never leaves permanent damage or stiffness.

Often no specific treatment is considered necessary and with bed rest the child gradually improves and the rash fades after about 2 or 3 weeks. Steroids may, however, be given if the erythrocyte sedimentation rate is high or if there is albuminuria. There is a tendency to recurrence.

Complications. Complications include nephritis and intussusception, which are dealt with in the usual way.

Nursing Care. Nursing care is symptomatic. Relief of pain for the affected joints may be given by applying pads of warmed cotton wool and in case of severe abdominal pain a well-protected hot water bottle might be used with special permission from the ward sister. Gentle massage may bring some comfort. A painful limb may be elevated on a small pillow and a bed cradle should be used to take the weight of the bedclothes. Pressure from the rim of a bed pan should be excluded by padding it with an air ring or by using a rubber pan.

Polyarteritis Nodosa (Periarteritis Nodosa)

Polyarteritis nodosa is an acute inflammation of the small arterioles, with aneurysm formation which can sometimes be quite easily felt as nodules under the skin. The damage to the arterioles may lead to thrombosis and to haemorrhage. The main signs and symptoms are fever, tachycardia, joint and muscle pains and proteinuria which may progress to renal failure. There is hypertension and a polymorphonuclear leucocytosis, and anaemia is common. Temporal arteritis may cause severe headaches and possibly cerebral haemorrhage. Renal and muscle biopsy will confirm the diagnosis.

Dermatomyositis

Dermatomyositis has an insidious onset. Muscle, skin and subcutaneous tissues become inflamed. The muscles are stiff, tender and swollen and become weak with atrophy, contractions and fibrosis. The heart muscle may be affected, causing myocarditis and tachycardia. There is a typical, violet-coloured rash on cheeks and eyelids, circumoral pallor, and an erythematous and sometimes urticarial rash on trunk, limbs and knuckles. The subcutaneous tissues become inelastic and there is a low grade pyrexia and progressive disability which may include muscles of respiration, speech and swallowing. The urinary creatinine levels are greatly elevated in the acute phase, and muscle biopsy and electromyogram confirm the diagnosis. The condition may become chronic with signs similar to scleroderma, but in spite of steroid therapy acute cases may die of cardiac or renal failure or intercurrent infections.

Lupus Erythematosus

The disseminated form of lupus erythematosus is rare in childhood, and has an even worse prognosis than in later life. The most characteristic lesion is a purplish-red, raised and indurated 'butterfly' rash over the cheeks and nose. All the mesenchymal tissues are affected, leading to hypertension, anaemia, pyrexia, painful swelling of joints, enlargement of liver and spleen, pleurisy, endocarditis, proteinuria and renal lesions. The bone marrow is depressed, causing leucopenia, and the blood sedimentation rate is very high. Atypical antibodies from the autoimmune reaction—lupus erythematosus (LE) cells—can be seen in blood tests and are specially diagnostic. Treatment is with prednisone 1–2 mg/kg/day initially, but other immunosuppressive agents such as azathioprine 2–5 mg/kg/day may be given.

Further Reading

BRIMBLECOMBE, F. S. W. & BARLTROP, D. (1978) *Children in Health and Disease*. London: Baillière Tindall.

JOLLY, H. (1976) *Diseases of Children*, 3rd ed. Oxford: Blackwell Scientific.

12

Diseases of the blood

ANAEMIA, the most common disorder of the blood in childhood, it is due either to a reduction in the quality or the quantity of red blood cells (erythrocytes). Apart from a decrease in the number of red blood cells or of the quantity of haemoglobin present, alterations in the shape and size of these cells may also occur.

Classification of Anaemias

1. *Deficiency anaemias*
   Decreased blood formation
   (a) Too few red blood cells.
   (b) Too little haemoglobin in red cells.
2. *Haemolytic anaemias*
   Increased haemolysis (blood destruction)
   (a) Due to production of abnormal red blood cells or
   (b) Abnormal destruction of red blood cells.
3. *Haemorrhagic anaemias*
   Due to blood loss, acute or chronic.

Anaemia, no matter what the underlying cause, produces a similar clinical presentation in the child.

Clinical Picture of Anaemia

When the onset is insidious mother often first notices the child to be listless, apathetic and tiring more easily than his playmates. The young baby often refuses feeds or may not complete them. The older child sometimes complains of headaches, giddiness and blurred vision. In the younger child pica (dirt eating) may be observed, this usually stops once the cause of the anaemia has been treated.

Mother will notice that the child is difficult over eating,

refusing previously well-liked foods. Episodes of sepsis and upper respiratory tract infections are very common, often necessitating frequent absence from school. In severe cases dyspnoea and some puffiness or oedema of the lower limbs may be present. On physical examination the doctor may hear a cardiac murmur.

Some children with anaemia appear pale, but this is deceptive as red cheeks or a dark skin may hide severe anaemia. The colour of the conjunctivae or of the mucous membrane are more important to observe, these will appear pale in the anaemic child.

When anaemia develops rapidly, e.g. after haemorrhage, the child will appear limp and breathless with a marked tachycardia within a very short time.

Whenever anaemia is suspected it is important that a specimen of blood is obtained before treatment is commenced in order that the primary cause of the anaemia be detected as quickly as possible.

Deficiency Anaemias

Iron deficiency is the most common of this group and of all childhood anaemias. Iron is essential for the production of haemoglobin and deficiency may be due to:

1. Insufficient iron in the diet;
2. To prematurity, multiple births or maternal anaemia before birth of the baby.
3. Failure to absorb iron in the gastro-intestinal tract following neonatal surgery or with malabsorption syndromes, e.g. coeliac disease.

Iron deficiency anaemia is most common in those infants fed on a milk-only diet after the age of 4 to 5 months, when all the reserves of iron stored in the liver have been used up. Premature infants are particularly at risk for the development of this condition as the stores of iron in the liver are built up during the last months of pregnancy. The onset is gradual. Increased susceptibility to infection is often the first indication that anaemia may be present.

In later childhood this anaemia follows infection especially of the gastro-intestinal tract. Intestinal parasites combined with infection and a poor diet will add to the iron deficiency.

Treatment. Prophylactic addition of iron to all premature infants from the age of 1 month.

Mixed feeding to all babies is introduced from the age of 4 months. Some paediatricians advocate iron supplements from the age of 12 to 16 weeks until mixed feeding is fully established. As with other medicines this should never be added to the milk feed but given separately.

Children often accept iron medicines more readily than they do pills. They can be given either through a straw or from a spoon. Older children should be encouraged to brush their teeth after taking the medicine, as in some cases they may produce some discoloration of the teeth. For all ages it is best to give the prescribed preparation before a meal.

As well as giving iron supplement the appetite should be stimulated with an attractive, well-balanced diet rich in iron containing foods:

Eggs	Liver	Chocolate	Dried fruits
Meat	Fish	Fruit	Wholemeal bread

It is important that adequate amounts of vitamin C, copper, folic acid and vitamin B are also present in the diet as these are also essential for the development of mature red blood cells.

The nurse should remember that anaemic children tire more easily than their friends, and will often need a rest during the day or a quiet play period instead of joining in more boisterous games.

In very severe cases a blood transfusion may be necessary to replace the missing haemoglobin and stimulate the bone marrow. Intramuscular iron is not now recommended, nor is intravenous iron necessary for most children.

When anaemia is associated with malabsorption syndromes the underlying cause must be treated with the addition of vitamin and iron supplements to the diet.

Hypoplastic and Aplastic Anaemia

Failure of the bone marrow to manufacture erythrocytes

completely is called *aplastic anaemia* but fortunately this is rare. *Hypoplastic anaemia* or under production of erythrocytes may occur. These conditions may be caused by certain drugs, e.g. chloramphenicol, but often the cause is unknown. Diagnosis is established by bone marrow puncture. The white cells and platelets are usually also reduced, so that these children suffer from infections and bleeding as well as anaemia.

Treatment consists in giving whole blood or packed cell transfusions in order to provide the mature red cells. These transfusions need to be given repeatedly and the consequent frequent admissions to hospital should be carefully considered. The child should be admitted to the same ward each time so that he returns to people and surroundings who are familiar to him and so eventually comes to accept this process as part of his normal routine. Steroids may be given and occasionally the bone marrow recovers spontaneously, but the disease is commonly fatal.

Haemolytic Anaemias

Haemolytic anaemias are due to excessive and rapid breakdown of red blood cells, and patients may become jaundiced, as the haemoglobin released from the broken-down cells is converted into the bile pigment, bilirubin. Treatment consists in repeated blood transfusions. The most important haemolytic anaemia in childhood is haemolytic disease of the newborn which is considered on p. 68.

Acute Haemolytic Anaemia

Acute haemolytic anaemia is characterized by a rapid destruction of red blood cells, so that haemoglobin and red blood cells fall dramatically in a very short time. The spleen is enlarged, petechial haemorrhages may occur in the skin, mild pyrexia may be present and the child is listless, fractious and acutely ill. Vomiting and diarrhoea may aggravate the condition. The illness is usually cured by blood transfusion, but may continue as a chronic acquired haemolytic anaemia which needs to be controlled by the use of steroids.

This disease may be caused by drugs, sulphonamides and

antimalarial agents in susceptible people who can be shown to have a deficiency of the enzyme G6PD (glucose-6-phosphate dehydrogenase) in their red blood cells. This deficiency is inherited as sex-linked trait, and is most common in people of negro descent, Italians, Greeks, Oriental Jews and Arabs.

Acholuric Jaundice (Hereditary Spherocytosis)

The cause of this haemolytic anaemia is the unusual fragility of the red blood cells resulting in rapid haemolysis producing jaundice. The spleen is enlarged and firm. Latent periods and exacerbations occur. Crises are often caused by infections and at such times the jaundice deepens the child may complain of severe abdominal pain, his general condition is poor and may even give rise to anxiety.

Blood transfusion may be needed during a crisis, otherwise a good diet with therapeutic amounts of iron as indicated by the haemoglobin level and prompt treatment of any infection is needed. Splenectomy may be necessary but should only be performed when the child is free from infection and able to tolerate operation. Removal of the spleen produces a clinical cure and prevents the risk of traumatic injury to the enlarged spleen.

Thalassaemia

Thalassaemia (or Cooley's haemolytic anaemia) occurs in families of Mediterranean origin. The cause is the failure of change from fetal haemoglobin to the more mature adult form. Severity of the disease is determined by inheritance.

In the homozygous child (inherited from both parents) anaemia is very severe marked by extreme fatigue and apathy; repeated infections occur. The child will be noticed to be 'pot-bellied' due to the enlarged liver and spleen and growth is stunted.

Treatment consists of frequent fresh blood transfusions with long-term desferrioxamine therapy to minimize the accumulation of iron in the tissues (haemosiderosis). Folic acid, 5 mg daily should also be given. The prognosis is poor due to heart or liver failure.

Thalassaemia minor occurs in the heterozygous child where the condition is inherited from one parent only, the child may be clinically unaffected or only suffer from a mild degree of anaemia, but on reaching adulthood may pass the disease on to the next generation.

Sickle Cell Anaemia

Sickle cell anaemia is common amongst negroes. In this disease the red cells contain an abnormal haemoglobin which distorts the cells so that they become 'sickle-shaped'. This haemoglobinopathy results in excess haemolysis and may occur in two forms. Inheritance of the recessive gene from both parents (homozygous) results in severe anaemia, jaundice with repeated attacks of pain and fever. The prognosis is poor. Treatment is aimed to allow the child to lead as normal a life as possible and protect against possible infection. Repeated transfusions of packed blood cells will be necessary in order to maintain the level of haemoglobin.

The minor form of sickle cell disease (heterozygous) may go undetected, but it should be remembered that the disease may be passed on to the next generation.

Leukaemia

Leukaemia is a disease affecting the white blood cells. It is characterized by the presence in the circulating blood of immature leucocytes. The cause is unknown. There are several types of leukaemia depending on the type of cell affected, by far the most common in childhood is *acute leukaemia.* The disease may occur at any age but is most common between 2 and 5 years.

Acute Leukaemia

Signs and Symptoms. Children suffering from leukaemia present a typical picture, they are listless and tire easily due to severe anaemia secondary to the disease. Their skin is extremely pale and usually has a yellow tinge and a wax-like transparent quality. The temperature is of a characteristically swinging type and varies between 37.2° and 39.4°C (99° to 103°F). Anorexia, constipation and vomiting are common. There is a general tendency to bleeding due to a low platelet count. Large bruises and petechiae appear on the skin and all over the body, pain and tenderness may be caused by subperiosteal haemorrhages. Haemorrhage into the retina may interfere with vision and bleeding into the renal tubules will cause haematuria. Bleeding from the gums, epistaxis, haematemesis and malaena are among the more distressing symptoms. The mouth may become sore and ulcerated, the lips cracked, the gums swollen and stomatitis may be severe in spite of careful oral hygiene. The lymph nodes are enlarged and tender, the spleen is palpable.

As the disease progresses the child may vomit and complain of headache indicating involvement of the central nervous system. Sometimes too, children complain of limb pains and this usually occurs in the terminal phase of the leukaemic disease. Infections become more common especially of the throat.

The diagnosis is confirmed by a blood count and by a bone marrow puncture.

Investigations. Investigations which are commonly carried out include blood picture and bone marrow puncture. The procedure for bone marrow puncture is similar to that carried out on adults but the site of the puncture is usually the crest of the iliac bone rather than the body of the sternum. In small babies the shaft of the tibia may be used.

The child should be told what is going to happen according to his age and understanding. A sedative is usually given before the procedure as the child may be very frightened and anxious. A nurse or the child's mother should remain with the child throughout the biopsy to comfort and support.

Drug Therapy. Without the use of modern drugs children with acute leukaemia would die within a few months but by using steroids and cytotoxic drugs, e.g. 6-mercaptopurine, methotrexate, vincristine and cyclophosphamide, remission of the disease may be obtained for a variable period of time. The effect may be quite dramatic; the child starts to eat well and takes part in all his former activities. It should be remembered that these drugs are also toxic to healthy cells and must be used with great care. The white cell count may fall considerably and therefore secondary infection may occur. For this reason prophylactic antibiotics may be ordered. The child as far as possible should be protected from infection and nursed in a cubicle. Frequent transfusions of blood, platelets and white cells will be required. Any vomiting may be controlled with the use of anti-emetics.

Relapses will occur necessitating re-admission and a further assessment of drug therapy. As far as possible the child should return to the ward and the staff with whom he and his family are familiar.

Intrathecal methotrexate together with deep X-ray therapy to the meninges are now accepted as part of the routine management of acute leukaemia. Epilation is unavoidable, but the hair grows again afterwards. Ten per cent of the children treated display the 'somnolence syndrome': about 6 weeks after irradiation the child becomes drowsy and feverish with leucocytosis. Nursing care is symptomatic and the condition usually resolves spontaneously after 10 days. The addition of C.N.S. irradiation to drug therapy has increased the average survival of these children from 2½ years to 5 years, and many of the 5-year survivors may be cured.

Side Effects of Drug Therapy. Side effect of drug therapy may be:

- Cushing's syndrome;
- Alopecia;
- Constipation;
- Infections;
- Mouth ulcers.

Nursing Care. The nursing of children suffering from acute leukaemia calls for a high degree of skill, observation and gentleness. It is the nursing of a helpless child who during relapse is restless, listless, to whom movements are often painful and who is disinclined to eat or play.

Care and understanding for the parents requires warmth of understanding, empathy and a recognition of the anxieties of this very difficult time for the whole family. The parents should be given the opportunity to discuss their fears and apprehensions with the ward sister and doctor in charge of the patient, in order that they can be of help and support to the child during his illness. Mother should be allowed to help with feeding, mouth toilet and other nursing care as in this way she will feel less helpless and may be able to nurse the child at home for a time if this should seem desirable. The medical social worker can be invaluable in helping the whole family during the illness with social as well as emotional problems as they may arise.

The child is best nursed in a semi-recumbent position or else sitting up well supported by pillows. His position should be changed from time to time, supporting him in the lateral position alternately. For as long as possible the child should be dressed in his own clothes even when he has to spend a large part of the day sitting on his bed as this will often make him feel happier. If he is to remain in bed for any length of time an air ring or soft pillow will add to his comfort.

A daily blanket bath should be given as this may induce rest and will refresh the patient who has a high temperature. Care must be taken when lifting or turning the child to avoid bruising, easily caused by slight pressure.

Oral hygiene needs to be carried out with special care and gentleness.

The mouth should be observed daily for the presence of ulcers and treated if necessary with 0.5 per cent solution of gentian violet. Thrush frequently occurs but responds well to the application of nystatin. Care should be taken that all feeding utensils are sterilized after use to avoid the spread of this fungal infection.

When bleeding has occurred, saline can be used to rinse the mouth. In many cases it is advisable to clean the teeth with cotton wool swabs securely held in a pair of forceps rather than use a toothbrush, as the gums are inclined to bleed and become sore. The lips should be kept from cracking and protected from crusts of blood by the application of a little vaseline several times a day.

The sudden and frequent epistaxes are frightening to the child and to any relatives who may be visiting. The nurse should remain calm, local application of chipped ice to the bridge of the nose and sedation may help control the bleeding; if this fails platelet or blood transfusion may be necessary.

A special diet is not needed in this illness but the child's nurse should take the trouble to find out what he particularly likes so that the child might eat. Mother should be allowed to bring in favourite dishes or tasty snacks from home to tempt the child. Loss of appetite may be countered by offering small, frequent and attractively served meals, extra milk drinks and special treats. Adequate fluid should be given and extra vitamins may be prescribed in order to try and prevent infection and to raise the general standard of health.

Diminished urinary output and haematuria should be reported and a fluid balance chart maintained. Fluids and fresh fruit in the diet will help to prevent constipation which may occur as a result of the use of cytotoxic drugs and by being confined to bed, this may be treated by the use of 'Blandlax', an aperient. Occasionally suppositories may be necessary. In addition to the specific drugs iron may be given in order to help combat the anaemia. Drugs given to relieve pain and induce rest and sleep include Nepenthe, phenobarbitone and Valium.

If hair fall out and alopecia occur as a result of the use of cytotoxic drugs great care must be taken to keep the thinning hair clean, using a mild shampoo. A soft brush only should be used to keep the hair neat and tidy. If hair loss becomes severe, a specially made wig can be prescribed and ordered through the National Health Service, as baldness can be most distressing to child and parents.

Hodgkin's Disease

Hodgkin's disease affects the lymphoid tissues of the body, causing enlargement of lymph glands. Any group (or groups) of glands may be affected but it is usually the cervical or axillary glands that are involved. The disease is rare, and is most unusual under the age of 5 years.

The child is listless, anaemic and progressively becomes more ill. Waves of recurrent low grade pyrexia or 'Pel-Ebstein' fever is usually present. Remissions may occur. There is no cure for this disease but life can be prolonged by therapy. Treatment includes deep X-ray therapy and the administration of cell-destroying drugs, e.g. cyclophosphamide and chlorambucil.

Acquired Methaemoglobinaemia

Methaemoglobinaemia may follow absorption through the skin of aniline dye from unfixed marking ink or from the ingestion of some marking pencils, paint removers and some drugs, e.g. phenacetin. Occasionally in times of drought there may be a concentration of nitrates in water. Mothers should be advised against the excessive boiling of water at this time, for those babies who are bottle-fed. The signs and symptoms are: cyanosis, respiratory difficulties, muscle twitching and hypertension. Treatment is by intravenous injection of methylene blue (5 mg) and ascorbic acid. Paint removers and marking pencils should be kept well out of the reach of small children to avoid accidental ingestion—it is the only sure way of averting a tragedy.

Purpura

Purpura may be the sign of an underlying disease rather than a disease in itself. Characteristic, spontaneous haemorrhages appear in the skin and mucous membrane of the body, causing bruising, petechiae and frank bleeding of the gums, kidneys, intestinal tract, conjunctivae and the brain. The causes of purpura in childhood may be classified under the following headings:

1. Purpura due to primary or secondary platelet deficiency;
2. Purpura due to vascular defects. This may be congenital (e.g. Ehlers–Danlos syndrome) or acquired (e.g. Henoch–Schönlein);
3. Purpura due to congenital defects of blood plasma, such as prothrombin;
4. Raised capillary pressure.

Purpura due to Platelet Deficiency

Idiopathic Thrombocytopenic Purpura. Idiopathic thrombocytopenic purpura (Fig. 41) occurs without a known cause. Repeated blood transfusions and in some instances platelet transfusions will be given in an attempt to treat the anaemia and control the bleeding which may be most severe and difficult to

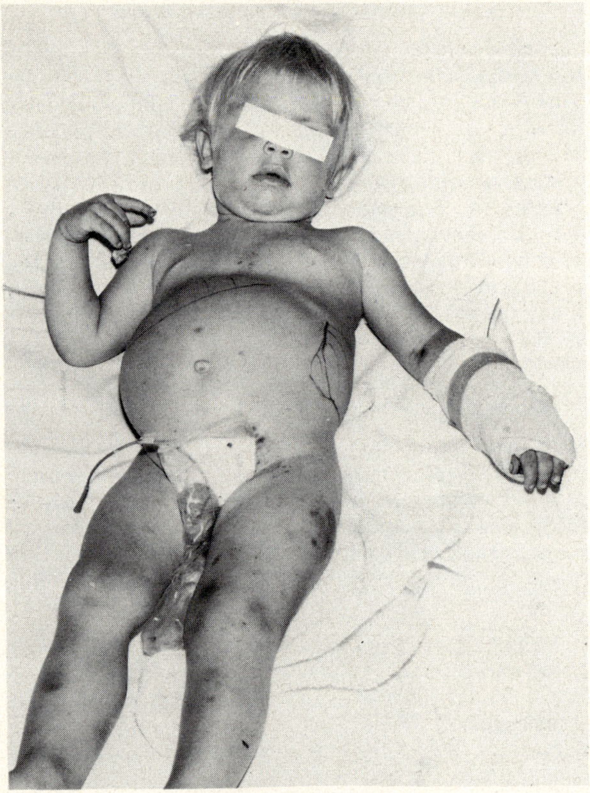

FIG. 41. A very ill child with thrombocytopenic purpura. Extensive bruising has occurred.

control. Steroid therapy and prophylactic antibiotics may be given. Some of the more chronic cases may respond well to splenectomy.

Symptomatic Thrombocytopenic Purpura. Symptomatic thrombocytopenic purpura occurs in such illnesses as leukaemia, aplastic anaemia, rubella syndrome, severe infections and some malignant diseases.

Familial Thrombocytopenic Purpura. One of the causes of haemorrhage in the newborn is familial thrombocytopenic purpura. Apart from giving platelet transfusions from time to time there is no curative treatment. Splenectomy may be performed, when the child is older and this gives good results (*see also* Haemolytic Disease of the Newborn, p. 68).

Purpura due to Vascular Defects

May be either primary or secondary. In primary cases it is thought that a hypersensitivity response may be present which causes temporary permeability of the capillary walls. Henoch–Schönlein's purpura is the most common of this type.

Among secondary types the causes include scurvy (p. 396), meningococcal meningitis and intolerance to drugs.

Purpura due to lack of Essential Constituents in the Blood Plasma

This occurs in haemorrhagic disease of the newborn and obstructive types of jaundice.

Disturbances of Clotting Mechanisms

Haemophilia

Haemophilia is a bleeding disease which occurs exclusively in males; the sex-linked genes are transmitted by unaffected females who are carriers. Clotting time is prolonged, so that even minor knocks, injuries or operations take on unusually serious proportions. Recurrent episodes of bleeding occur right throughout life and may produce deformity, e.g. of limbs or spine when bleeding into joint spaces arises. Death may occur from intra-cerebral haemorrhage, from extreme loss of blood, or from asphyxia due to bleeding into the tissues of the neck.

Treatment. Acute haemorrhage must be treated with fresh whole blood or plasma, 10 ml/kg at a rate of 1.5 to 2.0 ml/minute to initiate haemostasis. When blood loss has been severe, rapid infusion of plasma may first be needed to restore the blood volume and so prevent further shock.

Frozen anti-haemophilic globulin (cryo-precipitate) containing the missing factors is now available. This is given intravenously in a small fluid volume, so that the child may be treated as a day patient and avoid the need for repeated transfusions. Factor 8 concentrate is now available from a few centres only as it is expensive and in short supply. This preparation has the advantage in that it is given as a single intravenous injection which can be given by the parents at home whenever bleeding is suspected.

The patient and the family will need continual support and guidance throughout life. The child should be allowed to lead as normal a life as possible, with the avoidance of strenuous games. Long trousers should be worn, and the mother can sew a foam rubber pad on the inside to protect the knees. He should attend a school near to his home, and intellectual activities should be encouraged. Regular dental care and a well-balanced diet should be given. Orthopaedic care of affected joints is essential.

The child should carry suitable identification at all times in order to alert medical and nursing staff should accidental trauma occur away from home.

Christmas Disease

Christmas disease is very similar to haemophilia. The condition is inherited in the same way but is not confined to male sufferers. Heterozygous females may rarely be affected in the same way as males. Treatment is the same as that for haemophilia with the need for continual support and guidance for the family and the child throughout life.

Further Reading

GOLD, E. R. & BUTLER, N. R. (1972) *A.B.O. Haemolytic Disease of the Newborn*. Bristol: John Wright & Sons.

BRIMBLECOMBE, F. & BARLTROP, D. (1978) *Children in Health and Disease*. London: Baillière Tindall.

13

Diseases of the alimentary system

DAILY oral toilet is as important in young children as in the older ones and as in the case of adults. The popular belief that the first teeth are unimportant as they will soon be replaced by the permanent ones, is erroneous, and the nurse should make it her duty to teach the child—and through him the mother—good habits with regard to dental care.

Cleaning the teeth with an attractive toothbrush and nice-tasting toothpaste can be a pleasant part of the morning and evening toilet. Very young children are often reluctant to open their mouth, and so make effective cleaning impossible. It is therefore often best to let the child chew a piece of raw apple at least once a day as soon as the first teeth have come through—a most effective way of keeping the teeth healthy and clean.

The Mouth

Intelligent observations on the condition of a patient's mouth will often assist in diagnosis and treatment. Of special importance are the following points:

1. *Dry lips and tongue* which will be present in mouth-breathers and in those with high fevers and dehydration. At the same time the tongue will often be thickly coated.
2. *Herpes* which is often seen in patients with colds, high fevers and pneumonia. These small vesicles, grouped on a patch of inflammation around the mouth, are sometimes also called fever blisters.
3. *Pallor of the lips* which is caused by anaemia and may be a sign of loss of blood.
4. *Cyanosis* which signifies lack of oxygen and is seen in congenital heart disease, respiratory tract infections or obstruction and in some instances in newly born babies.

5. *An abnormally large tongue* which is characteristic of hypothyroidism.
6. *A constantly moving tongue* which occurs in chorea.

Important odours which a nurse should recognize include:

A sweet smell, where acetone is present;
The smell of stale blood in cases of bleeding from the tonsil bed or from the stomach;
Offensive smells which may be due to the presence of pus, as in retropharyngeal abscess and bronchiectasis;
A faecal odour in intestinal obstruction;
A urinary smell in uraemia;
A foul smell from the mouth occurs in the late stages of leukaemia;
Specific smells when poisons have been swallowed.

Treatment of any of these symptoms depends on their cause, but in all cases of sickness careful mouth toilet is an essential of good nursing.

Herpes Simplex

Herpes simplex is a virus infection which causes eruptions of vesicles. A common site is the lips in febrile illnesses causing swelling and blisters. The latter dry off and leave thick, uncomfortable crusts. The lesions are best treated by drying them up with dusting powder or applying Neocortef ointment. Dabbing the blisters with methylated spirit is painful and for that reason particularly unsuitable for children.

Catarrhal, Aphthous and Ulcerative Stomatitis

Catarrhal, aphthous and ulcerative stomatitis are varying degrees of generalized inflammation of the mouth. There is swelling and inflammation of the gums, coupled with ulcers on the mucous lining of the mouth. The tongue is coated and there is a foul smell. The patient seems ill, the temperature is often raised by two or three degrees Fahrenheit, he refuses his food and shows intense misery. Frequently these children are debilitated and come from poor homes.

A swab is taken to determine the causative organism. In

many cases of aphthous stomatitis, the cause is the ultramicroscopic virus of *herpes simplex*.

Treatment. The application of Vaseline will give some relief from this painful condition by protecting the ulcer from rubbing on the gums or teeth. Benzocaine lozenges to suck will also help. For persistent ulcers, a light touch with a silver nitrate stick may shorten the course of the ulcer. For Vincent's angina oral penicillin is usually effective, alternatively oral metronidazole (Flagyl) may be given.

Nursing Care. As these children dribble saliva because swallowing is so painful, the chin should be protected by applying petroleum jelly. A dish or a piece of absorbent material can often be arranged to catch the saliva. Very young children may have to have their arms restrained to prevent them from putting their fingers in their mouths. It is usual to carry out barrier nursing.

Bland, cool fluids containing plenty of glucose should be given at first and later the diet should contain extra milk and nourishment. Vitamins are important, but concentrated orange juice should be avoided as it stings on the open lesions. Groats are often enjoyed and can be fortified by addition of an egg. Teeth and tonsils should be inspected and, if necessary, treatment or tonsillectomy carried out to eliminate septic foci.

Gingivitis

Swollen, bleeding gums, may be present in general oral infections. They occur in ulcerative stomatitis, scurvy and in leukaemia, but sometimes may merely be due to poor oral hygiene. Careful mouth toilet and a well-balanced diet are essential. Certain drugs taken over a long period may also cause gingivitis.

Stomatitis

Stomatitis is fairly common in childhood and may vary in severity from simple swelling of the gums due to teething, to extensive inflammation and ulceration. The child is usually reluctant to swallow during the acute stages owing to the pain caused by the inflammation and ulcers, and there is therefore danger of aspiration pneumonia from inhaled saliva. Drainage of saliva during sleep should be encouraged by raising the foot end of the bed at night. Occasionally this has to be done also during the day, the saliva being allowed to drain into a kidney dish or a piece of absorbent material.

Teething

Gentle mouth toilet should be carried out. A mild analgesic, such as Disprin or a Junior Aspirin may be ordered for relief of pain and there is no point in withholding this simple analgesic. A little comforting and nursing will help to soothe these children. Teething rings, which the infant can bite on, relieve the discomfort and there is nothing against them, provided they are kept clean and safely tied to the cot to prevent them from falling on to the floor.

Thrush

Thrush is caused by the fungus *Candida (Monilia) albicans.* It is mostly seen in bottle-fed babies and is a highly contagious condition. White or grey patches appear on the inside of the cheeks and lips, on the roof of the mouth and on the tongue and cannot be removed without damaging the mucous membrane. The baby will be reluctant to take his feed.

Thrush can be prevented by scrupulous cleanliness, especially with regard to feeding utensils, and by keeping the mucous membrane moist in cases of high fever or dehydration. Babies on broad spectrum antibiotics are particularly prone to thrush because the drug kills the organisms which are normally present in the mouth and which can control the antibiotic resistant *Candida albicans.* Vitamin B should always be given with these antibiotics.

Treatment. Strict barrier nursing is essential. Feed bottles must not be returned to the common feed kitchen until sterilized. Milky feeds should be followed by a small drink of plain boiled water, in order to clean the mouth. The infection is treated by giving an oral antibiotic called nystatin. The usual dose is 1 ml (100 000 units) four times a day until all signs of thrush disappear. The solution can be added to the infant's feeds or dropped directly on to the tongue. It is important to know that nystatin should not be used for more than 7 days after it has been dispensed. If treatment exceeds this period a newly prepared solution should be ordered. Other means of treatment are: painting the mouth with a 0.5 per cent aqueous solution of gentian violet or Bradosol, or a 0.5 per cent solution of stilbamidine, or a 1:10 000 solution of thiomersal (Merthiolate), or a 1:1000 solution of benzalkonium chloride (Zephiran). The treatment is done three times a day.

Complications. Infection may spread throughout the gastrointestinal tract and cause thrush septicaemia, a very serious condition. Severe cases are treated by giving hydroxystilbamidine in a solution of glucose and saline by intravenous infusion. Buttock lesions should be treated with a local application of gentian violet, 0.5 per cent, and the baby nursed with exposed buttocks.

Nurses can assist in the prevention of thrush by teaching mothers adequate, easy methods of hygiene in infant feeding.

Tongue Tie

Occasionally a child cannot stretch his tongue sufficiently to make it protrude beyond the teeth. This may cause feeding and speech difficulty so that the fraenum has to be cut in a minor operation. Mild degrees of tongue tie usually right themselves as the child grows older.

The Oesophagus and Stomach

Vomiting

Vomiting in the neonatal period should never be treated lightly. If it is persistent, recurrent, forceful or copious, admission to hospital should be arranged at once. Immediate operation for an obstruction may be necessary, and expert observations may prove life saving. In childhood the causes of vomiting are very varied and some children seem to vomit at the slightest provocation and show little or no concern about it.

THE CAUSES OF VOMITING IN CHILDHOOD

Causes	*Age*	*Content of the vomit*	*Remarks*
Underfeeding	0–3 months	Recently taken feed.	The hungry infant cries, swallows air and gulps the feed when offered.
Indiscretion in diet	All ages	Undigested food.	Milky curd in infancy.
Congenital abnormalities (e.g. hiatus hernia)	Infancy	Milk, mucus.	Effortless or projectile.
Pyloric stenosis	2 weeks to 4 months	Curd, mucus, occasionally blood.	Projectile.
Gastritis	All ages	Food, mucus, blood.	Colicky pain often present.
At the onset of fevers	Young children	No characteristic.	Accompanied by rise in temperature.
Acute appendicitis	All ages	Food at first. Bile later.	Associated with abdominal pain.
Toxic illness	All ages	Food, gastric fluid.	Quickly causes dehydration.
Whooping cough	All ages	Food and mucus.	During or just after meals. After attack of coughing.
Diabetes mellitus	All ages	Food.	Heralds impending coma.
Renal diseases, (e.g. uraemia)	All ages	Fluid gastric contents	Mostly in late stages of the illness.
Poisoning	All ages	Gastric contents.	Must be saved with special care.
Intolerance to drugs	All ages	Gastric contents.	e.g. Salicylates. The drugs may have to be discontinued.
Nervous conditions	All ages	Watery.	Excitement, anxiety, habit.
Cyclical vomiting	After age of 2 years	Food at first, later gastric fluid only.	Severe, general disturbance. Ketosis, may last several days.

Causes	*Age*	*Content of the vomit*	*Remarks*
Mechanical	All ages	Gastric contents.	May result from finger sucking, enlarged tonsils, mucopus in nasopharynx, air swallowing.
Oesophageal reflux	Infancy	Feed, mucus, sometimes blood.	e.g. Hiatus hernia.
Intracranial pressure	All ages	Not related to taking food.	Gastric contents. Projectile, without warning. If associated with meningitis, constipation is often an accompanying feature.

None the less the nurse should remember that vomiting in most cases entails considerable effort and the child may feel dizzy, faint, cold and miserable. The nurse should always remain with the child. She should protect the bedclothes, place the patient in a comfortable position and, if possible, draw curtains around the bed. The patient may find it comforting if the nurse holds her hand on his forehead and supports any recent abdominal wound. When the attack is over, the patient should be given a mouthwash, or have his teeth cleaned, and be left comfortable. Persistent vomiting may cause considerable loss of fluid and replacement by a parenteral route is sometimes necessary.

The vomit should always be inspected before it is discarded and an entry should be made on the patient's chart. The amount should be measured, the reaction tested with litmus paper, and the time and relation to meal times recorded. The nurse should notice whether the vomit is effortless, or forcible and projectile in nature. The presence of curds, blood, excess mucus, bile or foreign bodies should be reported at once. The odour may also be of importance in arriving at a diagnosis.

Cyclical Vomiting

Cyclical vomiting is a distressing condition occasionally seen in a children's ward. The child affected is, as a rule, tall for his age and thin, his posture is poor. He may be highly strung, inclined to sleep-walking, car-sickness and vomiting due to excitement, and frequently he is above normal intelligence. Children usually outgrow cyclical vomiting at puberty but some develop attacks of migraine at that time.

Signs and Symptoms. Attacks start very suddenly. The child complains of severe headache and abdominal discomfort. He is irritable at first but soon becomes drowsy. Anything taken by the mouth, including plain water, is vomited immediately and signs of dehydration develop rapidly. The scanty amounts of urine are loaded with ketone bodies and the breath smells of acetone. The temperature may rise by one or two degrees.

This alarming state of affairs may continue for 3 to 4 days and may recur with regularity as often as once a fortnight or merely once or twice a year. In spite of the apparent severity, there is no serious danger and the distressed parents can be reassured.

Nursing Care. The child should be treated with firm sympathy. He is best nursed in a darkened room and sedatives should be given as soon as an attack is suspected. Glucose may be given either in fluids or in the form of barley sugar. If fluids taken by mouth are retained, they are best given as frequent sips of fruit juice and glucose in a saline solution. Acidosis is severe, and intravenous fluids are given accordingly to correct the blood chemistry and replace fluid loss. On recovery the child is given a light diet with restricted fat. Glucose, toast, honey, and sweetened tea are particularly suitable.

General Points. These children should be allowed extra rest in their daily routine. They should go to bed early and avoid undue fatigue. On the other hand, as little attention as possible should be drawn to the condition and the child should be kept fully occupied and his intelligence used to the utmost in order to keep him from self-centred interest.

The diagnosis of cyclical vomiting is usually made with great caution and such conditions as appendicitis, intestinal obstruction, pyelitis, meningitis and diabetic crisis have to be most carefully excluded. Vomiting due to excitement, as for instance before birthday parties, return to school or before an examination, is not true cyclical vomiting even though they may recur with certain regularity.

Gastritis

The causes of acute irritation or inflammation of the gastric mucosa range from unsuitable diet, swallowing infected material, e.g. pus from sinusitis, or dental caries causing incomplete mastication, to intolerance of drugs, swallowing an irritant such as a poison, gastro-enteritis or chronic dilatation, as in pyloric stenosis.

If old enough, the child may complain of discomfort or even pain, nausea and vomiting. The tongue is furred and the appetite is poor. The vomit may contain mucus, pus or altered blood. Vomiting frequently relieves the distension and discomfort.

Treatment. As gastritis is as a rule a symptom of some other disturbance, the underlying cause must be found and appropriately treated. In order to give the stomach a rest ordinary diet is omitted for a few days. Bland fluids and Bengerized milk are well tolerated. Lightly boiled eggs, soups, mashed potatoes, jellies and ice cream, toast and honey are all light and suitable as soon as the child is ready to have solid food. The return to a full diet should be gradual. Severe or long-standing cases may benefit from gastric lavage. The mouth toilet should receive particular attention.

Congenital Hypertrophic Pyloric Stenosis

Congenital hypertrophic pyloric stenosis is due to the thickening of the pyloric sphincter, causing a narrowing of the lumen. Signs of obstruction, gastritis and malnutrition develop.

Pyloric stenosis develops soon after birth and symptoms are first noticed at the age of 2 to 6 weeks. Mild cases or those which show late symptoms may improve spontaneously at the age of about 4 months, but early and severe cases require medical or surgical treatment.

Diagnosis. Diagnosis is often delayed as varying feeds are tried in an attempt to stop the baby from vomiting. At each change a temporary improvement may take place but vomiting and loss of weight soon recur and eventually the presence of pyloric stenosis is suspected.

Signs and Symptoms. The infant's appearance is typical. He is wizened and pale and has large, anxious and hungry-looking eyes. The skin is dry and the fontanelle sunken. The lips and mouth are red and dry but remain clean despite the vomiting. Even though there is marked wasting he remains bright and very active.

In the early stages vomiting may occur once or twice a day

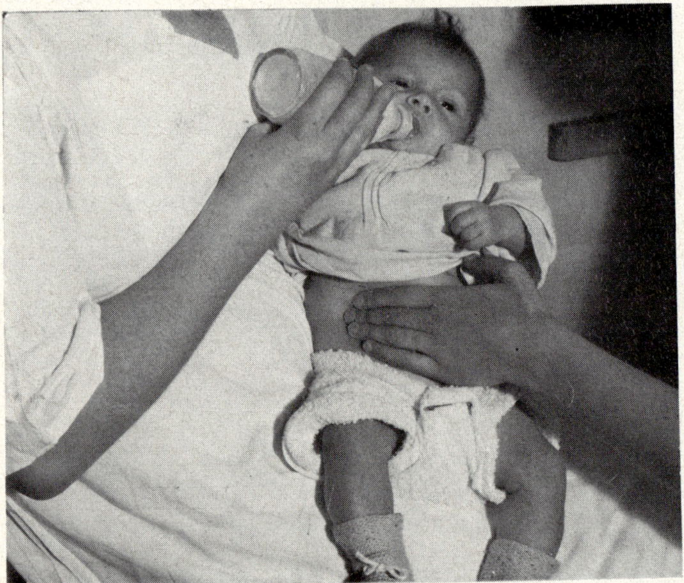

FIG. 42. Pyloric stenosis. The doctor is feeling the swelling and watching for visible peristalsis. Note the relaxed position and the way in which the abdomen has been exposed by the nurse, although the rest of the baby is being kept warm.

only, but soon it follows every feed. Curd from previous feeds may be present in the vomit. As gastritis develops, mucus and specks of blood are noticed. Vomiting may at first resemble regurgitation but it soon becomes projectile, that is to say it occurs suddenly and with so much force that it is rarely seen on the baby's pillow or bib but usually hits the floor. Starvation and dehydration make the urine dark and concentrated and the stools are small and constipated. They may be infrequent and are often green 'hunger stools'.

The loss of chlorides in the vomit has a serious effect on the blood chemistry. Plasma bicarbonates are high and there is an increase in the non-protein nitrogen in the blood and urine. This toxic state is known as alkalosis and must be rectified without delay.

Examination of the Patient. For examination by the doctor, the baby should lie on the nurse's knees in a relaxed position while taking a feed (Fig. 42). After the baby has taken 30 to 60 ml, peristaltic waves, resembling the movements of a golf ball, may be seen passing across the abdomen, just underneath the ribs and from the left to the right side. This is known as visible peristalsis. At the same time, the examining fingers can feel the hardening of the pylorus (the feel resembles that of the tip of the nose) immediately beneath the liver margin to the right side of the rectus muscle. A barium meal may help to confirm the diagnosis.

The treatment of choice may be medical in mild cases, frequently, however, surgical treatment is preferred, though the baby usually remains in a medical ward under the care of the paediatrician.

Medical Treatment. The principal points adopted in medical treatment of these children are:

1. A radical reduction of feed volume is made in order to reduce the vomiting from the start, and this is coupled with gastric lavage. For this normal saline is used.
2. A muscle relaxant drug of the atropine group is given 15 to 20 minutes before feeds. These include:

Atropine methonitrate 0·6 per cent alcoholic solution given from a pipette or dropper direct on to the tongue at the back of the mouth. Three to six drops are the usual dose.

This is an unstable solution and should never be kept longer than a maximum of 4 weeks.

As vomiting ceases, the feeds are gradually increased to the amounts appropriate to the infant's age and requirements. Another scheme in common may be prescribed instead. It is sometimes referred to as a Medical Pyloric Ladder Diet. Very small feeds which are gradually increased, combined with the relaxant drug 'skopyl'.

Surgical Treatment. *Rammstedt's operation* (division of the pyloric sphincter). Thorough preparation of the patient for this operation is essential. Blood is taken for analysis and any abnormality in the blood chemistry is corrected by intravenous infusion of normal saline with added potassium up to 10 mmol/kg/24 hours. During the pre-operative period, gastric lavage using normal saline may be performed once or twice daily and again before the operation. The wash-out not only serves to clear the stomach of stale milk, curd and mucus, but also helps in assessing the type of curd and the severity of the gastritis as well as forming part of the treatment. It is of vital importance to obtain completely clear fluid at the end of the pre-operative wash-outs as any stale material left behind in the stomach would pass into the intestine once the obstruction is relieved and might cause enteritis. Normal milk feeds should be discontinued and clear fluids only given by mouth.

Preparation for operation. General anaesthesia is now almost always used. The stomach should be washed out with normal saline and the tube left in situ, unspigotted after the washout. The umbilicus should be inspected and thoroughly cleaned. The infant should be dressed in an open-backed gown and wrapped in a cotton blanket. The baby can then be left to rest—atropine (0.3 mg) will be given a half-hour before operation.

Post-operative feeding. Details of feeding vary from one hospital to another but the fundamental principles remain the same. A typical post-operative pyloric feeding regimen is:

Hours post-operation

4–8	5 ml dextrose hourly
8–10	10 ml dextrose hourly
10–12	10 ml half-strength milk feeds hourly
12–18	15 ml half-strength milk feeds 2-hourly
18–24	30 ml half-strength milk feeds 2-hourly
24–30	30 ml full-strength milk feeds 2-hourly
30–36	45 ml full-strength milk feeds 2-hourly
36–42	60 ml full-strength milk feeds 3-hourly
42–48	75 ml full-strength milk feeds 3-hourly

Then give normal feeds according to expected weight. If the baby is breast-fed every effort should be made to help the mother keep the supply going. During the first 48 hours, the same type of schedule can be kept, but substituting half-strength expressed breast milk, and the baby should be put to the breast within 48 hours of the operation.

Nursing management. One or two vomits post-operatively are not uncommon, because although the obstruction has been relieved, there may be a little delay in establishing normal gastric peristalsis. This is usually resolved with a further stomach washout. The baby is usually well and gaining weight by 72 hours, and may be discharged home once he is taking full feeds for 24 hours. The steri-strip dressing may be removed from the wound in 5 or 6 days. Mother should be given an appointment for out-patients within 4 weeks of discharge. There are few paediatric conditions that offer greater satisfaction and opportunities for skill in nursing than pyloric stenosis. As the babies are often breast-fed, every attempt should be made to admit the mother with her baby. This gives a longer time for hospital staff to comfort and reassure the young mother, who is bound to find the thought of an operation on her baby distressing. There is no reason why the mother should not assist with the care of the baby and her own confidence and peace of mind will help to maintain a good supply of breast milk for her child.

While the nurse should be careful to prevent the parents from taking too grave a view of the condition, she should always remember to ascertain in advance whether the baby has been christened and, if desired, should arrange for a minister of religion to christen the infant in the presence of the parents.

Gastric Lavage

The equipment required for gastric lavage in young children differs from that used for adults only in some minor detail. As the nasogastric tube can be connected directly to the funnel neither extra length of tubing, nor a size 8–10 French gauge connection are needed. This eliminates extra weight to manipulate. To stop the flow the tube is often doubled back on itself instead of using a gate clip and the rate of flow is regulated by raising or lowering the tube and funnel. Instead of the open-type funnel a cylindrical upright glass funnel is used and any gastric contents or lavage fluid should be allowed to run back into the funnel and not emptied direct into a receiver or bucket. In that way a comparison can be made between the amounts run in and returned. This is important on account of the small amounts involved and the danger of causing distension and colic if too much fluid is allowed to run into the stomach or to accumulate there. A measuring jug should always be used. Suction is never employed (e.g. by aspirating with a syringe or a Senoran's pump) but instead the fluid is siphoned back by quickly lowering the funnel and tube just before the last fluid disappears at the juncture of glass funnel and tubing.

Gastric lavage in children is as a rule less upsetting than in adults but babies and young children should be securely wrapped in a blanket to avoid any struggle (Fig. 33) as little co-operation can be expected. The tube should be measured from the bridge of the nose to the lower end of the sternum to give an idea how far the tube needs to be passed in order to enter the stomach. The point is reached when the mark made on the tube after measuring, reaches the level of the dental arch.

Children cannot be expected to assist with the passing of the tube by swallowing or deep breathing and it is best to feed the tube gently, but firmly along the floor of the mouth after lubricating it with a little sterile water. The assisting nurse may steady the child's head (Fig. 37) or support the chin as this helps to reduce the tickling sensation and excessive retching. After seeing gastric residue rise in the funnel, or after testing some resting juice which has been obtained by siphon action for reaction on litmus paper, fluid [e.g. normal saline at a temperature of 37.2° to 37.8°C (99° to 100°F)] is run into the stomach. The amount will vary according to the age and size of the patient but in the majority of cases it is satisfactory to allow one funnel-full to run in at a time and then to siphon the fluid back. Gastric lavage in children should always be supervised by a trained nurse who will be able to give advice from her own experience as to the correct quantity of fluid which should be used. By raising or lowering the funnel, fluid can be siphoned back. At the end of the procedure the nurse should make sure that no fluid is left in the stomach.

When giving a feed by tube the technique and equipment are essentially the same but at the end of the feed the funnel should be allowed to empty down to the juncture of the funnel and rubber tube, before adding a small amount of plain water. This reduces the mixing of plain fluid and feed to a minimum and also ensures that the baby really gets all the feed. If the tube is withdrawn before it has emptied completely as much as 14 g of feed may be lost, a considerable proportion of the total if the small amounts sometimes involved in infant feeding are considered. Furthermore, as long as there is any fluid in the tube, there is always a danger that some may be aspirated into the trachea as the tube passes the larynx when it is withdrawn. As an additional safety measure and in order to prevent this from happening it is considered wise to pinch the tube whilst withdrawing it. The tube should always be withdrawn fairly quickly and in one steady pull.

The Intestines

Constipation

Infrequent bowel actions are unlikely to be harmful provided the stools are soft and passed without causing pain or distress. Few paediatricians are in favour of giving enemata or aperients and the 'weekly dose' is a deplorable custom which should be strongly discouraged. No medication is satisfactory unless used intelligently and as the need arises, and it is obvious that giving an aperient on a set day once a week cannot be classed as either an intelligent or a necessary measure. It is far more likely to cause resentment and a family scene if, for instance, Friday evening is set aside for the giving of an aperient, than to contribute to good health and good bowel training of the child.

True constipation, that is to say dry, hard faeces passed with difficulty, may be due to a long list of causes including those mentioned below:

In young babies: Underfeeding due to inadequate fluid or calorie intake or a failure of lactation. Insufficient sugar added to artificial feeds.

Congenital abnormalities may hold up the food or faeces or inhibit peristalsis. Among such conditions are congenital pyloric stenosis, intestinal atresia, stricture of the anus, Hirschsprung's disease, hypothyroidism, mental deficiency and atonia due to muscular dystrophy or debility.

Painful defecation may be due to local causes, e.g. anal fissure, which makes the child hold back the stool to avoid pain.

Parenteral causes include tuberculous meningitis and nephritis with oedema.

Psychological factors. These, or faulty habit training, may lead to infrequent bowel actions and so cause hard stools and painful defecation. Such psychological factors include maternal anxiety.

Treatment. Laxatives may occasionally have to be used for short periods until a regular routine has been re-established. In early infancy a teaspoon of milk of magnesia, given three times a day may be ordered. For older children Syrup of Figs, 2 to 15 ml daily, or Senokot, ½ to 1½ tablets daily, are suitable. Liquid paraffin should not be given as it interferes with vitamin absorption and because there is some danger of lipoid pneumonia from inhalation. Severe cases of long standing, may need initial treatment by colonic lavage or enemata. Special points arise in the case of:

Anal Fissure. The severe pain experienced on defecation

should be minimized by keeping the faeces soft with giving a correct diet and mild laxatives. Witch hazel ointment may be applied to the anal region and a small piece may be introduced into the anus several times a day. This assists the healing of the torn mucosa and relieves pain. Alternatively an anaesthetic ointment such as amethocaine may be used.

Constipation with Overflow. This is a term used for leakage of decomposed faeces around a mass of impacted faecal matter. The condition is mainly seen in children with psychiatric disturbances or children who are mentally handicapped. Treatment includes patient toilet training, aperients and, occasionally manual removal under anaesthetic. For treatment to be successful it is important to find out the underlying cause. In the meantime the patient's mother, exasperated by the constant soiling of clothes will need support and sympathy in order to gain her co-operation in treating the condition.

Complications of True Constipation. True constipation can be responsible for a number of symptoms such as furred tongue, anorexia and vomiting, poor general circulation and sluggishness, restless sleep and bedwetting.

As constipation is a symptom rather than a disease in itself, the underlying cause should be found and treatment given accordingly. Dietary adjustments may be all that is necessary. For infants this may mean additional sugar in the bottle feeds or drinks of boiled water in between ordinary feeds as well as extra orange juice. In older children a diet rich in roughage and adequate exercise and regular habit training should be encouraged. All-bran, wholemeal bread, fresh fruit, green vegetables and prune juice are palatable, suitable high roughage additions to the daily diet. Occasionally it is found that constipation has developed because the lavatory in the child's home is situated in a cold, dark or isolated part of a tenement building or at the bottom of the garden, so that the child is frightened of going there on his own. Alternatively, the toilet seat may be too high and, as the child's feet cannot touch the ground, he is frightened of falling in. Lack of time before leaving for school may be another, easily remedied cause of chronic constipation. Lack of exercise leading to poor circulation and muscle tone

TYPES OF STOOLS IN INFANCY AND CHILDHOOD

Description	*Usual occurrence*	*Colour*	*Odour*	*Consistency*	*Frequency*	*Composition*	*Reaction*
Meconium	First 2–3 days after birth	Tarry, changing to greenish-black	None	Semi-solid	3–6 daily	Normal	Neutral
Changing stools	Approx. 3rd–6th day of life	Dark green changing to yellow	None	Soft	5–8 daily	Normal	Acid
Breast-milk stools	In breast-fed babies	Mustard colour	Characteristic	Soft homogenous	5–6 daily	Normal	Acid
Cow's-milk stools	In artificially fed babies	A pale yellow-grey	Musty	Semi-formed bulky	4–5 daily	Normal	Alkaline
Mixed feeding	In toddlers	Brown	Slight	Formed	1–2 daily	Normal	Varies
Buttermilk feeding	In infancy	Olive-green	Characteristic	Soft	5–6 daily	Normal	Acid
High protein content	In infancy	Grey	Sour and offensive	Dry and crumbling	1–2 daily	Excess protein	Alkaline
High fat content	e.g. Coeliac disease	Grey, clay coloured	Offensive	Bulky greasy	Several daily	Excess fat deficient in bile	Acid
High carbohydrate content	In infancy	Green	Slightly offensive	Relaxed frothy	Frequent	Fermented faeces	Very acid
Soapy stools	Digestive disturbances	White	Offensive	Pasty	Several daily	Excess fat or deficient in bile	Neutral

Melaena	Swallowed blood, intestinal bleeding	Tarry-black	Characteristic sweet	Soft	Varies	Blood	Alkaline
Intestinal hurry	Gastro-intestinal infections	Bright green	Characteristic offensive	Fluid relaxed	Many times daily	Unconverted bile	Neutral
Hunger stools	Infancy	Dark green	None or sour	Small dry	Frequent	Large proportion of mucus-bile	Acid
Over-feeding	Infancy	Bright green	Offensive	Frothy fermenting	Frequent	Excess fat and carbohydrate	Very acid
Intestinal infections	Gastro-enteritis	Pale green	Characteristic offensive	Soft or liquid	Very frequent	Partially digested food, mucus	Varies
Fresh blood	1 Anal fissure 2 Ulcerative colitis 3 Dysentery 4 Rectal polyp	Bright red	1 none 2, 3 offensive 4 none	1 hard 2, 3 liquid 4 normal	1 infrequent 2, 3 frequent 4 normal	1 normal 2, 3 mucus bile, blood 4 normal and streaks of blood	Alkaline
Red currant jelly stool	Intussusception	Bright red	None	Jelly-like	1 or 2 isolated stools	Mucus blood	Neutral
Pea-soup stool	Typhoid	Green	Offensive	Liquid	Very frequent	Mucus, pus, blood	—
Pus, mucus	Pelvic abscess	Normal or green streaked with pus	Offensive	Relaxed	Once after rupture of abscess into bowel	Pus, mucus	—

should be corrected. Television viewing has contributed to physical inactivity in recent years and all types of sport should be encouraged as a healthy counterbalance.

Observation of Faeces

Although the observation of faeces is an important duty of every nurse it is of immeasurable value in paediatric nursing. Children are often unable to describe symptoms accurately and the abnormal stool, preserved for inspection by an experienced ward sister or medical officer may frequently lead to the establishment of a previously doubtful diagnosis. The nurse should note such points as the colour, consistency, the odour, shape and frequency of the stools. Any abnormal constituents such as blood, mucus or foreign bodies should be noted and any complaints of pain on passing the stool treated as being significant.

Collection of Specimens. The collection of faecal matter for investigation does not differ from that in adult nursing but, in the case of 24-hour specimens for very young children, a specially constructed chair may have to be used or the napkin lined with thin plastic or cellophane. The type of colostomy bag known as a 'Chiron' disposable bag can sometimes be fixed to the buttocks and the child allowed to run around without restriction while the faeces are being collected.

The handling of bedpans and pots should at all times be reduced to a minimum. Soiled napkins should be saved with the corners tucked underneath the part on which the stool lies when first taken off the baby, placed in a receiver and covered with a glass plate. It is now ready for easy inspection. Any doubtful stool should always be saved and kept available during the paediatrician's round (see p. 44).

Infantile Gastro-Enteritis

At one time gastro-enteritis was one of the killing diseases of infancy. Today, in this country, the illness remains serious and is a prolonged one with an anxious period for all concerned. Gastro-enteritis now occurs throughout the year, in contrast to the one-time high incidence during the summer months which gave the illness the name of summer diarrhoea. Premature babies are particularly prone to gastro-enteritis, but it is rarely seen in breast-fed babies or in any babies before the age of a month or after the age of 2 years.

The infection is as a rule due to various strains of *Escherichia* (*Bacterium*) *coli*, salmonella or dysentery bacillus, and possibly to some as yet unidentified virus. Other types are secondary to infection outside the gastro-intestinal tract such as middle ear infections, meningitis or the common cold. Symptoms similar to those caused by infective gastro-enteritis may be due to dietetic errors and disaccharide intolerance.

Signs and Symptoms. The symptoms of gastro-enteritis in infancy may vary from slight frequency of the bowel actions, relaxed stools and an occasional vomit, to a severe illness with gross dehydration and generalized disturbances. For the purpose of this chapter a severe, fully established case is described.

The infant with severe gastro-enteritis presents a pitiable picture. He is limp and lethargic, although often restlessly moving his head and beating his arms around. His cheeks may be flushed and his eyes sunken and surrounded by dark rings. The fontanelle is depressed. The abdomen is often distended and the infant draws his legs up as if in pain. The skin is dry and inelastic and feels hot to the touch. The temperature may be raised to 39.4°C (103°F) and the pulse is rapid and of poor volume. In severe cases convulsions are common.

The mother will explain that the infant has had increasingly frequent, loose and explosive stools with a characteristic, offensive smell and that his buttocks are becoming sore. She may have noticed traces of blood or mucus in the stools, or she may have seen bits of curd and free fluid. The colour may be green or bright orange. An observant mother may even have noticed that her baby is passing very little and rather dark urine, a sure sign of severe dehydration and incipient renal failure. She will say that the baby is wakeful, restless and constantly whimpering. Although he appears to be thirsty and to want his feeds, he is often unable to retain them and the vomiting may be forceful and copious and occur during or immediately after taking a feed. Vomiting, however, is not a constant feature and in many cases it is absent or develops as a late symptom. As he gets worse, the baby may refuse his feeds. It is obvious that loss of weight will be rapid and severe, and that all the signs of dehydration and loss of electrolytes will soon be present.

Investigations. A thorough examination of the child is essential in order to exclude any parental cause of the illness. Blood is taken for biochemical analysis and any electrolyte imbalance corrected without delay. In vomiting, chlorides are lost to the body and diarrhoea causes loss of sodium and potassium. These deficiencies must be made good by giving intravenous fluids urgently, as young infants deteriorate very rapidly. It is often necessary to start treatment without waiting for the result of the laboratory tests. The acid base upset may be severe and is usually corrected by giving modified Ringer Lactate (Hartmann's) solution or Molar Lactate solution. Serum protein deficiencies and anaemia may have to be corrected by blood transfusion. Anaemia may be severe, though haemoglobin readings may at first be high, due to haemoconcentration; the blood urea will also be raised.

A specimen of stool should be sent to the laboratory, while fresh. If a rectal swab is taken it may be moistened by dipping it in sterile broth solution, as used for blood cultures, before insertion into the rectum.

Special Observations. It is important that any complication should be noticed early because no time should be lost before appropriate treatment is started. Any change in the infant must be reported without delay and its significance understood. Starvation will be obvious through loss of weight, weakness, the appearance of ketone bodies in the urine. Babies up to 3 months need about 150 ml of fluid per kilogram of body weight to maintain hydration. The loss of 150 to 300 ml will cause a baby to look very ill. Fat babies however, may not look dehydrated even if they have lost proportionately more than that; particular attention must be paid to the sodium level in the blood, which in the case of dehydration is, of course high. Deep, rapid respirations are characteristic of acidosis, and an increase in the vomiting, spasms and convulsions are often signs of severe alkalosis. A diminished urinary output is a sign of impaired renal function or dehydration. Abdominal distension may be marked and is caused by gas formation in the intestines; pallor may be a sign of anaemia.

Treatment. Treatment aims at eliminating the underlying cause and replacing lost fluids and electrolytes; also at introducing suitable feeds very gradually after resting the gastro-intestinal tract. Pyelitis, otitis media and any other parenteral infections are dealt with in the appropriate manner and the giving of an antibiotic is usually part of the treatment.

Drugs. Neomycin, a broad-spectrum antibiotic, or gentamicin are at present the drugs of choice. Others used are succinylsulfathiazole and phthalysulfathiazole. Some Gram-negative pathogens respond best to Penbritin (ampicillin) and colomycin. They can be given in high dosage as they are not absorbed but remain in the bowel. Their use not only serves to shorten the course of the illness and reduce mortality, but by sterilizing the stools and so eliminating pathogenic bacteria, the risk of spreading infection is also reduced.

Once the electrolyte and serum protein losses have been corrected by intravenous therapy, oral feeding can be started and it is now rarely necessary to continue with intravenous or subcutaneous fluids for longer than 36 hours. If subcutaneous fluids are ordered, they are usually given with hyaluronidase to assist absorption but even so this method is rarely satisfactory if dehydration is severe, as the peripheral circulatory failure impedes absorption from the tissues.

The *prognosis* of severe infantile gastro-enteritis has recently changed completely, due to the better understanding and management of blood chemistry. Many infants can now be expected to make a good recovery.

Nursing Care. Strict precautions against spread of infection must be observed and where other infants are nursed in the same unit, ideally no nurse attending a case of infective gastro-enteritis should handle these or be allowed into the feed kitchen. Although lack of ideal conditions does not preclude excellent nursing care, the following facilities and equipment should be available whenever possible.

A cubicle equipped with a swing door, running water and good ventilation, two buckets or pedal-bins (one for napkins and one for clothes), a plastic apron, two barrier gowns, their outside plainly marked and hung on coat hangers when not in use, an adequate supply of masks, facilities for preliminary sterilization of feed bottles (e.g. a bowl of Milton solution 1:80), separate toilet equipment, stethoscope, auriscope, pencils for charting observations and a pulsometer. Some hospitals use only materials which can be easily boiled for bed linen, blankets and clothing. Cotton is ideal and with good heating and ventilation which excludes draughts, entirely adequate from the point of view of warmth. Separate cleaning utensils and materials must also be provided.

In addition, nurses should be meticulous in the care of their hands and finger nails and a hand lotion should be provided to avoid rough or cracked skin due to frequent hand washing.

Bearing in mind the symptoms of the disease and the complications already mentioned, the nurse will closely observe the following points: the infant's attitude in his cot and the degree of restlessness or lethargy, the condition of the skin, whether hot or cold, dry or clammy, pale, flushed, inelastic or even jaundiced. She will note whether the fontanelles are depressed or bulging and whether the mouth is dry, the lips cracked, the tongue unusually red or coated, and whether there are signs of thrush. She will watch to see whether the eyes are anxious, staring, sunken and only semi-closed during sleep and whether the abdomen is distended or sunken. She will make further observations on the state of the buttocks which may be raw and excoriated and of the extremities which may be blue and cold. She will note the amount of urine passed and the degree of its concentration and the number, frequency, size, colour and odour of the stools and she will watch for the presence of blood, mucus or free fluid.

The infant's eagerness or reluctance to feed is an important guide and, when temperature, pulse and respirations are taken, full observations should be made. The infant should be weighed daily even while parenteral fluids are being given and to make this possible the intravenous tubing should be long enough to allow for lifting the infant on to the scales. At first the gain should not be regarded as an absolute gain. When the intravenous infusion is discontinued there may be a temporary slight loss of weight or at least no gain until the body has regained its normal balance of hydration and until adequate intake by mouth and general improvement cause a real gain which will eventually be maintained.

Rectal temperatures should never be taken, as the irritation of introducing the thermometer into the rectum may cause unnecessary bowel actions. It is always necessary to correlate these observations and to judge the condition of the patient as a whole, when deciding on treatment and diet, instead of noting only the number and frequency of the stools.

Complications of Gastro-Enteritis. It is sometimes difficult to distinguish between the primary-parenteral illness which causes gastro-enteritis and the complications which result from the illness and the low resistance of the infant. Inhalation of vomitus causing pneumonia, inflammation of the middle ear and mastoiditis from vomitus tracking up the short, straight Eustachian tube are examples. Other complications include sore buttocks, thrush, convulsions, meningitis and circulatory failure.

Severe gastro-enteritis may result in disaccharide deficiency due to a transient intolerance of one or more of the following sugars: lactose, sucrose and maltose. The picture is that of a severely ill baby resulting from dehydration and the production of explosive, frothy acid stools. The baby often has a sore mouth and very excoriated buttocks. The condition will improve as the offending sugars are eliminated from the diet.

The Diet. In all but the mildest cases, milk feeds are discontinued for 24 to 36 hours and are replaced by boiled water and glucose 4.3 per cent or dextrose in $\frac{1}{5}$ strength normal saline solution. If the baby is being treated at home, a suitable mixture may be made by using one tablespoon of sugar to $\frac{1}{4}$ teaspoon of salt in 1 pint (0.6 litres) of boiled water. This gives a solution of approximately 5 per cent sugar in a $\frac{1}{4}$ strength normal saline. The amount of fluid required is based on the principle of giving 75 to 90 ml ($2\frac{1}{2}$ to 3 oz) of fluid per day for every 0.45 kg (1 lb) of the baby's highest known body weight and allowing up to

300 ml extra daily to make up for loss of fluid. Milk in dilution is gradually introduced until the infant's usual feed has been re-established. Expressed breast milk may be invaluable in some cases. Sugar is at first omitted and the fat content of the feed should be low as fat is not easily tolerated. Saccharin can be used as a sweetening agent and should not be withheld while the feeds are diluted as most babies object to unsweetened feeds and refuse them even though they may appear to be eager when they first start sucking.

Except in the case of planned schedule feeding, time should always be allowed to observe the effect of various stages of the diet and, as a rule, changes should be made once in 24 hours.

Disinfection of Feeding Bottles. After use, feeding bottles are rinsed under the cold tap and placed in a solution of Milton 1:80 in the infant's cubicle until the next feed. Care should be taken to fill the bottles to capacity with the Milton solution before immersing them. The pre-sterilized bottles are then dealt with in the usual way. Teats are rinsed under cold, running water and kept in a special teat jar filled with a disinfectant lotion such as Milton 1:80 in the cubicle.

Disposal of Napkins. Napkins used by gastro-enteritis patients should be soaked; Formalin 1:250 or Milton 1:80 solution are suitable disinfectants. After 1 hour, the napkins are rinsed and wrung out by a nurse wearing protective gloves and apron and are then disposed of in the usual way. Some hospitals allow these napkins to go to the laundry. In specially treated bags, that disintegrate in the washing machine when the water reaches a pre-set high temperature in other hospitals, disposable napkins are used; these can be placed in paper bags immediately they are taken off the baby and bag and napkins burned in an incinerator in the ward sluice room.

Health teaching in the home should ensure that mothers understand the need for cleanliness and that sterilizing solutions are made up in the correct strength and used effectively.

Intestinal Obstruction

Intestinal obstruction in childhood may be due to congenital abnormalities, strangulated hernia, intussusception, volvulus, a swallowed foreign body or pressure from a tumour. The classical symptoms are the same as in adults, namely vomiting, pain, absolute constipation and abdominal distension (Fig. 43). Urgent operation to relieve the obstruction is necessary otherwise there is danger that the constriction of the blood supply may lead to gangrene of the strangulated portion of gut, and the continued vomiting result in dehydration and loss of electrolytes. A nasogastric tube is passed and the stomach contents aspirated before giving an anaesthetic. An intravenous infusion will be necessary.

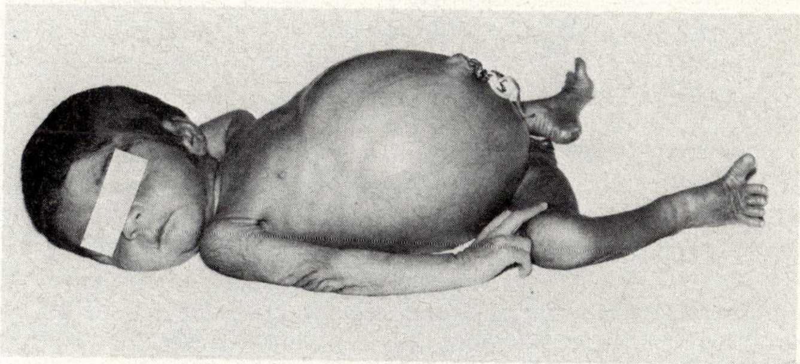

FIG. 43. Young infant with gross abdominal distension due to intestinal obstruction.

Volvulus

A different kind of obstruction occurs in volvulus when a loop of bowel gets twisted round itself causing complete obstruction, but symptoms and treatment are similar to the ones described above. After opening the abdomen the site of volvulus is sought and the gut untwisted and anchored to the peritoneum. Resection and anastomosis are rarely necessary.

Intussusception

In intussusception a partial or total obstruction of the bowel is caused by invagination of a piece of bowel into the bowel beyond it.

Intussusception is one of the most urgent emergencies of early childhood, though on occasions repeated attacks occur, which rectify themselves. Acute intussusception is seen usually at the time the infant starts on a weaning diet and it is possible that irritation of the bowel causes a small area of inflammation and oedema in the ileocaecal or ileocolic region which is the starting point of the telescoping of the bowel. A high proportion of children show signs of a recent virus infection causing oedema of the lymphoid tissue of the bowel. This swelling is then the starting point of the telescoping. A portion of the bowel becomes invaginated and is dragged onwards towards the rectum by peristaltic movement. If the diagnosis is doubtful, a barium enema may be ordered to confirm the diagnosis and on occasions this has the effect of reducing the intussusception, so that surgery becomes unnecessary.

Signs and Symptoms. The infant is as a rule a well-nourished healthy baby of 4 months to 2 years. The mother will explain that he suddenly seemed to have severe abdominal colic which made him draw up his legs and that these pains had been recurring at intervals, between which the baby seemed normal and contented. At first the pain may recur every hour or $\frac{1}{2}$ hr but it soon becomes more frequent and its severity causes shock, with pallor, sweating and a cold clammy skin. The baby soon becomes exhausted. At first a normal stool may be passed but this is followed by complete constipation due to the obstruction, except for the passage of blood-stained mucus—the typical 'red currant jelly stool'. Vomiting may occur but is not a constant symptom.

On *examination* a sausage-shaped tumour may be felt over the colon, while the right inguinal fossa feels empty as the caecum is drawn into the colon—the 'Signe de Dance'. On rectal examination the apex of the intussusception may be felt.

Operation. The child is prepared as for any other operation but a gastric tube is passed and the stomach contents aspirated to avoid inhalation of vomited food. An intravenous infusion may be started to treat the shock and to restore the electrolyte balance. An antibiotic such as Cephaloridine may be commenced to avoid the risk of septicaemia. The abdominal skin, the umbilicus and the groins are washed with soap and water or the child is bathed, if his condition permits.

No time is lost in starting the operation as the invaginated section of the bowel causes obstruction of the blood supply and if left too long would result in gangrene and toxic symptoms. A laparotomy is done, the intussusception found and the invaginated bowel gently drawn out, with a 'milking movement'. After reduction the bowel is sometimes stitched to the peritoneum to prevent recurrence of the intussusception. Special care is taken to ensure that the bowel is viable and that the blood supply is capable of complete recovery. Occasionally when resection of gut is necessary, a blood transfusion will also be required.

Post-Operative Care. Post-operative care is usually straightforward. Fluids are given in small amounts—some hospitals start on a 'pyloric schedule'—but in most cases the child can return to a light, normal diet within 3 or 4 days. Any vomiting, the passage of flatus and the first stool are reported as they are an important guide to treatment. The wound is often left exposed or covered with a small dressing and the stitches are usually removed on the eighth and tenth day respectively.

Restriction of Bowel. Whenever extensive resection of bowel has been carried out the child's diet will have to be carefully regulated as abnormalities of digestion and absorption result. Disturbances of growth, electrolyte balance, blood formation and vitamin absorption must all be prevented.

Acute Appendicitis

There are few conditions in childhood that present a more confusing picture than acute appendicitis. Among the conditions which may lead to this diagnosis erroneously are tonsillitis, mesenteric adenitis, urinary tract infections, pneumonia, diaphragmatic pleurisy, meningitis, anaphylactoid purpura, dysentery, gastro-enteritis, and premenstrual pain. Assessment of all symptoms and sometimes a period of careful observation will, however, establish the correct diagnosis. Because of the extensive examination that is necessary to establish the correct diagnosis the nurse may have to be prepared for an ear, nose and throat and a neurological examination, a rectal swab, a clean specimen of urine, blood picture and possibly a lumbar puncture and chest X-ray.

Signs and Symptoms. Acute appendicitis is rare before the age of 2 years and most common at 5 to 12 years. The onset may be insidious with ánorexia, listlessness, nausea or one or two attacks of vomiting and constipation. Alternatively the child may become acutely ill with little warning. The temperature may rise to 37.2° to 38.4°C (99° to 101°F), the pulse become rapid and the expression anxious. The tongue is furred and there is halitosis. The child is irritable and resents being touched or examined. If the appendix lies deep in the pelvis—pelvic appendix—the symptoms may include frequency of micturition and diarrhoea due to irritation, and if the appendix is retrocaecal the abdominal signs will be masked and diagnosis made very difficult.

Pain may be vague at first and may be intermittent to begin with but it gradually moves to the para-umbilical region and within 12 hours settles in the right iliac fossa.

On *examination* there is guarding and tenderness, and rectal examination causes the patient to flinch or cry out in pain as the finger points towards the right side. Abdominal rigidity may be caused by cold or general protest and for that reason it is particularly important in children that the doctor's hands should be warm and that a moment or two should be spent in gaining the child's confidence. Occasionally a sedative has to be given before a satisfactory examination can be carried out. If a white cell count is done, it is found to be raised to as much as 30 000 white cells/mm^3 (mainly polymorphonuclear cells).

Once diagnosis has been made, operation should not be delayed. Peritonitis occurs readily as the poorly developed peritoneum is less resistant to infection in a child than in later life, and infection does not localize well in childhood. The appendix wall is thin and the appendix perforates more often than in adults with more serious results. Operation and after-care are the same for children as for adults and in an uneventful case the child can be expected to be up for bedmaking on the first day and playing happily in the wards on the second day after operation.

Complications: Perforated Appendix. Acute appendicitis which cannot be diagnosed or treated in time may lead to perforation and set up peritonitis or form a pelvic abscess. When perforation has occurred, there may for a time appear to be some improvement in the child's condition. The pain subsides, he seems more relaxed and may fall asleep. However the temperature and pulse rate will rise and the rigidity spread and after a few hours, it becomes evident that he is seriously ill and in spite of operation, complications have now become unavoidable.

Peritonitis. The course of peritonitis is now usually controlled by chemotherapy, but severe cases do occur and merit description, as good nursing care has considerable bearing on a satisfactory outcome. Peritonitis may be caused by surgical emergencies such as a ruptured appendix, perforation of the bowel due to ulcerative colitis, by ascending infection from the vagina and by infection in the blood stream. In newly-born babies the infection may enter via the umbilicus. The causative organisms include the staphylococcus, *Escherichia coli* (bacterium), the tubercle bacillus, gonococcus and pneumococcus.

In the case of a perforated appendix the causative organism is usually the *Escherichia coli* and the fluid in the peritoneal cavity soon becomes infected. The onset is mostly very acute. The temperature rises to 39·4° to 40·6°C (103° to 105°F), the tongue is furred, the child vomits and complains of abdominal pain or draws up his legs. In very young patients this pain may not be localized as it is in older children. Respirations are rapid and shallow, the diaphragm being immobilized as the movements of the abdomen cause pain, but the arms are thrown out above the head in order to increase the respiratory capacity. The colour of the skin is grey, with a malar flush and the eyes bright but sunken and surrounded by dark rings. The legs are drawn up in 'frog position' in an attempt to relieve abdominal pain. Free fluid will be present in the abdominal cavity and the abdomen is rigid. The entire picture is that of severe toxaemia.

Nursing care. Children suffering from such a serious illness need expert and continuous nursing care. The mouth will have to be treated frequently, the position changed and pillows turned in order to encourage rest and sleep. Pressure areas need most careful attention. For bedmaking the child should be lifted rather than rolled from side to side so as to keep the intraperitoneal fluid localized. The upright position is adopted for the same reason and at the same time this will encourage deep respirations (Fig. 44). Hot fomentations may relieve abdominal

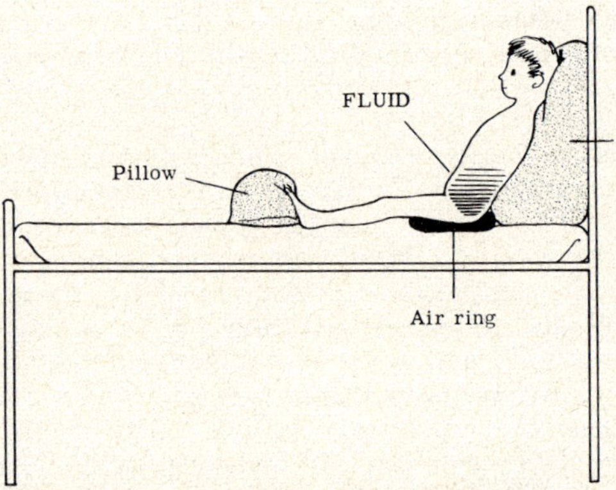

FIG. 44. Peritonitis, with free fluid in the peritoneal cavity. Sitting the patient in the upright position helps with drainage and localizes the fluid in the pelvic cavity. Children move around far more freely than adults so that danger from the use of pillows causing thrombosis of a deep vein is negligible.

pain and rigidity. Open windows and the use of electric fans help to reduce hyperpyrexia. Fluid balance charts are kept as well as 4-hourly temperature and accurate observation charts. The room or ward should be well ventilated and provided the child is warmly covered and that draughts are excluded only good can come from opening a window.

With the help of a stethoscope, the bowel sounds should be checked as the absence of peristalsis, flatus and bowel actions are signs of intestinal paralysis. A small blood transfusion is sometimes given to correct anaemia. It may also help to build up the patient's general strength and resistance.

At times the free fluid in the abdomen may fail to absorb and become infected. A generalized septicaemia may develop or in more favourable cases, the pus will localize and form a pelvic abscess. Adhesions may form between the convolutions of the bowel and later give rise to colic and obstruction.

Subphrenic Abscess. Rarely the pus localizes below the diaphragm causing an abscess which is difficult to palpate and diagnose. Treatment is by surgical drainage.

Pelvic Abscess. Pelvic abscess rarely requires surgical interference. The pus localizes and in the majority of cases the abscess eventually ruptures into the rectum. Pus and mucus are passed when the child has his bowels opened. This complication delays recovery by a week or two but is rarely very serious although the child may have considerable pain.

Paralytic Ileus. When the serious complication of paralytic ileus arises, peristalsis ceases and there is complete constipation; no flatus is passed and the abdomen is distended and resonant when tapped. Vomiting may be severe and continues even when the normal stomach contents have been vomited and the vomit consists only of gastric and intestinal secretions mixed with bile.

Treatment. This consists of resting the bowel completely until peristalsis is re-established. Continuous gastric suction (Fig. 45) or frequent aspirations by syringe through a nasogastric tube are carried out until there is no more aspirate and bowel sounds can be heard through a stethoscope.

Fluids are given only by the intravenous route until peristalsis is once more present. The child will need a good deal of nursing attention. He is usually restless and needs comforting. Hands and face should be sponged from time to time, the mouth treated regularly, the position of the limb into which the infusion is running adjusted and supported by small pillows and the hands restrained to prevent him from pulling out the aspiration tube. Thirst may be troublesome and occasionally it

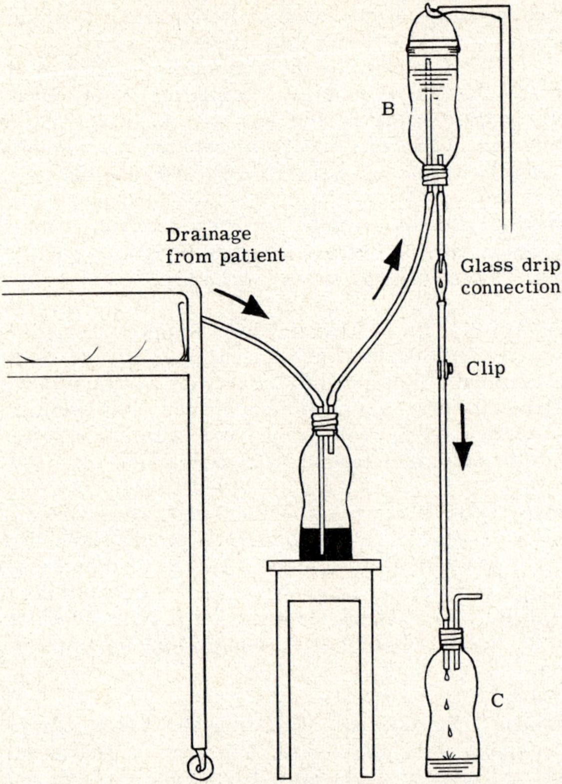

FIG. 45. Continuous gastric suction. The equipment is easy to assemble. Its gentle action makes this method particularly suitable for children.

is permissible to give sips of water even though they may have to be aspirated again. Once peristalsis has started again, recovery is rapid and the child is as a rule eager to have his meals and gains strength rapidly. Despite the serious manifestations of paralytic ileus, prognosis is good.

Drugs. Since the advent of modern drugs, particularly the broad spectrum antibiotics, most patients suffering from appendicitis with complications are now successfully treated. Appropriate antibiotics are prescribed according to the seriousness of the causative organism, determined by blood culture and from a swab of the discharging wound.

Rectal Prolapse

When a section of mucous membrane comes down and presents at the anal orifice, the condition is known as rectal prolapse. Only rarely do all the coats of the rectum come down in this way and if this happens the condition is called *rectal procidentia.*

Rectal prolapse is a common occurrence in children of about 9 months to 3 years. There are several underlying causes and each will have to be treated before improvement can be expected from either medical or surgical therapy. The following are the *usual causes*: poor muscle tone as in diseases of the nervous system; malnutrition and wasting disease in which the supporting fatty tissue is absent; stress from coughing, as in whooping cough; long-standing diarrhoea causing irritation of the lower bowel; general mismanagement, behaviour problems, poor toilet training, long periods spent sitting on the pot and finally mental handicap.

Treatment. When a rectal prolapse occurs it should be dealt with calmly and the prolapse gently reduced. In most cases it can easily be pushed back by steady pressure with a piece of damp cotton wool while the patient is lying on his back. Alternatively, very young children can be held up by their legs when gravity may cause the prolapse to reduce itself. It may help if, after reducing the prolapse, the nurse holds the child's buttocks together for a few minutes, while she distracts his attention by telling a story or playing with him.

Patients who have had prolapses over a long period of time may have to learn to defecate in a recumbent position. Sometimes a small toilet seat can be fixed over the adult lavatory to avoid the child adopting a squatting position. Good, consistent toilet training is a very important part of the treatment, but young children should not be allowed to sit on their pots for long, nor should undue importance be attached to a daily bowel action. A day or two missed will rarely be of consequence and is preferable to fussing over this point.

Operation. Intractable or long-standing cases may have to be treated surgically. The rectum may be fixed by inserting a stitch from behind and around the coccyx or alternatively by tightening the anal sphincter with a piece of chromic catgut. The latter method is the more painful of the two. Alternatively a fibrosing agent, such as hypertonic saline is injected into the rectal wall. The fibrosed tissue causes some constriction and gives support to the rectal wall. In either case there is no pre-operative treatment although some surgeons may order a rectal wash-out before the patient is sent to the theatre. Post-operatively the buttocks may be strapped together for 4 or 5 days. Extra fluids, a roughage free diet and liquid paraffin are given, to ensure soft stools and easy bowel action without straining.

Special Points. All young children are inclined to focus much attention on their excreta and the anal region. This is an entirely natural thing. It is, however, important to manage rectal prolapse and the attendant treatment with as little fluster as possible and to ensure that the discomfort accompanying the operation should not be regarded as a punishment by the young patient.

At times, a strong psychological factor is involved and the child of over-anxious or over-protective parents may learn to produce a prolapse at will, in order to call forth demonstrations of concern. In such cases the parents require reassurance and help. They should be told that the condition is a relatively harmless one and that their expressions of interest in the child should be directed into other channels. Proof of the psychological nature of the disturbance is that these children rarely have a prolapse in hospital.

Jaundice

Jaundice is the yellow staining of the skin and conjunctiva of the eyes by pigments absorbed from the blood instead of being excreted in the bile, as in a healthy person. It is therefore a symptom and not a disease in itself and there are several causes, some of which are dealt with in the appropriate chapter in greater detail. Jaundice arises if the breakdown of red cells is so rapid that the liver cannot cope with it. The unconjugated bilirubin in the circulation then rises. If in the case of babies it exceeds the normal level of 340 μmol/litre (20 mg/100 ml) of blood, bilirubin will be deposited in the ganglia of the nervous system, resulting in spasticity and mental handicap. Low birth-weight babies and those with haemolytic disease are at particular risk and frequent estimations of the serum bilirubin levels have to be performed and appropriate treatment given when danger point is reached. The main causes of jaundice in childhood can be grouped under the following headings.

The Haemolytic Types. These are due to excess destruction of red cells, i.e. at a greater rate than the liver can deal with. As these bile pigments are not excreted by the kidneys but are eliminated by the liver, stools and urine retain their normal colour. Examples are:

1. Haemolytic disease of the newborn (see p. 68);
2. Acholuric jaundice (see p. 229);
3. Transfusion jaundice.

Obstructive Jaundice. This is caused by an obstruction in the bile ducts so that bile pigment cannot reach the duodenum. Stools are pale or even colourless but the urine is heavily coloured, and the skin is tinged yellow to olive colour. Examples are:

1. Biliary atresia (see p. 83);
2. Obstruction from pressure of a tumour or a choledochus cyst;
3. Very rarely obstruction by gall-stones or roundworms.

Jaundice Due to Sepsis. The principal examples are infection spreading from the umbilicus of the newborn or general infection spreading via the blood stream and causing liver damage. In these instances the jaundice is rarely very deep.

Infective or Acute Virus Hepatitis. This type of jaundice frequently appears in epidemic form. Serum hepatitis comes under this heading and this is caused by contamination with virus-infected blood or needles used for injections and blood tests. The urine is dark while the faeces are pale or colourless. There is a similar neonatal 'giant cell' hepatitis.

Other conditions accompanied by jaundice are congenital syphilis, galactosaemia, cystic fibrosis of the pancreas, physiological jaundice and Weil's disease.

Infective Hepatitis
(Epidemic Hepatitis, Virus Hepatitis, Catarrhal Jaundice)

Infective hepatitis is an acute inflammation of the liver. It is caused by a viral infection.

Children are frequently admitted to hospital suffering from infective hepatitis and whole epidemics may sweep through schools and nurses' homes, as the long incubation period (2 to 6 weeks) makes the control of the infection difficult. The virus is present in the faeces and carriers may harbour the infection for many months.

Signs and Symptoms. The onset of an attack may follow one of several patterns. It may be acute, the temperature quickly rising to 38.4° to 39.4°C (101° to 103°F) and the patient feeling very ill. Alternatively there is a low pyrexia coupled with mild gastro-intestinal disturbances, malaise and gradually developing jaundice. In yet another variety there are few symptoms apart from general malaise, the first indication of the illness being the appearance of dark urine.

In the most typical cases of infective hepatitis the mother will have noticed almost complete loss of appetite, mild gastro-intestinal upset with occasional vomiting, a furred tongue, abdominal distension and possibly some diarrhoea (though constipation is an equally common feature). The child may complain of vague abdominal pain and tenderness particularly on movement and when lying on the right side. He is irritable and feverish and wants to be left alone. After 3 to 4 days the urine turns brown and shortly after that the temperature starts to subside. The faeces are now pale and constipated; the skin takes on a yellow tinge and the conjunctivae become jaundiced.

The child may complain of feeling cold, his pulse is sluggish and there is marked irritability and lethargy. As the jaundice becomes established, these symptoms usually improve. Irritation of the skin is not a common feature in children. Bile pigments are present in the urine in the earliest stages of the illness; often diagnosis can be confirmed by a urine test.

Nursing Care. Paediatricians differ in their wishes concerning the isolation of these patients. As a sound principle however, barrier nursing should be observed for 5 days after the onset of jaundice and the excreta disinfected for approximately 3 weeks.

The patient is kept on bed rest and the clothing should be warm, though wool next to the skin should not be worn as it may cause unnecessary irritation. Any itching may be treated with calamine lotion or ordinary dusting powder. Observation charts will mention particularly the colour of the stools and urine, the degree of jaundice present and the quality of the pulse. A series of specimens of urine are saved daily so that comparison of colour can be made throughout the course of the illness and tested for bile.

Diet. In the early stages of the illness there is almost complete anorexia. Fruit juices and abundant glucose (as much as 230 g a day) are given. Few paediatricians prescribe a rigid, fat-free diet and as a rule the best guide in the matter is the patient himself, who will accept fat as soon as he feels ready for it. Where a more definite diet is prescribed, tea, toast and honey or golden syrup, jellies, fat-free broth and skimmed milk dishes are offered. Adequate fluid intake should be ensured. Occasionally high protein intake in the form of Casilan or Complan may be ordered and often these have to be camouflaged skilfully to make them acceptable to the patient. Loss of weight may be severe during the acute stage of the illness but is usually made up rapidly during the convalescent stage.

The first signs of improvement may start a few days after the onset of the jaundice. The stools and urine gradually regain their normal colour. The patient feels better and the appetite returns and may soon become voracious. The child should, however, be kept in bed until all jaundice has cleared and is not discharged until all liver tenderness has subsided. Fatigue may persist for some time, and extra rest and a period of convalescence before return to school is highly desirable. Some paediatricians make a rule that convalescence should be double the time spent in bed. The total recovery may take from 2 to 3 months. The outlook is as a rule good, but patients may have to have treatment and be careful with fat intake for several weeks. On occasions permanent liver damage is caused and very occasionally necrosis of the liver, followed by death, may ensue. For this reason, the illness should never be treated lightly and adequate rest and treatment must be given.

Drugs. On the whole little drug therapy is employed. Occasionally, if constipation is obstinate, saline aperients are ordered. In chronic cases or where there is recurrence of symptoms, cortisone therapy may prove of value. Avomine, 12.5 mg (for 6 to 10 years old) given three times a day may lessen the feeling of nausea and reduce vomiting.

Complications. Severe attacks of hepatitis or recurrent attacks may lead to permanent damage of the liver structure. The prognosis of chronic hepatitis and cirrhosis of the liver is always grave although compensation in the liver function may stimulate permanent recovery. The symptoms of cirrhosis include jaundice, pale stools, the presence of bile pigment in the urine, portal hypertension, the formation of varicose veins in the oesophagus, haematemesis, ascites and mental changes. The breath takes on a sweet, faecal odour. Coma is common and eventually leads to death of the patient.

Intestinal Parasites

Threadworms (*Pinworms—Oxyuris vermicularis*)

Threadworm infestation is exceedingly common in children and entire families may be affected.

The threadworm normally inhabits the large intestine but the female migrates to the anal region where she deposits her eggs. Irritation, particularly during the night causes the child to scratch and reinfect himself through his finger nails. Sharing beds and towels is an obvious way in which infection is spread to others.

Signs and Symptoms. The most general symptom is itching and this in turn may cause restless sleep and irritability. Scratching and irritation may cause inflammation of the perineum, vulvo-vaginitis, bed-wetting and occasionally diarrhoea or rectal prolapse.

The tiny worms may first be noticed in the course of a toilet round, although the worms remain on the surface of the stool only momentarily and then disappear into its substance. Alternatively the mother may describe symptoms which suggest the diagnosis.

Diagnostic Test. In order to prove the presence of threadworms a simple test can be done. A piece of Sellotape (adhesive cellulose tape) 2.5 cm (1 in) wide and 7.6 cm (3 in) long is placed, sticky side down on the perineum immediately on waking. It is then transferred to a microscope slide, again sticky side down and labelled and sent to the laboratory. The threadworm ova are obvious under the microscope. As the procedure is such a simple one it can easily be carried out by an outpatient's mother.

Treatment. Careful hygiene is the first essential. Finger nails should be kept short and hand washing before meals be enforced. Pyjamas should be worn in preference to night gowns and both pyjamas and day knickers should be washed and boiled daily. At night cotton mittens can be worn to prevent infecting the finger nails. The local application of an analgesic ointment is useful to relieve rectal irritation.

Drug Therapy. Piperazine hydrate (0.25 to 2 g twice daily—for 7 days) may be given. Pripsen, a granular compound containing piperazine phosphate and standardized senna, as Senokot. It is effective when given in one single dose. However, in order to exclude possible reinfestation during the first 2 days after treatment, when occasional ova may still be present, a second dose is often given after a week or 10 days. Vanquin, another single dose anthelmintic, is equally effective. All members of the family should be treated.

Tapeworms (*Taenia saginata*)

The sight of long lengths of tapeworm may cause justifiable disgust and alarm to parents and they should be reassured about the comparatively harmless nature of the infestation.

Treatment can be carried out successfully as an out-patient by giving an oral dose of dichlorophen with a drink before breakfast on two successive mornings. The dose is from 2 to 4 g and the drug is well tolerated. This drug has a laxative action. The worm is digested in the bowel after destruction by the drug, so that no segments are passed in the stool. Alternatively niclosamide 500 mg (Yomesan) before breakfast followed by a second tablet 2 hours later may be given. Mepacrine 0.05 to 0.3 g according to body weight and followed by a saline purge 3 hours later is another effective form of treatment. Occasionally, however, there are side effects such as gastro-intestinal irritation, nausea and malaise.

Roundworms

The roundworm has a complicated life cycle and the fully grown worm can survive a number of years inside its human host. Roundworms resemble earthworms in shape and size and stools should be watched for their appearance, as this is the usual means of proving the diagnosis. Other signs and symptoms are uncommon, though furred tongue and halitosis may be present and in rare cases the worms cause intestinal obstruction or may even be vomited, or reach the lungs and cause collapse of a lobe, or jaundice due to blocking of the bile duct. Worms which have died within the host, may cause convulsions due to liberated toxins. Treatment with piperazine is usually successful. The dose is the same as for threadworms.

Toxocariasis (Visceral Larva Migrans)

Toxocariasis is an infection caused by the transmission of the visceral larvae migrans. These are deposited in the soil from dog and cat faeces. Children 1 to 4 years of age are the most likely to be infected, especially if they have a 'dirt-eating habit'. When the ova are swallowed, the larvae hatch in the intestine, pass through the intestinal wall and wander through the viscera. They pass first to the liver and then to other intestinal organs, where they may produce granulomas. These are most commonly found in the liver but can also occur in the kidney, heart, striated muscle, brain and eyeball. Common presenting symptoms are fever, skin rash with general malaise and anorexia. As the larvae migrate haemorrhage, granuloma formation, chest infections with enlarged tender liver and spleen occur. Ophthalmitis may occur in severe infections. There is an associated eosinophilia. Diagnosis is difficult although a standardized skin test is available. With many children a spontaneous improvement is common. Treatment is symptomatic.

Prevention is the most effective weapon against this infection. All pet dogs and cats should be given regular periodic anthelmintics. Dogs should not be allowed to foul children's playing areas or foot paths.

The Colon, Anus and Rectum

Megacolon

Megacolon means enlarged colon. It may be:

1. The result of chronic constipation.
2. Due to a narrowing of the rectum.
3. Caused by an absence of the parasympathetic ganglia of the rectum, as e.g. in Hirschsprung's disease.

The treatment of the first two causes may require the initial manual evacuation of the rectum under general anaesthesia and frequent rectal washouts, using normal saline and aperients, such as Senokot. These measures must be combined with toilet training to redevelop normal bowel habits. In cases where the megacolon is secondary to chronic constipation the nurse should appreciate that there may be also present quite a severe degree of psychological disturbance and the help of the psychiatrist may be needed.

Hirschsprung's Disease

Hirschsprung's disease (Fig. 46) is due to the absence of the parasympathetic ganglia in the rectum and occasionally farther along the large intestine perhaps even beyond the sigmoid colon. As peristaltic action is initiated and maintained by these nerve

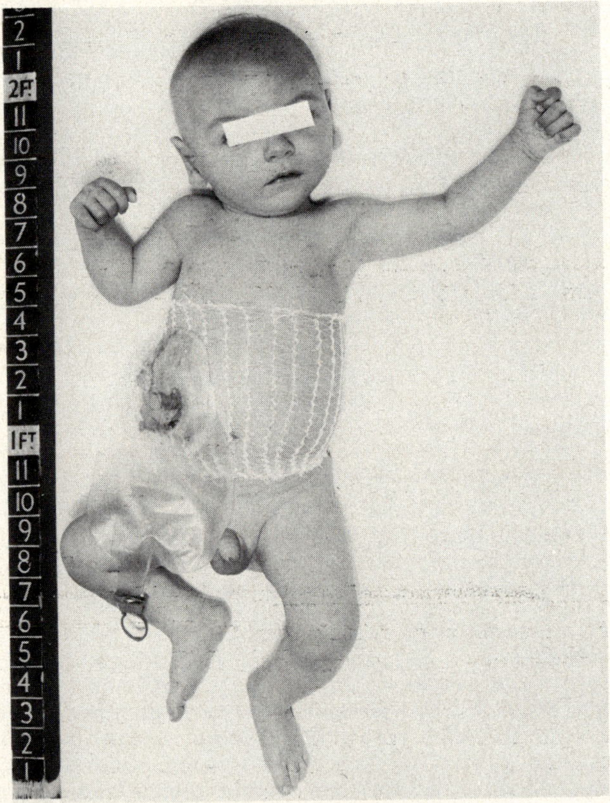

FIG. 46. Young infants with Hirschsprung's disease. Colostomy performed. Major surgery involving a radial pull through delayed until after the age of 6 months.

cells, normal bowel movements do not take place and the intestine above the affected part becomes grossly dilated, while the rectum is as a rule empty, smaller than usual and frequently in spasm.

The disease is present at birth, but delay in diagnosis may occur depending on the length of the aganglionic segment. Constipation is the presenting symptom, and there is often a delay of passage of the first meconium stool, which in the majority of normal babies is passed in the first 24 hours of birth. It is often associated with Down's syndrome.

Signs and Symptoms. Children with Hirschsprung's disease look miserable and unhappy with thin wasted limbs in contrast to the big distended abdomen. The baby is often reluctant with his feeds, and will be inclined to vomit. As the condition progresses visible peristalsis may be observed across the drum-like abdomen. Occasionally foul-smelling flatus and thin 'ribbon-like' stools are passed. Characteristic rumbling noise can be heard; these are known as borborygmi. At intervals the mucous lining of the bowel becomes inflamed and the stagnated, putrified, offensive bowel content is passed. This enterocolitis can at first be mistaken for gastroenteritis and may rapidly lead to a dangerous loss of body fluids requiring intravenous replacement. Characteristically, the distension and constipation may be relieved by digital examination of the rectum or by irrigation, and the child's condition will improve for a short period. Chest complications are common as the distension of the abdomen impedes respiration by pressure on the diaphragm. Babies suffering from Hirschsprung's disease cannot thrive unless treated, surgery being the only hope of survival. Commonly, if the affected segment is a relatively short one, the child will present at a later age as a failure to thrive, appearing puny and stunted in growth. It is through good nursing observations and reporting that the lead to Hirschsprung's disease can often be given. Accurate recording of the number of bowel actions and the nature of any stools passed will bring abnormalities to the notice of medical staff at an early date. The putrified smell often associated with bouts of diarrhoea, and the abdominal distension which causes the umbilicus to evert, and the abdominal veins to be unusually prominent are often first observed through daily handling and nursing care of the patient.

Diagnosis. *Barium enema,* will show the characteristic features of the collapsed aganglionic segment and the proximal dilated bowel. Before this examination, when Hirschsprung's disease is suspected, the normal bowel preparation must be omitted, because the 'deflation' will relieve the contrast between the two segments and may lead to mis-diagnosis.

Rectal biopsy, a submucous biopsy is taken to demonstrate the absence of ganglion cells. This can now be obtained with a special instrument using suction which avoids the need for general anaesthesia.

Ano-rectal manometry demonstrates the absence of the normal reflex inhibition of the internal anal sphincter on rectal distension and is useful as a screening test.

Treatment. If the diagnosis is made in the neonatal period, a colostomy will be performed and surgery delayed until the child is aged between 6 to 12 months, when he will be better able to withstand major surgery. When the diagnosis is made in the case of the older child a colostomy may not necessarily be performed. Treatment with saline washouts for a sufficient time to clear out the stagnant faecal material from the bowel before operation will be required. The two most common operative procedures for Hirschsprung's disease are Swenson's (Fig. 47) and Duhamel's (Fig. 48) operations. Each involves laparotomy, mobilization of bowel, resection and reconstitution of the lower alimentary tract and often a temporary colostomy for the post-operative period.

Prior to operation a course of phthalysulphathiazole is given to sterilize the bowel. Any anaemia is treated and blood taken for grouping. The immediate pre-operative preparation is the same as for any other major operation. An intravenous infusion is set up, and a nasogastic tube passed.

Colostomy. The colostomy is usually retained for a further 2 or 3 weeks to allow for healing. Following closure, careful

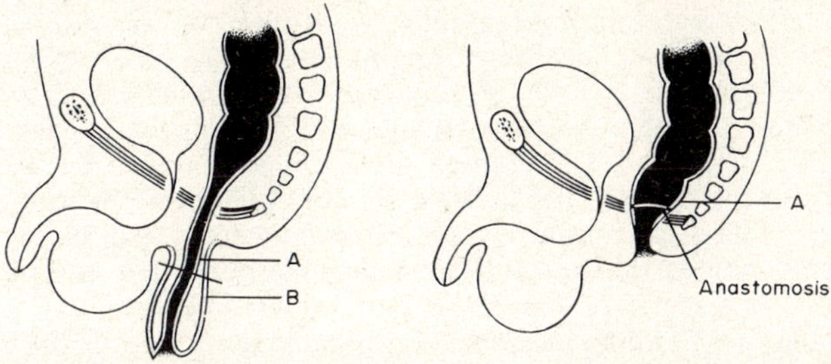

FIG. 47. Swenson's operation. *Left*: the colon is mobilized, the rectum prolapsed through the anus allows an anastomosis. *Right*: completion of the operation with the bowel returned to the pelvis, the ganglionic bowel (A) is anastomosed to the rectal stump.

regular bowel training is necessary at first. The mother is taught to give her child an adequate intake of roughage and fluids to avoid constipation. At first careful, regular bowel training will also be necessary and the occasional laxative or even enemata may have to be given.

General management of a colostomy in children differs little from that in an adult. In the immediate post-operative period there is danger of bleeding from the bowel and this is best

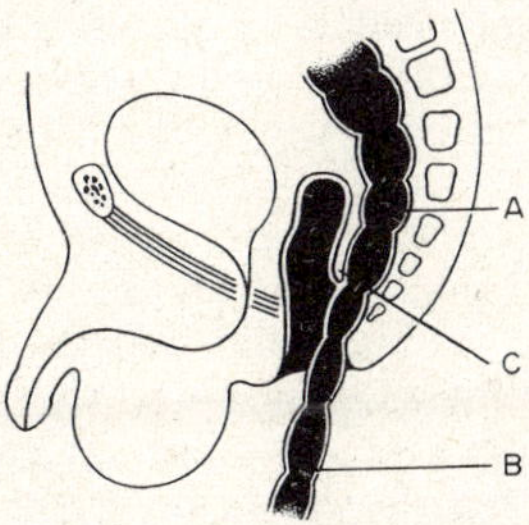

FIG. 48. Duhamel operation. Aganglionic bowel (B) is pulled down behind the closed rectum through the internal sphincter until the normally innervated bowel (A) is pulled through and fixed to the distal rectum. The aganglionic section that is pulled through is excised and the spur (C) is crushed with a clamp applied at the end of the operation.

stopped by the application of a firm bandage and a gauze pad soaked in a solution of adrenaline 1:1000. Occasionally the protruding bowel becomes strangulated and the opening in the abdominal wall has to be enlarged. A loop of bowel may prolapse through the incision and if this happens a pack of warm, sterile saline is applied until the patient can be taken back to the theatre. The delicate skin of children needs particularly careful attention. The surrounding area and buttocks should be washed frequently and no soiled pads left on longer than necessary. A barrier cream should be applied. The protruding bowel is protected from damage by a layer of tulle gras. If washouts are ordered they are done with a very soft catheter for fear of perforating the bowel.

With care the bowel can be so regulated as to produce a semi-formed stool which is easily passed but not too messy, and bowel actions can be reduced to twice daily. Extra nourishment and vitamins should be given, keeping in mind the fact that absorption can take place only in part of the length of the digestive tract.

The *psychological aspect* of a colostomy is of little importance in children of this age but it is important to remember the effect such an operation may have on the mother. As a rule she can be reassured that the colostomy is merely a temporary measure. Permanent colostomy, performed for a congenital abnormality of the lower bowel will of course cause greater distress to the parents and they will need a long period of adjustment and sympathetic support. Children with a permanent colostomy can be fitted with a colostomy belt and a normal life should be possible.

Post-operatively. Intravenous therapy will be needed for the first 24 hours or so, as the child will be allowed nothing by mouth. During this time careful mouth toilet will be required to keep the mouth moist. Frequent observations must be recorded including a quarter hourly pulse rate. If the pulse rate is rising a doctor should be informed, as in Hirschsprung's disease this is often a sign of fluid loss from an inflamed bowel. A naso-gastric tube will be in position and should be aspirated two-hourly and providing the aspirate volume is low, feeding with clear fluids only can be commenced 24 hours after operation,

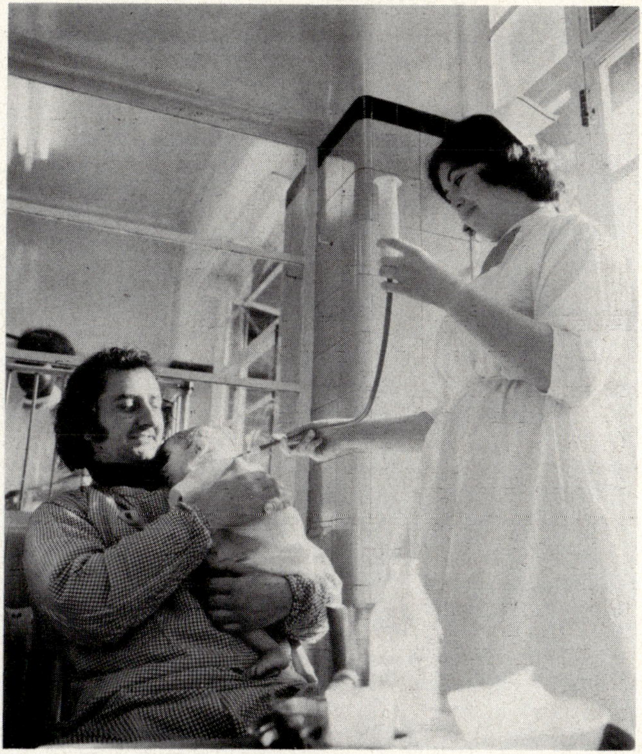

FIG. 49. Proud father holding infant son during naso-oesophageal feed.

and the intravenous infusion may then be discontinued. Care of the colostomy is described on page 284. Gradually, over the next few days a normal diet is introduced. The peri-anal skin may become sore, and should be washed frequently and a barrier cream applied. As the child's condition improves ambulation can be encouraged. Sutures are removed about the eighth post-operative day if the wound is well healed. The child with a colostomy has it closed about 2 weeks later.

Prognosis is excellent for these children with the majority

achieving normal bowel function although a few may require anal dilatations in the post-operative period to prevent stenosis.

Umbilical Hernia, Inguinal Hernia

A hernia is a protrusion of an organ from the cavity in which it is normally contained. The following pages describe two types of hernia, commonly met with in children.

Umbilical hernia is a very common condition of childhood. It is entirely harmless although it is unsightly but may cause parents much worry and may be thought by them to be the cause of such disturbances as wind and colic. The defect consists of a small, oval-shaped weakness in the linea alba through which a loop of gut protrudes, and in the majority of cases it disappears spontaneously during the first three or four years of life. Small umbilical hernias rarely call for treatment but larger ones resolve more rapidly if surgical treatment is given. This is a simple repair of the hernia and can be done as a minor operation as an outpatient or as a day case. Trusses, adhesive strapping and elastic bandages are useless.

Supra-Umbilical Hernia

Sometimes the hernia is just above the umbilicus. As this type of hernia does not cure itself it is important to make a careful assessment and diagnosis.

Inguinal Hernia

Inguinal hernias are due to a developmental weakness in the abdominal wall and are usually first seen when the child cries, strains at stool, or coughs (particularly during the paroxysms of whooping cough). A small lump appears just lateral to and above the crest of the pubic bone. Occasionally this lump spreads down into the scrotum. It usually disappears when the child is at rest, or he is held with shoulder and head lower than the rest of the body. In the majority of cases operation is the treatment of choice. The operation is a minor one, consisting of locating and excising the hernial sac, and can be carried out in an outpatients' theatre, or the child admitted as a day case. Post-operatively the child is allowed the freedom of the cot as soon as he feels like it, and he can be allowed up on the day after the operation.

Inguinal hernias occur more frequently in boys than in girls because in development before birth, or in some cases during infancy and early childhood, the testes migrate through the inguinal canals into the scrotum. There is therefore a certain weakness in the abdominal wall in boys due to the fact that the inguinal canal is patent and the track through which the testes descend has not become obliterated. If either of the testes remains undescended it has to be brought down into the scrotum by a surgical operation (orchidopexy). Often at operation for undescended testicles, a hernial sac is also found and a herniotomy performed.

If an inguinal hernia is sufficiently large or the neck of the hernial sac very narrow, the hernia can become *irreducible* and there is a danger of intestinal obstruction. As the child draws up his legs in pain and cries, the abdominal pressure increases and so aggravates the state of affairs. A sedative should be given and the buttocks and foot end of the cot raised. Occasionally the child is put into a warm bath or is nursed in a gallows-type of extension. Alternatively an ice bag is suspended over the area to reduce the engorgement caused by the constriction of vessels in the inguinal canal. As the child relaxes, gravity causes the intestinal loop to slip back into the abdominal cavity and the hernia reduces itself. Once this kind of situation has arisen, operation and repair should be carried out at an early date. If the hernia cannot be reduced by any of these methods, an operation should be carried out before a *strangulated hernia* occurs, as if this happens, the blood supply to the loop of gut is cut off, and this leads to gangrene of the loop.

Ectopic Anus

Occasionally a child may be born with the anal opening in an abnormal position. Various types may occur, and one of the most severe and common of these is the type often referred to as rectovaginal fistula. In this anatomical abnormality the anus opens into the posterior wall of the vagina and just inside the vaginal orifice. Faeces may leak through the fistula but in rare cases there is a fairly satisfactory sphincter action. Treatment consists of plastic repairs which aims at producing as normal a function as possible. Although there is an ever-present danger of infection, these patients can often lead a perfectly normal life in spite of their abnormality.

A comparable condition occurs in boys. The ectopic anus may open on to the skin surface at the juncture of penis and scrotum and in this case the condition is left untreated. Occasionally faeces are discharged per urethram. In these cases surgical repair is attempted but results are as a rule disappointing. Occasionally no apparent anal orifice can be found. A variant of imperforate anus is fully described on page 82.

Meckel's Diverticulum

A Meckel's diverticulum is a remnant of the vitello-intestinal duct which connects the ileum with the umbilicus. In the majority of cases there are no symptoms, but occasionally there are complications which necessitate surgical treatment. The diverticulum may become inflamed and produce symptoms similar to those of appendicitis. It may become the starting point of an intussusception or it may cause intestinal obstruction. Painless bleeding (often severe) is the most usual symptom. Some patients have a faecal discharge through the diverticulum in the region of the umbilicus.

Mesenteric Lymphadenitis

Children often complain of abdominal pain for which there is no obvious explanation. The pain is not usually severe and neither guarding nor tenderness on examination are marked. There may occasionally be vomiting. The condition resolves itself without treatment and recurs from time to time. Although the symptoms are unconvincing, laparotomy is sometimes performed in order to exclude acute or subacute appendicitis. It will then be seen that the mesenteric lymph nodes are enlarged. It is thought that the enlargement is due to a generalized reaction of lymph tissue to infection. The condition is not a serious one but because of the possibility of appendicitis or renal tract disease, it should never be taken lightly.

Further Reading

BLACK, D. A. K. (1968) *Essentials of Fluid Balance*, 4th ed. Oxford: Blackwell Scientific.

NIXON. H. H. & O'DONNELL, B. (1976) *The Essentials of Paediatric Surgery*, 3rd ed. London: Heinemann.

RICKMAN, P. P. & JOHNSTON, J. (eds) (1969) *Neonatal Surgery*. London: Butterworth.

YOUNG, D. & WELLER, B. F. (1971) *Baby Surgery*. London: Harvey, Miller & Medcalf.

14
Disorders of metabolism and absorption

METABOLIC DISORDERS should be suspect when there is mental handicap, abnormal hair or skin texture or colour, abnormal urine output or colour, excessive thirst, abnormal appetite and failure to grow. With such conditions the urine and the blood should be examined. Special biochemical tests can be carried out. A number of these diseases originate from an absence or abnormality of an enzyme which is essential for a particular metabolic process.

Rickets

Rickets occur as a result of lack of fat soluble vitamin D in the diet and from lack of sunshine. Calcium and phosphorus metabolism fail and serious, typical signs and symptoms occur.

High standards of living and nutrition and a well-developed welfare service have caused rickets—once known as the English Disease—to become a rare condition in the British Isles. The cases seen occur as a rule in over-crowded, industrial cities where little sunlight penetrates the atmosphere and the children are often kept indoors while their mothers go out to work, and vitamin supplements are often not given. Amongst the Asian immigrants and their families special problems arise. Very often the vitamin content of the traditional diet is low, and may even be neglible if strict vegetarianism is adhered to.

Active Rickets

Active rickets is often due to dietary deficiencies and the groups at risk are infants, toddlers and young adolescents. It is caused by lack of vitamin D, which is essential for the utilization of calcium and phosphorus for good bone growth. Neither human nor cow's milk provide sufficient vitamin D for the baby's need after the first weeks of life. The deficiency may also be produced by prematurity, lack of exposure to sunshine, faulty diet and inability to absorb the fat soluble vitamin D in diseases such as coeliac disease. The risk period for vitamin D deficiency is during the winter, especially in northern cities where the daylight hours are shorter than in the south.

Signs and Symptoms. In severe cases the entire bony system of the body can be involved. The sutures and fontanelles of the skull are late in closing and together with bossing of the forehead give the skull the so-called 'hot cross bun' effect. Thinning of the cranial bones causes a resilience known as *craniotabes*. Dentition is delayed and the teeth are defective. The affected infant sits up and walks late, the bones are soft and arms and legs are bent and the epiphyses enlarged. Respiration causes sucking in of the softened ribs which results in a horizontal groove, known as *Harrison's sulcus*, running round the anterior aspect of the chest. At the same time beading at the juncture of the ribs and sternal cartilages forms the *rickety rosary*. The pelvic bones may become flattened and the angle of the neck of the femur on its shaft alters and eventually leads to limping and in girls to obstetric complications in later life.

The abdomen in children with rickets (Fig. 50) is protuberant and there is a tendency to respiratory tract infections, sweating, and diarrhoea and vomiting. The child is often miserable and sleeps little. Tetany, carpopedal spasm and laryngismus stridulus, are all now rare complications.

Treatment. This consists of giving adequate amounts of vitamin D and minerals in the diet which should be rich in milk, dairy butter, fortified margarine, fresh eggs, green vegetables, meat and oily fish.

The diet should be supplemented by vitamin D concentrates. Daily doses of 5000 to 50 000 I.U. (international units) of vitamin D or of calciferol by intramuscular injection or by mouth may be ordered in the active, acute stage. Ultraviolet

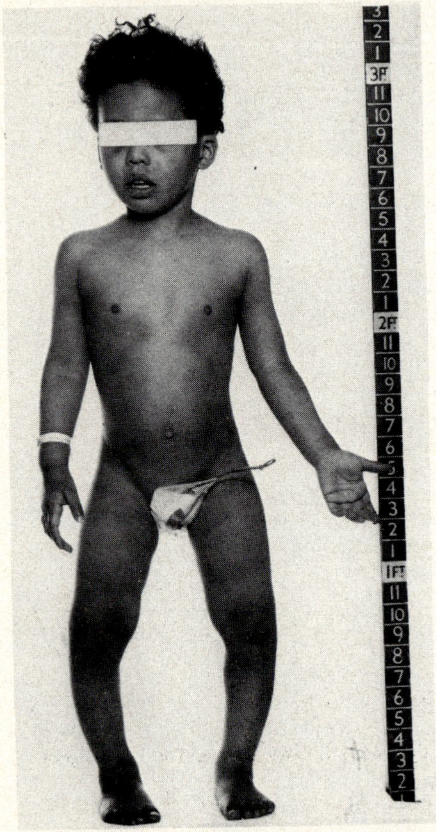

FIG. 50. A child with well-developed rickets. Urine bag in position for collection of specimen.

ray therapy may assist treatment where access to natural sunlight is difficult.

General Care. This aims at improving the child's health. Plenty of fresh air and sensible clothing, and a well balanced diet is often all that is needed. The wearing of thick napkins should be avoided as they may cause bowing of the femora by holding the legs apart. Deformities are prevented by restricting walking and crawling in the acute stages and by nursing the infant on a firm flat mattress. If admission to hospital is necessary the risk of cross infection is minimized by admitting these children to cubicles.

It is important that the correct dose of vitamin D should be given to the child.

If splints are worn, they are taken off daily and the skin washed and powdered to avoid pressure sores.

Prevention

1. A well-balanced diet with vitamin supplements up to the age of 5 years.
2. As much time as possible spent in the sunlight. Exposure of the baby's cheeks to sunlight for even a few hours is said to be sufficient for a day's requirement of vitamin D.
3. Co-operation between doctors, midwives, health visitors, teachers and nurses to identify children at risk and those showing the early signs of tiredness, pain and weakness in the lower limbs and often with a poor posture. Emphasis on the value of sunlight and vitamin supplements should be made to newly arrived Asian immigrant families, with the help of the local community leaders and translators to overcome any language problem.

Hypervitaminosis

Up to recent years it was thought to be impossible to give harmful amounts of vitamins. This theory, however, was recently disproved when a condition known as hypervitaminosis D was described. The symptoms are seen in very young infants who have been given fortified dried milk foods and fortified baby cereals as well as the usual amounts of vitamin D preparations such as cod-liver oil.

The manifestations are anorexia, failure to thrive, constipation, abdominal colic and eventually renal failure leading to death. The blood calcium level is raised.

Scurvy

Scurvy is a disease caused by deficiency of vitamin C in the diet. This may either be due to a lack of fresh fruits, potatoes and green vegetables or faulty cooking methods causing destruction of vitamin C.

Scurvy is now rarely seen in the United Kingdom. Better wages mean generally better nutrition including greater consumption of milk and fresh fruit, and more housewives know how to cook vegetables correctly.

Signs and Symptoms. These are due to abnormal permeability of the capillary walls, causing subperiosteal bleeding, bruising, haematuria, anaemia and in extreme cases cerebral haemorrhage. The gums may be swollen and bleed when touched and occasionally teeth may become loose and drop out. At times there is bleeding into the kidneys, bowels and the orbits of the eye.

The exquisite tenderness of the limbs make the child lie perfectly still so that it is easy to mistake the condition for a form of paralysis. The hips are abducted and the lower legs partly flexed. Any movement, jarring of the cot or picking up causes the child to scream with pain. There may be moderate fever, pallor and listlessness.

X-ray pictures show up the sub-periosteal haemorrhages and occult blood may be found in the stools and red cells in the urine. A vitamin C absorption test confirms that an abnormal amount of the vitamin is absorbed. The test is based on the knowledge that vitamin C taken in excess of normal storage is excreted in the urine. Vitamin C (3000 mg) is given orally. Urine is collected in a bottle made of dark glass and the amount excreted is analysed and compared with the test dose.

Prognosis. Scurvy responds rapidly to treatment and cure is complete. Treatment consists of giving vitamin C both in its natural form and as ascorbic acid. There is no known toxic effect.

Nursing Care. This aims at reducing any handling to a

minimum on account of the pain. The infant is washed and fed in his cot, clothing should be of a pattern that makes changing without too much movement possible and small, soft pillows are used to support the swollen limbs. As the gums are tender and inclined to bleed, the diet should be soft and should of course have a high vitamin C content.

All artificially fed babies should have vitamin C in the form of orange juice or other preparations such as rose hip syrup, or vitamin drops. Milk should be brought to the boil in a saucepan but not allowed to continue to boil. Green vegetables, tomato juice, fresh fruit and fresh orange juice should be introduced into the diet as soon as the child is old enough to be weaned. A dish high in vitamin C content and at the same time soothing to the gums and easily prepared is creamed potato. The floury part of the potato and particularly the part underneath the skin is mixed with milk and butter after baking the potato in its jacket. This meal is usually greatly enjoyed.

Phenylketonuria

Phenylketonuria is an inherited metabolic disorder, in which there is a failure to metabolize the amino acid phenylalanine. This is due to the absence of the liver enzyme phenylalaninase.

The majority of children with phenylketonuria are fair, with blue eyes, a marked tendency to eczema, a small head, large alveolar arches and widely spaced teeth. Their growth is stunted and they are late in sitting up. There is a peculiar musty odour to the urine of these patients. These children often suffer from epileptic fits.

The basis of treatment lies in the dietary limitation of phenylalanine. Some of this essential amino acid must be given for normal tissue growth and repair, but not enough for an abnormal accumulation to develop in the blood. For treatment to be effective it must commence between the age of 2 to 6 weeks. Therefore the early detection of phenylketonuria is of utmost importance, if mental handicap is to be prevented.

The Guthrie Test. A drop of blood is taken from a heel prick direct on to a filter paper and sent to the laboratory for specific culture tests which will show whether there is an increased level of phenylalanine in the blood. The normal phenylalanine level is 0.06 to 0.12 mmol/litre (1 to 2 mg/100 ml).

The test is reliable after the first week of life.

Phenistex. This is a simple test but it is only reliable in 80 per cent of cases. This test is carried out by squeezing the Phenistix between a wet napkin. The urine must have been freshly passed.

The incidence of this treatable condition is about 1 in 15 000 live births, i.e. about seventy-five new cases annually in England and Wales.

Treatment. The diet is complicated, expensive and unpalatable, which makes it difficult for parents to persevere with. An initial loss of weight must be expected.

The Diet.* The essential amino acid phenylalanine is carefully controlled according to body weight, about 25 mg/kg body weight in older children and 50 mg/kg body weight for babies.

For the young child this is given in the form of cow's milk. (30 ml contains 50 mg phenylalanine). Cereals, potatoes, fruits and vegetables may be given to older children in carefully measured amounts to meet their essential phenylalanine requirements.

Synthetic Preparations Used

First year of life — Minafen (Trufood)

This, plus the measured amount of cow's milk, will ensure all the protein requirements of the infant.

Older children — Cymogram (Allen & Hanbury)

The changeover from Minafen to Cymogram should be made slowly. The child should be weaned at the normal age (8 weeks to 3 months) and gradually introduced to solids.

* It is easy to make grave mistakes in the diet. Detailed dietary instruction. can—and should—be obtained. They are supplied, e.g. at The Hospitals for Sick Children, Great Ormond Street, London W.C.1.

Foods Allowed

Low phenylalanine bread
Low phenylalanine cakes and biscuits
Vegetarian jellies
Kosher, pure vegetable margarine
Honey, jams and boiled sweets

Note: Fish, meat, eggs, butter, cheese and some vegetables *must not* be given.

As the diet which can be offered contains little solid food the child should be given raw apple and whole carrots to chew in order to develop the teeth and dental arches.

Because the diet is so synthetic vitamin supplements must be given. These made by Paines and Byrnes are given in the form of Ketovite tablets and Ketovite liquid.

Careful monitoring of the serum levels of phenylalanine must be carried out, the aim of the dietary treatment is to keep phenylalanine levels below 0.30 mmol/litre (5 mg/100 ml) when it is thought that normal intelligence is most likely to be preserved.

The age at which the diet can be discontinued is thought to be after adolescence, but it should be remembered that maternal phenylketonuria gives rise to mentally retarded children unless the diet is controlled during pregnancy.

Both the special foods and the vitamins are expensive but they can be obtained on a National Health Service prescription.

Galactosaemia

Galactosaemia is a familial disease caused by an inability to metabolize galactose and so leading to intoxication of the body and brain cells. The result is mental deficiency, cataract and cirrhosis of the liver. The baby fails to thrive, is drowsy, refuses his feed and vomits. Jaundice may be present from the first day of life. Oedema may give a false impression of a satisfactory gain in weight. The stools are loose and the liver becomes enlarged. The death rate is a high one.

Treatment. Treatment must be started at once if it is to be effective. It entails substituting all feeds containing galactose or lactose by special preparations such as Nutramigen or Galactomin. Where these are not available, soya bean 'milk' to which Casilan, cane sugar, coconut oil, minerals and vitamins can be added, may be given.

Diagnosis. Whenever there is a familial history of the disease a simple test can be carried out on the cord blood, or alternatively a urine test will show the presence of galactosuria. Any finding of sugar in the urine must always be reported at once so that more specialized laboratory tests can be carried out. It is important to note that testing with the usual reagents will show sugar present in the urine, as the reaction is due to glucose. However tests with Clinistix will not detect the galactose which may be present, and specific tests have to be carried out.

Glycogen Disease
(Von Gierke's Disease)

Glycogen disease affects both sexes equally. It is a familial condition, due to an abnormality in the metabolism of glycogen. The first symptoms usually appear in the first 2 years of life.

Signs and Symptoms. Glycogen is deposited in the heart, liver and kidneys causing signs of heart failure, cardiac murmur, a large firm liver and ketonuria. There is no sugar present in the urine and the fasting blood sugar is low and does not rise when a test dose of adrenaline is given. Hypoglycaemia convulsions may occur. Obesity is common.

Treatment. There is no known cure and treatment remains symptomatic. The diet should be placed to maintain a reasonably constant flow of glucose into the blood, so preventing ketosis and hypoglycaemia.

Prognosis. Although most of these children lead invalid lives, death may not occur for many years.

Disorders of Lipoid and Glycogen Storage

This group of diseases includes such rare conditions as xanthomatosis, Schüller-Christian syndrome, Gaucher's disease, Niemann-Pick disease and lipoidosis. In the last, abnormal amounts of various lipoids are stored in the reticulo-endothelial system. The chief damage is in the brain cells, but in spite of this, diagnosis can be confirmed by a simple rectal biopsy involving approximately 1 cm of full thickness bowel wall.

Hypogammaglobulinaemia (Immuno-Deficiency Disease)

Hypogammaglobulinaemia is a rare condition mostly seen in boys and the principal manifestation is a marked tendency to infections, as the lack of gamma globulin prevents antibody formation.

Treatment. Gamma globulin is given by weekly injections and in some cases prophylactic antibiotic treatment is ordered.

Steatorrhoea

Steatorrhoea is a symptom rather than a disease in itself and by it is meant the passage of fluid or excessively soft stools containing an unusual amount of fat.

Steatorrhoea may be caused by some disturbance in the function of the small intestine and the amount of fat present in the stools may vary from amounts so small that they are only found in the process of careful analysis to visible, oily globules on the surface of the stools.

Causes. Causes include the following:

Absence of bile salts as in obstructive jaundice and infective hepatitis.
Absence of pancreatic enzymes as in fibrocystic disease of the pancreas.
Disorders of absorption as in coeliac syndrome.
Tuberculous peritonitis and mesenteric adenitis.

Ulceration of the bowel.
Lamblia intestinalis infection.

Some young infants suffer from mild fat intolerance causing fatty diarrhoea but this is readily treated by dietary measures and not necessarily due to disease.

Signs and Symptoms. The stools have a characteristic, highly offensive smell. Their appearance is putty-coloured, unformed and bulky and their frothy quality suggests the presence of fermentation. Occasionally fatty globules can be seen on the surface. The frequent loose evacuations may alternate with periods of constipation. Abdominal distension, redness around the anus, excoriated buttocks and rectal prolapse often accompany the steatorrhoea.

The affected child fails to thrive.

The abnormal fat losses and frequent stools may cause secondary symptoms such as a voracious appetite and tetany due to loss of calcium, which in turn results in a low blood calcium level, dehydration, stunted growth and lassitude.

Investigations. Investigations depend on the suspected, underlying cause and may include:

Mantoux test and X-ray of abdomen (tuberculosis).
Barium meal and X-ray (congenital abnormalities affecting the gut).
Glucose tolerance curve (this is a flat one in coeliac disease).
Analysis of duodenal secretions and stools for tryptic activity (fibrocystic disease of the pancreas—see page 307).
Sweat tests (fibrocystic disease of the pancreas—see page 307).
Examination of stools for ova, cysts, starch granules and excess of fat.
A fat balance will probably be done as one of the investigations.

Method. The fat balance is as a rule done over a period of 3 days. During that time a diet containing a known quantity of fat is given. At the end of the first 3 days a so-called marker is given (e.g. a capsule of indigo carmine) which colours the stools red. The diet is continued for a further 3 days and a further marker given at the end of that period. The collection of stools is stopped as soon as this marker has been passed. The fat content of the stools is analysed in the laboratory.

Not even the smallest amount of faeces must be wasted and it is useful to line the bedpan with cellophane paper or plastic material during the test period. The stool can then easily be lifted out and sent to the laboratory without wastage. The same can be done with a baby's napkins without causing much discomfort. Ways of collecting faeces in infants are given on page 258.

Care must be taken to ensure that the child has nothing by mouth beyond the prescribed diet (e.g. no chocolate brought in by visitors) and the parents' co-operation is essential. The nursing staff should keep them fully informed about the dietary restrictions. Any food not eaten, must be returned to the diet kitchen (including leftovers on the plate) and the fat content estimated and taken into account in the calculations. In a healthy individual 90 per cent of fat should be absorbed.

The Coeliac Syndrome

Coeliac disease is a chronic condition affecting young children. Children thus affected have grossly distended abdomens and pass large, pale offensive stools with a high fat content. They are generally wasted and growth is retarded. Periods of remission alternate with crises if the condition is left untreated.

The coeliac syndrome usually becomes established in the first year of life, frequently at the time of weaning. It is caused by malabsorption of food from the intestines and there is an abnormal sensitivity to gluten, found in wheat and rye.

Signs and Symptoms. Children with coeliac syndrome are stunted in growth and underweight and X-ray examination reveals osteoporosis (rarefaction) and immature development of bone due to poor vitamin absorption and calcium deficiency. Excess gas formation caused by fermentation of malabsorbed food causes abdominal pain and vomiting. The patient has a large, protuberant abdomen. The buttocks are wasted and the skin hangs in loose folds. The stools are bulky, putty coloured, unformed and greasy and have a characteristic, putrified smell. The child may have his bowels opened several times a day.

The child himself looks frail, stunted, pale and wizened, and usually utterly miserable, though the face may at first look round and well. The hair is sparse and dry, the limbs thin as drumsticks and cold to the touch. Poor muscle tone reflects itself in bad posture and rectal prolapse is common. Anaemia is a usual feature and sometimes a small blood transfusion or a course of Imferon will improve the child's condition considerably.

The appetite is very poor and capricious. These children often have the strangest whims and their feeding may tax the ingenuity and patience of the nurse to the utmost. The patient may insist on a special way of being served, on being fed by a particular person and on always having the same plate and feeding utensils. He may 'order' a particular dish and refuse it when it arrives. The slightest change in the accepted routine may cause a complete refusal of meals. These patients are negative in every way and often take an almost morbid interest in their illness. They are emotionally unstable, unhappy, and both apathetic and irritable at the same time.

Treatment. Relapses are now uncommon if parents can be persuaded to follow a diet free of gluten.* The child rapidly becomes happier, more comfortable and therefore less temperamental and the figure takes on normal lines and proportions. At first fat intake is restricted and extra protein is added to the diet. However, if all foods containing any product made from wheat and rye are omitted, a normal amount of fat can soon be taken. Gluten free bread, cakes and rusks can be obtained and gluten free flour can be made into cakes, bread, biscuits and puddings. A satisfactory diet can, however, be given without much extra work if foods made of maize (corn), oats, rice, sago and tapioca (not semolina) are substituted for those made of wheat and rye. Extra vitamins A and D, folic acid and iron should be given.

* Welfare Foods Ltd, Stockport, Cheshire; Vestric Ltd, 60 Graham St, London N.1.; Energen Food Company, London N.W.10.

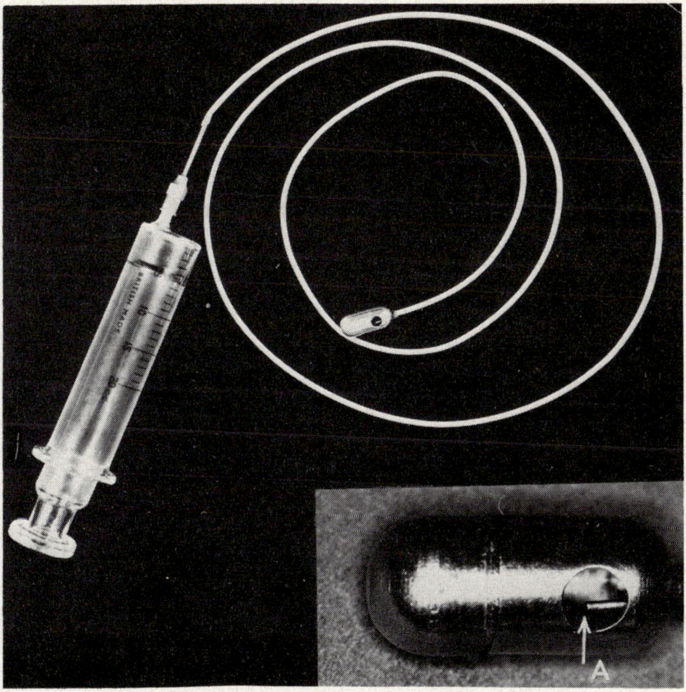

FIG. 51. A Crosby capsule, used to obtain small specimens of intestinal mucosa. (A) Mechanism fired to obtain specimen of intestinal mucosa.

Investigations. Analysis of stools, fat balance (see page 302), a complete blood count, a glucose tolerance test, a xylose excretion test and jejunal biopsy may all be performed. The fat balance will show that only 65 to 80 per cent against the normal 92 to 98 per cent of fat is absorbed, resulting in large amounts of split fats being excreted in the stools. The glucose tolerance tests show a flat curve. The jejunal biopsy is done with the aid of a Crosby Capsule (Fig. 51) and may reveal characteristic flatness of the mucosa of duodenum and jejunum.

Prognosis. With modern treatment, the prognosis should be favourable and improvement may be rapid. The stools soon become less bulky and offensive, the appetite improves and the child gains in weight and is happier.

Complications. Complications include intercurrent infections; oedema due to low serum protein; rickets and tetany due to impaired absorption of the fat soluble vitamins.

As excess amounts of potassium and fluids are lost in the large stools 'coeliac crises' due to electrolyte depletion occasionally call for urgent action. The child suddenly becomes severely dehydrated, lethargic and collapsed. The temperature may rise by several degrees. Intravenous therapy may be necessary to correct both the blood chemistry and the dehydration.

Nursing Care. Admission cannot always be avoided but the stay in hospital should be cut to a minimum while investigations are carried out and treatment is established.

Occasionally these children are acutely ill and during that time need careful nursing care. Because of emaciation, skin and mouth require special attention. Mouth toilet is carried out frequently and pressure areas are treated 4-hourly. Even slight wrinkles in the sheet, crumbs or a damp bed may cause bed sores which do not heal easily. After a bath the skin should be dabbed dry and a good dusting powder applied to the skin folds. The child should never be left sitting on a pot longer than is necessary, for fear of causing pressure sores and encouraging rectal prolapse.

Much can be done to reduce the bulk of the stools by adding a 5 per cent solution of Aroban in water to the food and chlorophyll tablets, taken orally, diminish their unpleasant odour.

As soon as possible, these children should be allowed to get up and lead a normal life. Schooling or play therapy are important in stimulating interest and speedy recovery. Frequent visiting will not only help the young patient but will also teach the mother much about the handling of her child and about the special diet. The mother must be told that even minor deviations from the prescribed diet may cause a serious relapse. The child may even need to persevere with the special diet well into adult life.

Cystic Fibrosis (Mucoviscidosis)

This condition is characterized by a disturbance of exocrine gland function, resulting in raised levels of sodium chloride in the sweat and thick mucous secretions from the secretory glands. In this country it is the most common of the inborn errors of metabolism, with an incidence of 1 in 2000 births. More than one child in the family may be affected as the disease is transmitted as a recessive gene carried by each parent.

The production of the abnormal mucus results in chronic lung infections, pancreatic insufficiency and intestinal obstruction in the newborn (meconium ileus).

Signs and Symptoms. Unlike the child suffering from coeliac disease, children with cystic fibrosis are friendly and good tempered. The appetite remains good in the absence of general infection but in spite of this there is failure to gain weight, growth is stunted, the abdomen is distended giving the child a 'barrel-like' appearance. The stools are pale and bulky, bowel actions are frequent and the smell is characteristically offensive.

When the disease is well established at birth intestinal obstruction results due to the failure to pass meconium. This is because the enzyme which would normally liquefy the meconium is absent. This serious condition requires urgent treatment either by surgery or treatment by Gastrografin enema under X-ray control.

Specific Investigations. Cystic fibrosis can be diagnosed at birth by the appearance of a bright blue colour at the end of the Boehringer meconium strip after smearing evenly with meconium and placing in water. This is due to the high albumin (over 20 per cent) content of cystic fibrosis meconium. Children with cystic fibrosis excrete increased amounts of sodium chloride in their sweat, and this fact is used as the basis for diagnostic tests. In a rapid screening test suitable for outpatients, the excess sodium chloride may be detected by placing the child's fingers on an agar plate containing silver nitrate and potassium chromate. If there is an excess of chlorides in the sweat, the impression shows up clearly as a grey fingerprint. The child's hands must have been washed half an hour before the test to remove excess sodium chloride and the results compared with those from a normal child.

For a more accurate test a sample of sweat may be collected on a weighed piece of filter paper (free from sodium chloride) after inducing local sweating by pilocarpine iontophoresis. The filter paper is taken to the laboratory in a sealed container for chemical determination. A child with cystic fibrosis usually excretes more than 80 mmol of sodium chloride per litre. In older children, rapid wrinkling of the skin of the fingers in water is a curious phenomenon due to the excess salt binding water in the surface tissues.

Duodenal Intubation. A Ryle's tube is passed into the stomach after the child has not had anything by mouth for at least 4 hrs, the tube is directed towards the pyloric sphincter. The child lies in the right lateral position to aid the tube to gravitate into the duodenum. Specimens are aspirated at frequent intervals and tested with litmus paper. A change from acid to alkaline reaction indicates that the tube has passed into the duodenum. Duodenal juice can now be withdrawn a minimum of 3 ml obtained, then immediately sent to the laboratory packed in ice whilst in transit.

As this procedure may take some considerable time, a nurse or the child's mother should sit with the child to amuse and comfort him.

Alternatively the tube may be passed in the X-ray department and screening will indicate that the catheter is actually in the duodenum; the juices are then aspirated.

Treatment. This aims at correcting pancreatic deficiencies with the replacement of pancreatic enzymes and dietary control to improve absorption. Pancreatic preparations may be given in the form of granules, powder or enteric coated tablets. The granules and powder have a strong taste and smell but many of the children learn to accept this very readily as part of their routine, some of the children prefer to take the preparation in cold milk or with cereal. Whatever preparation is prescribed by the paediatrician it must be taken before all main meals and snacks to be effective. The amount of pancreatin prescribed for the child must not be regarded as a fixed dose, parents are usually able to adjust the amount of pancreatin according to the fat content of the meal. Smaller low fat snacks will require a smaller dose of pancreatin than a main meal. Occasionally some irritation of the lips, chin or buttocks occurs, the dose should then be reduced for a short period.

In order to reduce the risk of chest infections a healthy open-air life away from crowds and air pollution should be encouraged. Long term antibiotic drugs may be prescribed therapeutically especially during the winter months.

Diet. These children require a high-calorie and high-protein diet in order to achieve a satisfactory growth and weight gain. Extra calories can be given in the form of sugary drinks, boiled sweets, chocolate and cakes made with honey, these are usually all enjoyed and prove popular with the children! Protein is absorbed badly, but the more the child takes the better in order to achieve normal growth and development. Those children with a low fat tolerance or who cannot take large doses of pancreatin need to have a fat restricted diet. In order to meet basic needs medium chain triglyceride fats (M.C.T. 34.7 J/g*) can be given and provide a useful source of calories. Roughage is best avoided in an attempt to reduce the bulky stools.

Vitamin supplements must be given regularly to all children with cystic fibrosis as deficiencies may quickly occur particularly of the fat soluble vitamins A, D, E and K.

In order to encourage the child to accept this diet, it should be served attractively and in small amounts. It is better to serve small frequent meals tempting to the appetite than two or three large meals a day. It must be remembered that pancreatin should be taken even with small snacks.

In hot climates salt supplements are advised in view of the excessive amount of sodium chloride lost in the sweat. This is not usually necessary in this country, but if the family are going abroad to a warmer climate they should be advised to take salt supplements with them. In any case it is a good idea to encourage the child normally to take added salt in normal amounts with all meals apart from that used by the mother in her cooking.

*1 Calorie = 4.18 Joules

Nursing Care. When intercurrent infection necessitates admission to hospital the child should if possible be admitted to a cubicle and away from any other infections that may be in the ward.

Oxygen therapy is frequently needed to relieve respiratory distress. The humidity of the tent may be increased by the use of a nebulizer through which compressed air is driven. Plain water is used or, alternatively, preparations such as Alevaire or Acetylcysteine can be added several times a day, this has a mucolytic effect making it easier for the child to expectorate the thinner secretions. Regular physiotherapy is an important part of treatment to aid expectoration of sputum and lung expansion. Physiotherapy should be continued throughout life. The child's parents are taught to take an active part in this treatment with encouragement and training in postural drainage, tipping and tapping, and breathing exercises.

Remembering the chronic nature of the illness, general attention should be given to the mouth and pressure areas. Clean linen must be given frequently with daily blanket baths as the child often feels sweaty and sticky. Deodorant talcum powders are much appreciated by the older child as an aid to freshness. To eliminate any odours as a result of the bulky offensive stools deodorant aerosols or wick should be used in the cubicle.

The prognosis of children with cystic fibrosis has much improved during the past few years as a result of vigorous treatment and care to combat respiratory infections which in the past resulted in death usually during adolescence. Parents need a great deal of help, to be able to support their child with this chronic condition, especially as they often feel guilty owing to the inherited nature of the disease. The medical social worker will be able to help and advise the parents with the many social and emotional problems that arise. Schooling and education must proceed according to the individual child, the accent being on his creative and intellectual talents rather than physical abilities.

Genetic counselling should be arranged in order that the parents understand the risks to future siblings if they wish to increase their family. Many parents obtain a great deal of help and support from the Cystic Fibrosis Society, a voluntary organization of parents (see p. 461).

Further Reading

CYSTIC FIBROSIS SYMPOSIUM (1964) London: Chest and Heart Publications.

FRANCIS, D. & DIXON, D. (1969) *Diets for Sick Children.* Oxford: Blackwell Scientific.

HOLTON, J. & TYFIELD, L. (1975) *The Child with Phenylketonuria.* London: National Society for Mentally Handicapped Children.

15

Diseases of the endocrine system

DISEASES of the endocrine system are comparatively rare in childhood but where they occur they may have a serious effect on mental and physical growth and maturation.

Those diseases which are so rare that they are unlikely to concern the nurse in training are omitted in this text.

The Thyroid Gland

Thyrotoxicosis

Over-secretion, causing thyrotoxicosis, is very uncommon in childhood. If it occurs, methyl thiouracil, carbimazole or potassium perchlorate and very occasionally surgery are employed in its treatment, in much the same way as for adults. Treatment by irradiation or radioactive iodine is considered unsuitable in children.

Hypothyroidism

Under-secretion of the thyroid gland causes cretinism in children. The condition, though congenital, is sometimes missed at birth as the infant carries a small amount of thyroid secretion from the maternal circulation. As the amount decreases, general metabolism is slowed down and symptoms appear.

Signs and Symptoms. All cretins have certain, typical characteristics. Their skin is cold, coarse and dry with a yellow appearance. The hair is brittle, sparse and lacks lustre and the hair line grows low down on to the constantly puckered brow. A broad, flat nose with a depressed bridge lies between the small widely spaced eyes. The lips are thick and as the tongue is apparently too large for the mouth, it protrudes. The abdomen is large, and constipation and umbilical hernia are common features. Pads of fat over the clavicles make the neck appear short. As bony development is retarded, the fontanelles are late in closing, the head seems disproportionately large and the first teeth are late in coming through. The entire appearance is heavy, coarse and dull. As general metabolism is suppressed, the temperature is subnormal and the pulse rate slow. Anaemia is common. Speech develops late and some cretins achieve only an elementary vocabulary. The voice is croaky and unmelodious. All milestones are late and, if left untreated, the child will be mentally severely subnormal, unable to look after himself.

Although not all these characteristics are noticeable at birth, a nurse will soon learn to recognize cretins at an early age. She may first notice the umbilical hernia and the constipation and, if she is alert and well-informed, may link these symptoms with the low temperature and sluggish pulse. Most cretins are poor feeders, at least partly due to the abnormally large tongue which makes sucking difficult and also causes attacks of suffocation. An observant nurse or midwife can contribute greatly to a good prognosis as early treatment is the key to success.

Investigations. The ones likely to be carried out are: blood cholesterol and serum lipid levels, both of which tend to be raised, creatinine and protein-bound iodine levels, which are abnormally low, X-ray of bones to estimate the bone age, electrocardiogram and blood picture. The basal metabolic rate is difficult to estimate in children but, if done, shows readings much below the normal.

Treatment. Treatment should be started without delay and will have to be continued throughout life in order to replace the thyroxine which the abnormal gland cannot produce. Treatment may be so successful that the child develops normally and cretins have been known to reach scholarship level. However, a great deal depends on the age at which treatment is begun. The treatment consists in giving Thyroxine in dosages just below the point at which signs of intolerance appear. The initial dose for infants is 25 μg daily and this is increased until tachycardia, diarrhoea and wakefulness suggest that the dosage has passed the tolerance level. Tolerance may be higher during the cold season than in the summer months. The maintenance dose is fixed slightly below the maximum reached during the stabilizing period.

Nursing Care and Observations. During the initial stage nursing care is symptomatic. The infant should be kept warm and the nurse feeding the baby will have to be both experienced and very patient. Suppositories or milk of magnesia will have to be given for the constipation and the skin should be kept supple with baby creams or lotions. Care must be taken when the baby is placed in his cot and it is safest to lie him on his side to guard against the danger of respiratory obstruction caused by the large tongue.

Once thyroid therapy has been started the nursing observations will be the principal guide in determining the maintenance dosage. Signs of response, such as an increased pulse rate and a rise in the body temperature, are all due to an increase in the metabolic rate. There is an improvement in the infant's colour and activity and a drop in weight due to the disappearance of the excess fat. The bowels will start to act regularly. The infant will begin to look around and play and will become more interested in his feeds.

The nurse should keep full and accurate observation charts. The feeds may have to be large for a time to satisfy the newly found appetite and to supply adequate nourishment for the sudden progress. As growth is rapid, extra vitamins should be given. It is well worth while to arrange for a little extra attention by the mother or nurse to encourage every attempt at play and to help the infant devélop his activities and mental achievements.

The Pituitary Gland

The chief importance of the pituitary gland is probably its influence on the other ductless glands. Abnormalities of the anterior lobe cause gigantism if there is over-secretion, dwarfism if there is under-secretion. Abnormalities of the posterior lobe cause *diabetes insipidus.*

The abnormalities may be congenital or may be caused by pressure from intracranial tumours or by inflammatory conditions such as encephalitis. None of these conditions are sufficiently common to warrant description in a small handbook and the reader is referred to larger text books for greater detail.

The hormone activity of the gland, however, is of great interest. The pituitary gland produces adrenocorticotrophic hormone (ACTH) which makes the adrenal cortex produce hormones with three effects:

1. On carbohydrate metabolism;
2. On mineral metabolism affecting blood electrolytes;
3. On growth and maturity including masculinization if there is excess in the female.

In addition excessive amounts can damp down inflammatory reactions by interfering with antigen–antibody reactions and can cause the production of ACTH to be lowered.

Cortisone or similar preparations such as prednisone, prednisolone or Triamcinolone can be given by mouth and hydrocortisone by injection for the following purposes:

1. To make up for deficiency of the adrenal activity as in shock or in Addison's disease;
2. To suppress the production of ACTH in cases of precocious sexual development of a masculine type;
3. To suppress antigen antibody reaction, as in rheumatic fever, rheumatoid arthritis, some types of nephritis, asthma and haemolytic anaemia.

ACTH may be given by injection for the last purpose (3) but would be useless in (1) and harmful in (2). If any of these drugs are given it may be necessary to counter their effect on mineral metabolism by giving potassium or calcium.

The Adrenal Glands

Diseases of the adrenal and suprarenal glands are extremely rare in childhood and are usually due to tumours, injury at birth resulting in haemorrhage, or infections such as tuberculosis. Both the diagnosis and treatment are difficult, though the discovery of cortisone has contributed much to the understanding of the diseases caused by over- or under-secretion of the glands.

Tumours of the medulla are often malignant and cause metastases in the liver, lungs and bone tissue. Surgery in the less malignant type of tumours however carries a hopeful prognosis. The adrenal medulla produces adrenaline and noradrenaline which, like cortisone, have a place in the treatment of asthma and shock.

Over-activity of the adrenal cortex leads to sexual precocity in both sexes and to virilism in the female. The over-activity may be present before birth and in this case causes pseudo-hermaphroditism (see below). In the young child over-activity causes sexual precocity and virilism and if the anterior pituitary gland is secondarily affected, Cushing's syndrome will result. True Cushing's syndrome is rare in childhood but it is often simulated when a child is having too large a dose of steroids. The child characteristically becomes 'moon-faced', looking flushed and bloated. Obesity develops with pads of fat accumulating on the upper part of the back, producing a 'buffalo hump' together with a fat abdomen and hips. In contrast the limbs remain thin. Growth of hair occurs on the face and body, together with purple striae on the trunk. Acne is common. Hypertension is usually present, and the child may complain of headaches. Glycosuria may also be found on routine ward testing.

Adrenogenital Syndrome

Very occasionally in some children there is difficulty in determining the sex of the child, owing to the malformation of the external genitalia in the male or masculinization of the genitalia in the female. This occurs as a congenital or as an acquired disorder. For a correct sex determination to be made it is necessary for chromosome studies to be carried out. To avoid distress to the parents and to the child in subsequent development it is important in all these cases that necessary examination of the blood, urine and smears from the buccal membrane are undertaken before the birth is registered.

Great understanding and tact is needed in helping the parents to understand and adjust to the condition of their child. Cortisone therapy and plastic surgery may be beneficial to some of these children. Nurses should see to it that these children are not subjected to unnecessary examinations as even very young children are sensitive to handling of the genital area, and repeated examination of this region may produce morbid introspection on part of the child.

The parents of children who are receiving steroid therapy should understand the need to adjust the dosage under stress and infections; failure to do so may result in acute adrenal crisis.

The Parathyroid Glands

There are four parathyroid glands and they are situated behind the thyroid gland. Their function is concerned with the regulation of calcium and phosphorus levels of the body.

Low activity of the gland may be due to damage or removal during the operation of thyroidectomy and may produce tetany, convulsions, osteoporosis and repeated fractures. The blood calcium is low. Treatment consists in giving high doses of vitamin D (calciferol) and a high calcium and low phosphorus intake in the diet.

Excessive activity of the gland may be due to a tumour or hyperplasia of the glands. Large amounts of calcium are excreted in the urine and calcification of the kidneys may occur. Sometimes characteristic cystic lesions are seen on X-ray examination of the bones. Treatment is surgical.

Diabetes Mellitus

Diabetic patients suffer from deficient insulin action caused either by a diminished insulin excretion by the islets of Langerhans in the pancreas, or due to the presence of insulin antagonists which render any insulin produced ineffective for carbohydrate metabolism resulting in glycosuria, ketosis and eventually coma.

Even newborn infants may occasionally suffer from diabetes, and apnoeic or cyanotic attacks in premature or ill-nourished infants should always be investigated. The disease, however, is very rare under the age of 2 years. In about a quarter of all cases there is a family history of diabetes. The basic cause of the disease is similar to that in adults. Insulin has to be given in most cases as severe dietary restrictions may impede the normal growth of the child, even in mild cases. The disease is frequently severe and dangerous fluctuations in blood sugar levels due to variable activities and childhood illness are common.

In children, the onset of diabetes is usually very sudden and, although never actually responsible for the disease, infections such as tonsillitis or measles, and emotional stress seem to act as the trigger starting off the symptoms.

Signs and Symptoms. Most obvious, and therefore often first noticed, is the sudden excessive thirst coupled with frequency of micturition or the onset of enuresis in a previously clean child. The output of urine is large but in spite of this it is of high specific gravity. The child grows listless and fractious. As dehydration occurs, his skin becomes dry and he is constipated. The breath may smell of acetone. The tongue is dry but, as a rule, it remains clean but abnormally red. Loss of weight may be rapid and considerable and a proportion of children develop an unusual appetite.

The penis or vulva is often red and irritating due to the high sugar content of the urine, and the child may complain of abdominal pain. As ketosis increases, vomiting sets in and may hasten the occurrence of diabetic coma. The urine contains sugar and acetone.

Investigations. These include testing of urine, blood sugar estimation and glucose tolerance tests, similar to those done for adults. If possible, tests involving pricks and fasting should be spaced and not all done the first day after admission, as it is important to preserve the young patient's confidence since he will probably be starting on a lifetime of daily insulin injections. In testing for acetone, many physicians prefer the ferric chloride test to Rothera's test as the latter is extremely sensitive. If the ferric chloride test is positive for acetone there is a definite danger of diabetic coma. A quick alternative test can be done with Acetest tablets. It is important to remember that the test may appear positive if aspirin has been taken.

Treatment. Some specialists like to treat these children as out-patients as they feel that the child should be assessed and stabilized under his usual living conditions. The majority feel, however, that the child should be admitted to hospital so that the investigations and the initial stabilizing can take place under controlled and known conditions. The fact that in hospital the child's activities are of necessity restricted should always be borne in mind. The mother should be asked about the child's normal routine and exercise should be given so that the child's usual energy output is maintained. He may for instance be allowed to accompany the ward orderly on errands. Diabetic children should never be kept in bed unnecessarily. From the start, a healthy attitude and interest should be fostered and any special diet should be accepted as a natural part of the young diabetic's routine. It is interesting to note how upsets such as home sickness can cause variations in the blood sugar levels and also that acetone is most frequently found in the urine of children who have failed to settle down happily at boarding school or in hospital.

The Diet. With the present-day insulins, which are very stable and long acting (e.g. the Lente group), the child, once stabilized, can be kept free from reactions by allowing his appetite to regulate his blood sugar levels. It will be found that if he has been unusually energetic he will also be very hungry, and if he has sat quietly for a time his appetite will decrease. Periodic tests to estimate the serum cholesterol levels are done. If the level rises, foods containing cholesterol are omitted from the diet (e.g. eggs) as a persistently raised serum cholesterol level predisposes to vascular changes in later life. Children receiving an unrestricted diet are much less likely to have the psychological problems which children who are placed on a restricted diet tend to develop. However, some paediatricians continue to advocate a strictly controlled diet on the grounds that it lessens the chances of future vascular complications. For children who are learning about the importance of diet, playing cards, charts and games which help to memorize food values, exist.

Insulin Therapy. The dose of insulin will have to be readjusted until the condition is stabilized. This may not happen until some weeks after discharge home. Adjustment will usually become necessary when the child has an infection or any severe emotional upset, as he grows and increases in weight and especially at the time of puberty. The aim is to find the dose which will enable the child to live a normal life on a diet adequate for growth, energy and enjoyment of life.

Operations such as tonsillectomy or even major surgery can be safely carried out providing they are done under controlled conditions. Glucose, equal to the normal diet in carbohydrate value, is given at any time when a meal has to be omitted.

Cortisone, owing to its action on carbohydrate metabolism, is not a suitable drug for use in diabetic patients.

It is here assumed that the reader has already a sound understanding of the types of insulin available and of the various syringes and their markings, as well as of the principles involved in insulin therapy. In these aspects there is no difference when dealing with young diabetics as compared with adults, but the approach to the problem of diabetes in childhood is important and specialized.

Both the parents and the child should be taught how to give injections and test the urine and, as far as they are capable, they should be taught to understand the principles involved. They should also be taught confidence and the child himself should take a healthy interest in his illness. By the age of 8 years it should be possible to teach a sensible patient to give his own insulin and to draw up the dose himself, even if it is still checked by his parents (Fig. 52).

The site of the injections should be as varied as is possible in order to prevent thickening of the tissues and local fat atrophy which, though harmless, causes unsightly depressions and irregularities in the contours of the limb. The injection should be given fairly deeply with the needle almost at right angles to the skin. Alternatively, a Palmer mechanical injector, shaped rather like a pistol, can be used.

General Points. Both the young patient and his parents should be helped to come to grips with the disability and the latter not allowed to make the child into an invalid by misplaced solicitude. Both the parents and the child, once he is old enough, should be taught the fundamentals of the illness and should be allowed to practise urine testing and the giving of injections well before discharge, so as to gain confidence and dexterity in so doing.

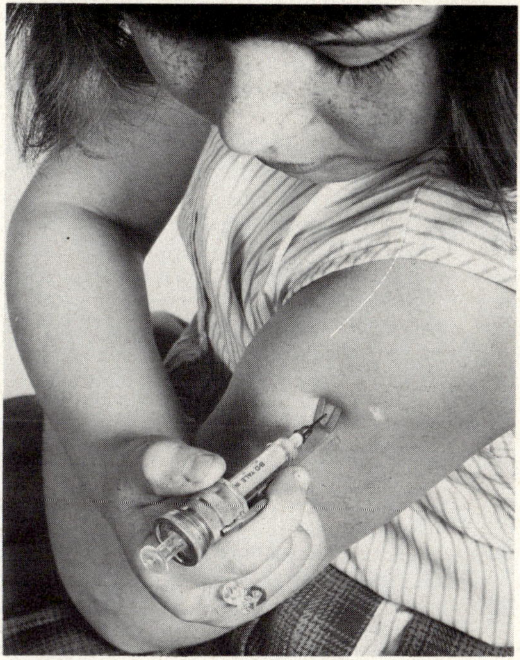

FIG. 52. Diabetic child giving own injection of insulin using automatic injector.

It is a good plan to allow the child to experience one or more insulin reactions while still under supervision in hospital so that after his discharge he will be able to guard himself in good time against any serious hypoglycaemic reaction.

Most diabetic children can attend normal schools provided the teachers know of their condition. Hypoglycaemic reaction is often heralded by naughty or unusual behaviour, and glucose or a lump of sugar may correct the hypoglycaemia without much disturbance. Teachers should have sugar or glucose available, but as soon as he is old enough the young diabetic should be made responsible for recognizing and dealing with a hypoglycaemic reaction by taking sugar from his own supply It is possible to allow diabetic children to have the usual school meals, as the high carbohydrate content of school puddings supplies the extra amount needed during the exertion of the afternoon games period.

For holidays, under controlled conditions and supervision, the Diabetic Association runs holiday camps which have the added value that the children meet other diabetics, often learn much from each other and come to realize that they are not alone with their abnormality.

Parents should be advised to let the child carry a card or disc with his name and address, particulars of his disease and the emergency treatment required. Undesirable food or sweets should be kept out of temptation's way but on the whole a normal outlook and existence should be encouraged.

Hyperglycaemic or Diabetic Coma

The signs of oncoming coma are essentially the same in children as in adults, but a child's behaviour may differ according to his age. Thus a very young child may demand to be put to bed or may curl up in a corner and fall asleep. Shock and dehydration often come on very rapidly and both may be severe.

Hypoglycaemic or Insulin Coma

Insulin coma comes on even more suddenly than diabetic coma. It often happens that the child is hard to wake in the morning and, when roused, looks pale and apprehensive and shows a peculiar emotional behaviour.

Points of Importance. If there is any doubt about the nature of the reaction, the child should be given some glucose as little harm can be done by hyperglycaemia, while insulin coma may require urgent relief. It is useful to remember that 2 slightly heaped teaspoonfuls of sugar in water equal approximately 10 g of carbohydrate.

Further Reading

FARQUHAR. J. W. (1975) *Notes for the Guidance of the Parents of Diabetic Children*, 2nd ed. London & Edinburgh: Churchill Livingstone.

HAMILTON, W. (1972) *Clinical Paediatric Endocrinology*. London: Butterworths.

16

The genito-urinary system

THE KIDNEY excretes waste products of metabolism, and acts as a filter and re-absorbs certain substances necessary to the body. A nurse who understands the importance of any abnormalities in the urine and who uses her powers of observation to the full should not find the toilet round a boring routine but will appreciate her responsibility in this respect. Her careful reporting may help the physician who relies on the accuracy of her reports and tests.

Observations should be recorded clearly and accurately on the patient's chart and abbreviations should be avoided as they may easily lead to misinterpretations or misunderstandings. The presence of albumin for example should be charted as being a trace, a moderate, or a large amount and not merely charted as one, or several + signs.

Methods of Collecting Clean and Ordinary Specimens of Urine

Even newborn babies may show signs of renal damage due to abnormalities present in utero, e.g. back pressure caused by inadequate relaxation of the bladder neck or sphincter or inadequate muscle action in the bladder wall or ureters. Such damage is usually irreversible.

Infection in infancy, caused by ascending bacterial invasion or by deformities such as double ureters, neurogenic bladder, horseshoe kidney, etc., may lead to permanent renal damage in later life unless treated at the earliest possible moment. Careful collection of urine for examination is therefore of very great importance.

Accurate measurement of the urinary output and drainage is of paramount importance as it may be an aid to diagnosis and lead to the prevention of serious complications. Where appropriate the nurse should state whether the urine came from a nephrostomy, perineal or supra-pubic or urethral catheter or if it was passed normally per urethram.

It may be difficult to collect urine from babies and toddlers. The container should be of appropriate size for the amount of urine collected (e.g. 10 ml bottles are quite adequate for babies). Special plastic urine collecting bags may be used both for boys and girls (Fig. 53). Where these are not available the following techniques can be used:

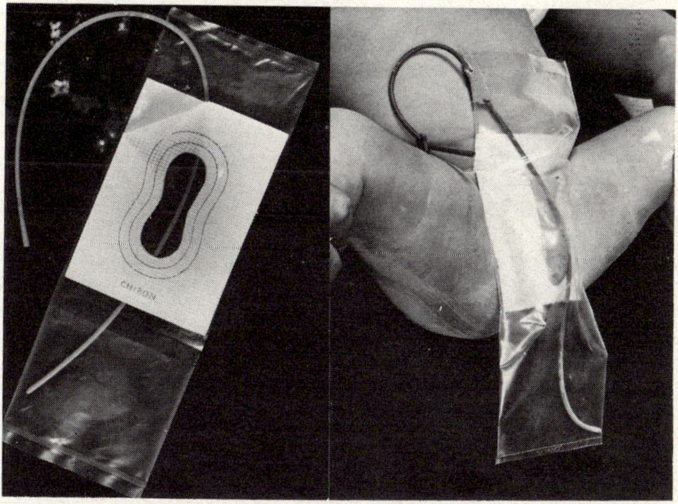

FIG. 53. Urine collecting bag (*left*), in position (*right*). The bag may be used for either boys or girls for obtaining single specimens, or for 24-hour collections.

Baby boys. Urine may be collected by strapping a test tube or Paul's tubing to the penis. If the specimen is for bacteriological investigation, an aseptic technique should be used. A tray with receivers and sterile cotton wool swabs, saline or a mild antiseptic solution, such as 1 per cent cetrimide, a sterile test tube or Paul's tubing, and four lengths of 6 mm ($\frac{1}{4}$ in) strapping is required. The penis is well cleaned, where possible the foreskin retracted and the glans gently swabbed before fixing the tube in position. Paul's tubing, previously sterilized, is easy to use and very effective.

Baby girls. Baby girls present a much more difficult problem. It may be advisable to wash and swab the buttocks and genitalia carefully before commencing a feed and then to sit the baby on a sterile receiver while she is feeding. Babies often pass urine during a feed.

Alternatively, a sterile receiver may be placed inside a well fitting air-ring and the baby nursed sitting upright over the opening. If these methods fail, the baby may be placed in a 'hiatus hernia chair' with a hole in the seat.

Specimens obtained in this way, are usually accepted for bacteriological examination but sometimes a catheter specimen is required for absolute reliability. In some units where metabolic beds are available, these may be used when 24-hour specimens are required. In view of the difficulties often encountered when collecting specimens of urine from young children, it is essential that such specimens should, once obtained, go to the pathological laboratory without delay.

Catheterization. Catheterization in young children should be avoided whenever possible. Sometimes catheterization may have to be carried out for diagnostic purposes, to relieve retention of urine, in preparation for operation and in certain post-operative cases. In the two last instances the catheter may be left in situ for several days.

Basically the requirements are the same for children as for adults. It is, however, essential to have at least one assistant who will ensure that the child maintains the correct position without struggling and who can reassure and talk to the child.

Little girls should have their buttocks raised on a sand bag. When the buttocks are thus elevated the catheter should be directed downwards rather than at right angles to the perineum, as it would be with an adult. As the urethra is short urine should be obtained after passing only 2.5 to 5 cm (1 to 2 in) of the catheter. It is important to wash the groins, thighs and genitalia with soap and water before starting the actual catheterization. When the procedure is completed the surrounding skin should be carefully dried and powdered. A pot or bedpan should be offered as catheterization leaves the patient with a feeling of irritation and an apparent desire to pass urine.

Supra-pubic aspiration in order to obtain sterile urine specimens is often now carried out instead of catheterization. This procedure is performed by a doctor with a fine needle and syringe. By this means the specimen obtained is not contaminated with other organisms, and there is less likelihood of introducing infection into the bladder.

Mid-Stream Specimens. With older children, capable of co-operation and control in passing urine, this method can replace catheterization in many cases. After cleaning the genital area in the method described above, the child is asked to pass some urine in order to flush the urethra. After approximately 30 g (1 oz) has been passed the stream is interrupted and the remaining urine collected in a sterile container with clear indication that the specimen was a mid-stream one.

Twenty-Four-Hour Specimens. To estimate accurately the volume of urine passed in 24 hours, the following procedure is adopted.

The patient is asked to empty the bladder at 08.00 hours and this urine is discarded. All urine passed in the following 24 hrs is then collected. The patient is asked to pass urine at 07.55 hours the following day and this specimen is added to the total collected.

Early Morning Specimens. Specimens of urine taken on waking are usually highly concentrated.

Retention of Urine

This, irrespective of the cause, may produce restlessness in unconscious patients and may disturb sleep. Simple nursing measures may relieve retention. The nurse can partly fill the pot or bedpan with warm water, she can irrigate the pubic area with warm water, sit the patient in a warm bath, allow small boys to stand up while using a bottle, and run a near-by tap. Such nursing attention is infinitely worth while and may make painful, complicated measures such as catheterization unnecessary.

Investigations of the Urinary Tract

Investigations involving X-rays are often unavoidable, but in all cases exposure to X-rays is reduced to a minimum remembering hazards caused by X-ray radiation.

Intravenous Pyelography

Intravenous pyelograms are done to outline the urinary tract and demonstrate the efficiency of renal function. Fluids are withheld for the 12 hours preceding the test. In some hospitals a vegetable aperient is ordered. Charcoal biscuits or tablets may be given during the morning to help absorb gas in the intestine. Children tend to swallow much air and to have more intestinal gases than adults and it is often difficult to obtain a satisfactory pyelogram. The following scheme may be used with some success. The child is given a bottle of fizzy drink and instructed to drink it through a straw. The fizzy drink tends to distend the stomach which in turn displaces the small intestine in a downward direction. A clear picture of the renal pelves and upper ureters can now be obtained. This procedure can be adopted with quite young babies without any harm, but it is obviously not useful if the lower portions of the ureters are to be shown up. If the child is well enough he should be allowed to be up and to run about as, together with abdominal massage, this may help to rid the bowel of stagnating gases which might obscure the radiograph. The patient should be asked to pass urine just before going to the X-ray department.

A straight radiograph is taken first, in order to ascertain that no gases will obscure the picture. If this is satisfactory a radio-opaque dye is then injected into a vein. In most cases the median basilic vein is chosen for the injection but with babies it may be necessary to use another vein or to give the dye intramuscularly. In that case hyaluronidase is used in conjunction with the dye,

SOME ABNORMAL SUBSTANCES WHICH MAY BE PRESENT IN THE URINE IN CERTAIN DISEASES

BLOOD *Haematuria*	SUGAR *Glycosuria*	ALBUMIN *Albuminuria*	BILE *Biluria*	PUS *Pyuria*	DIACETIC ACID OR ACETONE *Ketonuria*	HAEMOGLOBIN *Haemoglobinuria*
Nephritis	Diabetes mellitus	Nephritis	Infective hepatitis	Cystitis	Diabetes mellitus	Severe burns
Pyelonephritis	Low renal threshold	Pyelitis	Congenital obliteration of the bile duct	Pyelonephritis	Starvation	Severe infections
Tuberculosis	Excess carbohydrate intake	Cystitis			Severe vomiting	Incompatible blood transfusion
Calculi *Wilms's tumour* *Polycystic kidneys* *Trauma*		Fevers Congestive heart failure In the presence of pus			Infections Emotional causes After operations	*Note*: There are no red cells present
Foreign body in the bladder		In the presence of blood				
Purpura		Orthostatic albuminuria				
Leukaemia		Emotional causes				
Haemophilia *Sulph. therapy*						

Note: Red urine may be caused by urate crystals in infancy, by certain sweets and by beetroot. Other abnormalities may occur but they are rare and are not included in this table.

in order to speed up and facilitate absorption. The dye is rapidly excreted by the urinary tract.

Pictures are taken after 3, 8, 15 and 30 minutes, and the progress of the dye is watched. Any abnormalities in the filling of the renal tract or in excretion are demonstrated on the radiograph.

Micturating Cystogram

Co-operation will be needed from the older child during this procedure, so the nurse should carefully explain what is involved prior to catheterization. If the mother is accompanying the child, she too should clearly understand the procedure. A small child may have the examination carried out under a general aneasthetic. The child is usually catherized in the ward, before transfer to the X-ray department. Following introduction of the contrast medium through the catheter, which is then removed and the child encouraged to pass urine. As the bladder contracts X-rays are taken. If the cystogram is being carried out under a general anaesthetic, supra-pubic pressure is needed to empty the bladder.

Cystoscopy

Cystoscopy is exactly the same as with adults except that children are given a light anaesthetic. Cystoscopy is usually done to examine the bladder, urethra, and ureteric openings into the bladder for congenital abnormalities.

Retrograde Pyelography

For this procedure a light anaesthetic has to be given but otherwise preparation is the same as for intravenous pyelogram, and the procedure is similar to that used in adults.

Cystography

Cystography may be done in order to determine the capacity and outline of the bladder or to demonstrate the presence of urethral valves and vesico-ureteric reflux.

Urea Clearance Test

A comparison is made between the amount of urea present in the circulation and urine respectively. The test demonstrates the extent of healthily functioning substance in the kidney, following disease.

Investigation for Tuberculosis

For tuberculosis investigation, an early morning specimen of urine is sent to the laboratory on three successive days and injected into a guinea-pig. Four to 6 weeks later the guinea-pig is killed to see if it has developed tuberculosis.

Diseases of the Genito-Urinary Tract

Vulvovaginitis

Vulvovaginitis is a fairly common condition, especially in little girls from 3 to 10 years old.

Causes. These include lack of cleanliness, strongly acid urine, diabetes mellitus, eczema, threadworm infestation, gonorrhoea or foreign bodies. The latter may be particles of clothing 'sucked into the vagina' and lodged in the post-hymenal recess, or they may have been pushed into the vagina as young children do into any body orifice.

Signs and Symptoms. The child will frequently complain of soreness between the legs or alternatively the mother will notice a reluctance to let her touch and wash this area. She may also notice that the knickers are stained with discharge. On examination the labia are found to be red and oedematous, they may be stuck together and there is a ropy mucoid discharge.

Treatment. This will depend largely on the underlying cause. The area should, however, be washed frequently, dried by gentle dabbing with a soft towel. Antiseptic baths are soothing and speed up treatment.

General Care. The patient is frequently debilitated and efforts should be made to build up general health. The mother may be given advice about general hygiene.

Barrier Nursing. It is usual to nurse these children with barrier precautions for the first few days until the discharge has cleared. A swab is sent to the laboratory to determine the nature of the infection. Gonorrhoea should always be considered, and treated if present.

Special Points. Despite their age, these little girls are often very sensitive about their condition. Examination should be tactful. Screens should always be used when treatment has to be carried out, in order to ensure privacy. Vaginal douching is considered unsuitable during childhood, mainly on account of the psychological trauma which may be caused.

Early symptoms of urinary infection in very young infants are easily overlooked. However, symptoms such as anorexia, fever, vomiting, apathy and failure to thrive should alert the doctor and nurse, and a clean specimen of urine should be sent to the laboratory. Catheter specimens are usually unnecessary and are to be deprecated (see page 326).

Acute Pyelonephritis (Pyelitis)

This is essentially an infection of the renal parenchyma and the pelvis of the kidney. The disease is a very common one in childhood, affecting girls rather more often than boys and it occurs frequently in very young infants.

Mode of Infection. The infection may reach the kidneys via the blood stream, from the bowel via the lymphatic system or as an ascending infection from the bladder and urethra. In many cases the infection is caused by a malformation in the urinary tract, such as a kink in one of the ureters which causes the urine to be dammed back, to stagnate and to become infected.

In about 70 per cent of cases the causative organism is the *Escherichia coli* (bacterium), but streptococcal and staphylococcal infections also occur.

Signs and Symptoms. As a rule the onset of the disease is a very sudden one. One of the earliest symptoms is vomiting, soon followed by a rise in temperature to 39.4° to 40.6°C (103° to 105°F); rigors and meningism are common. The child is pale and ashen in colour, with flushed cheeks and dark rings round the eyes. She is irritable and there are signs that she is suffering from spasmodic, colicky pain, which is a constant feature. With young babies diarrhoea occurs and this together with the vomiting soon causes dehydration. The urine is scanty, strongly acid and may have a curious fishy smell. The tongue is dry and thirst is marked. If old enough to do so the patient complains of a burning sensation on micturition.

Complications. In extreme cases head retraction is present, a squint may develop and convulsions occur. It is in fact not always easy to distinguish the symptoms from those of meningitis on account of the meningismus, or of appendicitis on account of the abdominal pain and vomiting.

Investigations. Examination of a clean specimen of fresh urine under the microscope will reveal the presence of pus cells, albumin and organisms. The prognosis is as a rule a good one, recovery taking place in 3 days to a week. Recurrent cases are often due to malformations in the urinary tract and therefore X-ray investigations are carried out. The prognosis depends on the underlying cause.

Nursing Care. The nursing care in the case of an attack of pyelitis is mostly symptomatic. In order to reduce the temperature, the bedclothes are cradled and a fan may be used to cool and circulate the air. Tepid sponging is soothing but must not be done without medical permission. If the patient is incontinent the buttocks should be washed frequently as the acid urine is liable to excoriate the skin. Zinc and castor oil cream should be applied. The mouth easily gets dry and dirty, and careful mouth toilet is essential.

Temperature, pulse and respirations are taken and recorded 4-hourly and a strict intake and output record is important. If vomiting persists and dehydration becomes marked, fluids may have to be given intravenously.

Constipation may be marked and may have to be treated. Local applications of heat over the loins may help to relieve the pain.

Drugs. According to the sensitivity of the causative organism, various drugs such as: sulphonamides, nitrofurantoin, cephaloridine, colistin.

Diet. In the majority of cases the patient should be given liberal amounts of fluids especially while on sulphonamide therapy. For babies milk is withheld as long as vomiting persists. Once the acute stage of the illness is passed, the children quickly regain their appetite and no special diets need be given.

Cystitis

Cystitis (inflammation of the bladder) is rarely seen as a primary disease but is frequently associated with inflammation in other parts of the urinary tract. The cause may be infected, stagnating urine as in paralyses, infection following catheterization or malformation of the bladder and rectum.

Signs and Symptoms. The child complains of frequency and of burning pain on micturition. The temperature may be raised. On examination the urine is found to contain pus, mucus and occasionally blood.

Treatment. The nursing care is similar to that for pyelitis. Alkali mixtures, sulphonamides and antibiotics may be given. Bladder wash-outs may be ordered and a liberal fluid intake is essential.

Orthostatic Albuminuria

Orthostatic or postural albuminuria is a harmless condition which often is discovered only accidentally, for example in the course of a School Medical Inspection.

Signs and Symptoms. The albumin is present only after the child has been in the upright position for some time, hence early morning specimens are free from albumin. Children with orthostatic albuminuria commonly show signs of generalized poor tone. They have poor posture, lordosis is common and they are thin and frequently suffer from chilblains.

Prognosis. Parents may be reassured about this condition and the child should be treated as normal.

Nephritis

A variety of classifications of nephritis have been used in the past, but the term nephritis is now used for those conditions in which inflammatory changes predominate in the renal substance. Nephrosis or nephrotic syndrome is characterized by degenerative changes in the renal tubules. Sometimes it is difficult to draw a distinction between the two conditions and in the subacute phase the term 'nephrotic-nephritis' may be used.

	Nephritis	*Nephrotic syndrome*
Onset	Very sudden	Insidious
Cause	Streptococcal infection 10 to 14 days previously in 75% of cases	Unknown in many cases in others associated with renal disease
Age	Commonly 3 to 8 years, rarely in infancy	All ages
Haematuria	Present	Rarely present
Proteinuria	Moderate degree	Considerable
Urinary output	Diminished	Variable
Oedema	Of short duration if it occurs	Persistent
Blood pressure	Raised at onset	Usually normal
Diet	Restricted protein. Low salt if oedema present	High protein, low salt

Nephritis

(Ellis type I; Acute post streptococcal glomerulonephritis; acute haemorrhagic nephritis.)

Definition. A disease of sudden onset, usually following a streptococcal infection (most commonly tonsillitis) 10 to 14 days prior to onset of haematuria, hypertension and acute renal inflammation.

Pathology. Both kidneys are affected, but are of normal size. Microscopical appearance shows minute haemorrhages blocking the glomeruli which means that the filtering capacity of the kidneys is interfered with; small areas of necrosis may also be seen.

Age. Affects most commonly the age group 3 to 8 years; rarely in infancy.

Clinical Presentation. The passage of blood-stained urine is often the presenting symptom, it may be very obvious or only minimal giving a 'smoky' appearance to the urine. This may last for a few days or for many weeks. Urinary output at onset of the disease is usually diminished. The child appears 'off colour', disinterested in his normal play activities and very lethargic. Headache and vomiting frequently occur at onset of the disease. Oedema is common, and is especially noted in the eyelids and the pendant parts, but is of short duration. It is associated with an increase in weight. In cases of streptococcal infection the anti-streptolysin titre is raised. The temperature is elevated and the blood pressure may remain normal but more commonly it will also be raised.

Investigations. These will include daily ward tests of urine, quantitative daily albumin estimations may also be recorded. Laboratory examination of the urine to detect the presence of cells and casts will be required at frequent intervals, but less often once the haematuria has disappeared. As the kidney cannot clear the waste products in the normal way, the blood urea level may rise above 7.47 mmol/litre (45 mg/100 ml) or more, and creatinine and phosphorus levels are also higher than usual. Culture of throat swabs and a full blood count will also be made. X-ray of the sinuses and examination of the tonsils and teeth are carried out in order to discover any foci of infection.

Treatment. Diet, rest and good nursing care are the main forms of treatment. Penicillin may be prescribed for any latent streptococcal infection. Anaemia is treated with iron therapy. Sulphadimidine 1 g daily may be ordered as a prophylactic measure against infection.

Nursing Care. Children suffering from nephritis are kept on bed rest, until urinary output and blood pressure are normal, and the haematuria has subsided. The child should be kept warm, and nursed in a semi-recumbent position so that he is comfortable, resting, and yet able to watch the life of the ward around him. A daily blanket bath is given and the pressure areas treated 4-hourly. Mouth care is particularly important, and is carried out frequently. If constipation is troublesome a mild aperient may be given.

The nurse should make time to play and read with her patient in order to relieve the monotony of bed rest. Parental visiting should be encouraged to enable the child to maintain his family contacts, and to adjust to hospitalization. Later, the child will be able to take part in the activities of the hospital school.

Observations

1. Temperature, pulse and respirations are recorded 4-hourly initially as any change may be the first indication of complications developing, e.g. further infection.
2. Fluid intake and output should be recorded with accuracy.
3. Frequent recordings of the child's weight are made; it is most useful to chart this as a graph to show progress, as it is a good guide to the amount of oedema present.
4. Blood pressure readings are taken twice daily initially, then less frequently if good progress is made. Any rise in the blood pressure readings must be reported immediately.
5. The appearance of an early morning specimen of urine should be noted daily.
6. Note of the child's general appearance must also be made, e.g. how he looks and if he appears to be more or less interested in his surroundings. Any observation of

twitching of the limbs should be reported immediately as this may be an indication that hypertensive encephalopathy, a serious complication, is developing.

Diet. In order to rest the kidneys the fluid intake is usually restricted during the initial phase; the amount allowed varies according to the child's weight.

Examples of the Amount of Fluid Allowed in 24 hours

5 years	18 kg (40 lb)	Basic allowance	360 ml (12 oz)
10 years	30 kg (66 lb)	Basic allowance	480 ml (16 oz)

Added to the basic allowance would be an amount equal to the volume of urine passed during the previous 24 hours.

For the first 3 or 4 days the child's diet consists of fresh fruit drinks with added glucose. Orange juice should be avoided in view of its relatively high potassium content. The nurse should remember that the child will enjoy variety, and hot drinks as well as cold should be offered to relieve the monotony of the fluid diet. When diuresis occurs a light diet is gradually introduced, the protein of which is restricted until the urine tests show an improvement in the cell count. While any oedema is present, salt intake too will be restricted.

Prognosis

1. The majority of cases are uncomplicated and usually resolve in about 6 weeks.
2. Rarely hypertension may lead to cardiac failure and encephalopathy. A few patients progress into the nephrotic syndrome. If anuria develops the outlook is grave.

Nephrosis, or Nephrotic Syndrome

(Lipoid Nephrosis, Sub-acute Nephritis.)

Definition. This condition is manifested clinically by insidious onset of gross generalized oedema, and by proteinuria, associated with low plasma proteins.

Pathology. Both kidneys are affected and appear very pale and swollen.

Age. Pure nephrosis or lipoid nephrosis, starts in children below the age of 5 years. Nephrotic syndrome, associated with a variety of other kidney conditions is seen in older children.

Clinical Presentation (Fig. 54). The mother will tell of a gradual onset of oedema involving the face, extremities and later the whole body. She will also have noticed a gain in weight, and reduction in urinary output. The oedema may involve the peritoneal cavity (ascites) and the pleural cavity

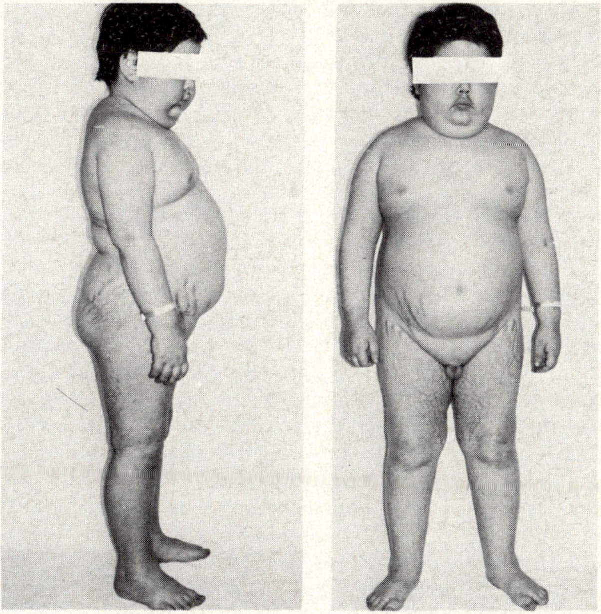

FIG. 54. A child with nephrotic syndrome who is also Cushingoid from the effect of over-treatment with steroids.

(hydrothorax) so that the patient may complain of dyspnoea. The child looks extremely pale as there is an associated anaemia, and he appears listless and distinterested in food.

The oedema which is gravitational may be so gross that the child is unable to open his eyes, and with boys swelling of the penis and scrotum may become very distressing. The urine is highly concentrated with a low sodium content and it is passed in small amounts. Hypertensive encephalopathy may ensue and this is treated by the use of hypotensive drugs, e.g. reserpine.

Investigations. Daily ward testing of urine and estimation of the amount of protein lost in the urine. Frequent laboratory examination of the urine for cells and casts, also culture for evidence of infection in the urine is required. Blood investigations needed will include a total blood picture, urea levels which are normal until the terminal stages, total plasma proteins which are low, serum cholesterol which is usually raised, and the ESR which may be elevated. Serum electrolytes should be estimated frequently. Renal biopsy may be performed to confirm the diagnosis if there is any doubt about this.

Treatment. In addition to that already described for nephritis, treatment also aims at relieving the oedema. Paracentesis abdominis may have to be performed if ascites is very marked and pressure on the diaphragm is causing respiratory embarrassment. This is done in the same way as for adults but with children emptying the bladder before starting the procedure, and preventing shock from lowering of the intra-abdominal pressure as the fluid is drained off, is even more important. With young children the trocar and cannula are sometimes replaced by a Southey's tube connected to fine rubber tubing. Drainage of subcutaneous tissues may have to be carried on for several hours or days, or may be repeated periodically.

The treatment though not a painful one may at first be alarming for the child, but soon the older child appreciates the relief obtained and will co-operate. For very young children, wrist restrainers may have to be used in order to prevent interference with the drainage tubes.

Drugs. Steroid therapy in the form of prednisone or prednisolone is of great value to the child with nephrosis; initially doses are high, the amount given being reduced after 10 days until a maintenance dose is reached to prevent the return of proteinuria. This maintenance dose may need to continue for as long as 6 months, but unfortunately relapses are common so that a return to higher dosages may be necessary. The long-term effect of steroids is to produce dwarfism, obesity and adrenal failure. The child receiving long-term steroids may need to receive antibiotics as a prophylactic measure as these children are especially prone to infection. In order to balance the low serum sodium level and the high serum potassium, an ion exchange resin (Resonium A 15 g to 30 g) may be given either orally or per rectum.

In cases where steroid therapy has failed to bring relief of oedema by producing a diuresis, the diuretic chlorothiazide may be combined with spironolactone (Aldactone A) in dosage of 25 mg four times daily. Potassium chloride should be given during therapy with chlorothiazide to prevent a potassium deficiency occurring. Cyclophosphamide (3 mg/kg) is sometimes combined with steroids for those children liable to relapse. The child and the parents should be warned that this drug may produce baldness, but that the hair will quickly grow again once the course of treatment has been completed. Meanwhile a wig can be worn if necessary.

A blood transfusion is given occasionally to correct anaemia and to improve the child's general condition.

Nursing Care. The basic nursing care is the same as that for the child with nephritis, but as the oedema may be causing respiratory embarrassment the nurse will have to use her skills in making the patient comfortable with extra pillows. Support for the scrotum may be necessary if the patient is a boy. As the child with gross oedema will be unable to move much, conscientious care of the skin and pressure areas is important. Small pillows and bed cradles should be used to prevent foot drop and to take the weight of the bed clothes off the patient's limbs. An air ring may be valuable as an aid to comfort and to prevent pressure sores. The peripheral circulation is often poor and oedematous limbs may be cold and discoloured; warm blankets and woollen socks may help to keep the feet warm. Care must be taken not to use hot-water bottles as the oedematous limbs are relatively insensitive, and burns could occur easily.

Because of the loss of gamma globulin together with oedema, there is a great tendency to infection and evidence of sepsis such as septic spots on the skin should be reported immediately.

Observations. Observations are the same as for the child with nephritis except that it is not usually necessary to record the blood pressure as frequently unless it is found to be raised.

Diet. As a great deal of protein is lost in the urine, a high protein diet is given as soon as the child is well enough to eat it. Estimations of the blood urea will act as a guide to tolerance of this régime; if the blood urea rises excessively it may be necessary to restrict protein intake. Restriction of salt to less than 2 g daily is also necessary while there is evidence of oedema. Paediatricians vary as to the need to restrict fluids, some allow 600 ml a day, others relate the fluid intake to the urinary output, while others do not restrict fluids at all.

Anorexia is frequently a problem, and the nurse needs to use skill and ingenuity to tempt the child's appetite by serving meals as attractively as possible. When a precise amount of protein is sent up from the diet kitchen the amount of food rejected should be recorded after every meal, so that the amount of protein refused can be accurately measured.

Prognosis. The long-term outlook is not good despite the use of steroids. Approximately 30 per cent of patients die from complications, e.g. intercurrent infections or peritonitis. Some children after a variable period become symptom free, in others the oedema persists.

Point of Interest. An attack of measles may bring about a long remission or even a cure. The reason for this is not yet understood.

Renal Rickets

Renal rickets or dwarfism is a rare complication of chronic kidney disease. Renal inefficiency causes large amounts of calcium to be excreted in the urine and this in turn causes delayed and incomplete bone formation which resembles the lesions in rickets due to vitamin deficiency. Polyuria is marked and the urine is pale and of low specific gravity. It often contains albumin. The skin is dry and thirst may be troublesome.

Treatment. Massive doses of vitamin D are given together with alkali therapy if acidosis is present. The increasing use of renal and peritoneal dialysis offers hope to these children as life can be prolonged with these procedures. For some children where a suitable donor kidney can be tissue matched and not rejected by the host, transplantation will enable the child to lead a full and normal life.

Renal Failure

Renal failure occurs when the kidneys are unable to maintain regulation of the composition or the volume of the body fluids. With acute renal failure the child's condition deteriorates rapidly in a few days. The chronic form of renal failure may take several months. The main causes of renal failure are:

1. Shock associated with major injury or haemorrhage;
2. Burns involving more than 15 per cent of the body surface;
3. Gastroenteritis resulting in severe dehydration;
4. Septicaemia;
5. Renal disease;
6. Obstructed urinary flow;
7. Mismatched transfusion, ingested poisons, anaphylactic shock.

Signs and Symptoms. The usual presenting symptom in acute renal failure is oliguria, but occasionally the child will be observed to pass dilute urine in large quantities. Drowsiness, headache, loss of appetite, pallor, vomiting, sore dry mouth, pyrexia, diarrhoea and convulsions are all common and may occur simultaneously or at different times. Blood pressure and intracranial pressure are high and there may be visual disturbances and retinal haemorrhages. The pulse rate is rapid and the volume poor.

Treatment. Uraemic children are particularly prone to infection, and the appropriate antibiotics will be ordered. These may need to be given in reduced dosage, as some reach dangerous blood level concentrations if given in the normal amounts when the kidneys are not properly functioning, e.g. gentamycin, streptomycin, kanamycin and the sulphonamides. Intravenous fluids will be required for some children depending on the primary cause of the renal failure. For the severely anaemic child blood will be required and will usually be given as packed cells in order to avoid overloading the circulation. Peritoneal dialysis or haemodialysis is sometimes indicated if the child's condition continues to deteriorate and the blood urea level rises above 65 mmol/litre (400 mg/100 ml). Haemodialysis is the most effective method but requires special facilities that are not available in all units. For most children peritoneal dialysis is effective and can be used even in young children. Kidney transplant operations in children have now been carried out most successfully in a few specialized units. This offers a new life to these children but unfortunately there are not yet enough suitable donors and there are still many technical problems to overcome.

Nursing Care. The aim of nursing care throughout this illness is to make the child comfortable by anticipating needs, alleviating symptoms and providing the nurse's prescription of t.l.c. (Tender Loving Care).

Accurate records of the intake and output must be carefully maintained. The basic fluid intake should be totalled together with the output of the previous 24 hours and calculated to allow for insensible loss through the skin and lungs which the nurse should remember will be greater during a heatwave or if the child is pyrexial. Because of the poor kidney function only small amounts are allowed. An average daily fluid intake allowance would be:

Infants	12 to 15 ml/kg/24 hours;
Older children	10 ml/kg/24 hours.

The mouth will be dry and careful mouth toilet is essential. For the older child frequent mouth washes can be given providing he knows not to swallow any of the glycothymoline or whatever fluid is being used. Sucking fruit pastilles slowly, will also help to keep the mouth moist as well as providing extra calories. Adequate calories must be given in the diet to minimize further protein breakdown. A pleasantly flavoured glucose concentrate such as 'Hycal' (25 ml = 60 calories approx.) can be given. Some first-class protein will also need to be provided in the diet to prevent further breakdown of body protein and so increase the blood urea. Occasionally if the child is comatosed 'Aminosol' or 'Intralipid' will be given intravenously to meet essential nutrition requirements. Daily weight should be recorded ideally using a weighing bed, taking care that the bedclothes remain the same weight. Temperature, pulse and blood pressure readings should be recorded frequently and any changes reported.

Peritoneal Dialysis. The procedure should be carefully explained to the child before the treatment commences. The child should also empty his bladder and be weighed. A sedative may be required. Strict asepsis is observed throughout the procedure. The abdominal skin is cleaned and the doctor will infiltrate a local anaesthetic of 1 per cent lignocaine into the skin midway between the umbilicus and symphysis pubis. A stab incision is made through which a 'Trocath' is introduced and a catheter is pushed gently into the pelvis and connected to the previously prepared dialysing set. The amount of dialysing fluid run in depends on the age and weight of child. Small infants will accommodate 150 to 200 ml each run, but a child of 12 years may take as much as a litre. The first run is drained immediately but in subsequent cycles the fluid is allowed to remain in the peritoneal cavity for 30 minutes. Dialysis is used continuously until the plasma electrolytes are more or less normal. Throughout this procedure the nurse must observe the child most carefully, noting any difficulty in respiration, nausea or vomiting. Care should be taken to prevent kinking of the tubing. If the flow diminishes it can often be rectified by changing the child's position or repositioning the catheter. If the catheter becomes blocked, the doctor will need to syringe it through with heparinized saline, or replace it with a new one.

Surgical Conditions of the Genito-Urinary Tract

In childhood the majority of operations performed on the genito-urinary system are done to correct congenital abnormalities. These are often the cause of recurrent urinary tract infections, colicky pain, and failure to thrive. In extreme, untreated cases, uraemia and death may result.

In investigations and treatments of the urinary tract the danger of ascending infection must constantly be borne in mind. Catheterization, the use of in-dwelling catheters and bladder lavage are consequently only ordered if there is no other alternative. When drainage tubes are in use it is the task of the nurse to watch the tube carefully. Kinking or compression of the tube may lead to damming-back of urine and as a child is unlikely to voice his complaint it is the nurse's responsibility to appreciate that there is something wrong by noticing the patient's restlessness or by noticing an abnormal output of urine. Accurate measurement of the urinary drainage and output is most important if serious complications are to be prevented. Operations on bladder or kidney may result in bleeding and clot formation. Morphine may be given to lower blood pressure and relieve pain and lavage may have to be employed to dissolve clots and prevent the child from straining in an attempt to pass the clot per urethram. At operations which may be expected to cause post-operative bleeding, the surgeon usually stitches a drainage tube into the wound, the substance of the kidney or the bladder to allow blood to escape. These tubes or drains call for careful nursing attention and vigilance.

Movement of the patient need not be restricted and change of position from side to side is helpful in promoting drainage and preventing chest complications.

Congenital Abnormalities and their Treatment

Agenesis of the Kidney

Failure of development of the kidney is as a rule unilateral. In that case the other kidney may hypertrophy and take over the total renal function and no treatment is necessary. Bilateral agenesis is incompatible with survival beyond the neonatal period.

Horseshoe and Double Kidney

A horseshoe kidney is formed by the union of the lower poles of the two kidneys, and may remain symptomless. The abnormality may be found accidentally in the course of a routine abdominal X-ray examination, or in other instances the child has recurrent urinary tract infections or attacks of pain and vomiting. A double kidney shows up plainly when pyelography is performed and it is often associated with double ureters. In long-standing cases hydronephrosis may develop. One of the ureters may have a kink or stenosis and if this is the cause of the recurrent infection or pain, it is removed.

Hydronephrosis and Mega-Ureter or Hydro-Ureter

Recurrent infections, obstructions and congenital abnormalities of urethra, ureters or renal pelvis may cause dilatation of one or both ureters or renal pelves. The patient suffers severe, recurrent pain and vomiting. The obstruction may be due to abnormally situated blood vessels which press on the ureters, stenosis of the ureter, ureteric or urethral valves, obstruction in the bladder neck and neurological causes. The obstruction may be unilateral or bilateral. If the cause of the obstruction can be removed, the ureters may regain their tone and return to a normal size. Nephrostomy and pyeloplasty are performed to relieve the condition (see page 355).

Vesico-Ureteric Reflux

Some infants suffer from a maldevelopment of the ureteric

orifices leading into the bladder. Every time the bladder contracts as the patient passes urine, urine flows back into the ureters and kidney causing disease and infection. The condition may rectify itself as the structures grow larger, alternatively operation of re-implantation of ureters has to be carried out.

Urethral Valves

Urethral valves occur only in boys. They may obstruct the urinary outflow and eventually cause renal failure. The bladder becomes distended and in babies this may cause a grossly enlarged abdomen. There is a constant trickle of urine so that the napkins are wet all the time. This may lead to the condition being missed for some time. The baby may, however, be observed to strain on passing urine and later there is enuresis both day and night. A catheter can be passed quite easily as the valves merely act as an obstruction to the outflow. Urinary tract infections are common as the bladder cannot empty adequately.

The presence of valves can best be demonstrated by carrying out a voiding urethrogram. A catheter is passed into the bladder and a radio-opaque substance run in. After removing the catheter radiographs are taken while the patient voids urine and dye and empties the bladder.

In some cases the urethra can be sufficiently dilated to relieve the obstruction, but often the valves have to be excised via a perineal urethrostomy using diathermy. The prognosis depends on the amount of renal damage caused through infection and back pressure.

Neuromuscular Incoordination of Bladder and Bladder Neck

Neuromuscular incoordination causes incontinence, back pressure of urine and eventually hydronephrosis. If the hydronephrosis is bilateral, it may be necessary to transplant the ureters into a resected loop of ileum opening on to the abdominal wall. A well-fitting appliance is made to fit over the stoma and urine is collected into a bag. The mother and child must be taught to keep the stoma clean and dry. The surrounding skin needs protection by painting it with tincture of benzoin. The bag should be emptied every 4 hours and the appliance renewed as necessary and at least once a week. The bag should be washed in soapy water in order to eliminate odour. The mother is given several bags to use and told to report to the hospital if the urine becomes scanty or offensive, or if the child seems off colour or is vomiting.

Ureterocele

It sometimes happens that part of the mucous lining of the bladder prolapses into it and causes obstruction of ureteric or urethral openings. This leads to stagnation of urine, back pressure, hydro-ureters and hydronephrosis. Treatment consists of diathermy to the prolapsed mucosa through a cystoscope or cutting and re-emplanting the ureters.

Sclerosis of the Bladder Neck

In this condition the bladder neck is fibrosed and hardened and so interferes with the normal contractions of the sphincter and causes urinary incontinence. Excision of a wedge of muscle may bring about the desired improvement but often repeated dilatation of the urethra may still be necessary.

Circumcision

Surgical removal of the foreskin is done either if it is abnormally tight (phimosis), for recurrent balanitis or for religious reasons. In the neonatal period the prepuce normally adheres to the glans penis and only begins to separate after some months. Attempts to retract the foreskin routinely at bath time should therefore not be made during the first 2 or 3 years of life as forceful retraction may cause tears, infection and scarring.

Circumcision should always be carefully considered. Some authorities believe that any operation in this area should be avoided if at all possible on account of the psychological implications. Post-operatively, severe haemorrhage occurs easily and irritation of the glans, ulceration of the urethral opening from friction, ammoniacal dermatitis and meatal ulcers causing scarring and stricture are complications which result fairly frequently.

In young children the operation is often carried out in the out-patient or minor operations' theatre and the child admitted to hospital as a day patient only. He is discharged towards evening and the mother is instructed to call her own doctor or bring the child back to hospital in the event of bleeding or if the child fails to pass urine.

Post-operatively the wound edges are often covered with ribbon gauze soaked in compound tincture of benzoin and left in place for approximately 1 week. After that time it is soaked off in a bath and routine washing and dusting with some antiseptic powder are all that are required. Very occasionally the ribbon gauze has been put on too tightly and congestion and oedema of the glans result. This requires urgent relief by sitting the patient in a warm bath of potassium permanganate (two crystals to each half-litre of water) and peeling the dressing off gently. Failure to do this may result in gangrene. Some surgeons leave the penis uncovered but spray the wound with Nobecutane, allowing the child to have a bath as usual from the second day. Others apply antibiotic ointment or powder instead.

During the immediate post-operative period these children are often very restless and miserable a sedative should be given. The mother or a nurse should be available to pick the baby up and comfort him as much as possible. In uncomplicated cases there is no difficulty of micturition but the first time the child passes urine should always be noted.

Paraphimosis

Occasionally children are brought to hospital with a grossly swollen or discoloured penis caused by a tight foreskin which has been retracted but could not be returned to its normal position. Relief is a matter of urgency as the blood supply is partly cut off. Cold packs or a bath may make it possible to reduce the condition and circumcision may be undertaken at a later date. Alternatively immediate operation may be necessary if other methods fail. The skin is divided and the constriction relieved. A watch should be kept for retention of urine.

Hypospadias

Malformation of the penis and urethra may cause the urethral opening to be somewhere on the undersurface of the penis and in extreme cases it may be at the juncture of penis and scrotum. Plastic surgery aims at straightening the penis and making a new urethra from flaps of skin. The operation is usually done in two or three stages and not started until the child is about 18 months old, although meatotomy may have to be performed sooner to enlarge the urethral opening. Oedema following operation may be severe and for that reason an incision is sometimes made on the dorsum of the penis to prevent constrictive swelling and the formation of a haematoma, by allowing for adequate drainage.

The stitches are as a rule left exposed and are kept dry by dusting with an antiseptic powder. Some surgeons secure the sutures with glass beads. During the second stage, when the urethra is newly constructed, the site of operation is kept dry by the use of an in-dwelling catheter which is passed into the bladder through the perineum immediately behind the scrotum. The catheter and tubing, leading to the underwater drain containing a mild antiseptic solution, should be watched for any kinking and drainage has to be carefully measured morning and evening. The drainage bottle is changed and replaced by a sterile one at least once in 24 hours to minimize the danger of ascending infection. Bladder lavage with a mild antiseptic solution such as potassium permanganate, sufficient to colour the sterile water pink, may be ordered. When the draining catheter is disconnected for treatment or for changing the drainage bag, it is spigoted off with a sterile spigot.

After 8 to 10 days the patient is allowed to pass urine through the urethra while the catheter is still in position, but spigoted and as soon as he can do so satisfactorily the in-dwelling catheter is removed. The perineal wound heals without suturing.

Following any operation on the penis or urethra, the urinal used by the patient, should be sterile until the wound can be expected to have healed.

All operations on the penis are extremely painful and distressing and every effort should be made to alleviate apprehension and discomfort. Sedatives should be given generously, penis and scrotum carefully supported by small pillows, the weight of the bedclothes taken by a cradle and great care taken not to pull at the catheter during bedmaking. Pressure areas need careful attention and the bowels should be watched as constipation is common and causes additional discomfort. Extra visiting and plenty of occupation will help to take the child's mind off his condition.

Undescended Testicle

The testes undergo migration in fetal life from a position high up in the abdomen through the inguinal canal and into the scrotal sac. They usually reach this final position by the time of birth. In some cases, however, migration is incomplete on one or both sides. On examination it is usually possible to determine the exact position of the testicle and the length of the spermatic cord. In many cases the testicle is retractile, that is to say it lies subcutaneously near the opening of the inguinal canal and can be brought down without difficulty. Although it may retract again it can be expected to descend by the time puberty has been reached. In other cases it is ectopic and has to be brought down by operation and stitched into the scrotal sac. This is usually done at the age of 6 to 8 years and always before the onset of puberty. Unfortunately the testicle may be malformed and atrophic. In these cases it is removed as there is a danger of malignancy if this is not done. There may be an associated hernia, which can be repaired at the same time.

Post-operatively a few days' bed rest is necessary but other nursing care presents no problems. If bilateral and if left untreated, undescended testes cause sterility and in later life malignant changes may develop. Sometimes hormone therapy replaces operation but not all cases are suitable for this method of treatment and some authorities consider it to be altogether undesirable.

Exomphalos with or without Ectopia Vesicae

If the anterior abdominal wall is absent or if fusion of the abdominal muscles is incomplete, the abdominal and pelvic organs may be only thinly covered by amnion or peritoneum or even lie on the surface at the time of birth. The pubic bones are separated and the hip joints are abnormal. Malformation of this kind may be associated with malformations of the penis or the vagina and with absence of the urethra or bladder wall or eversion of the bladder. If this is the case, the ureteric openings can be plainly seen and there is a constant trickle of urine. Ammonia dermatitis and excoriation of the surrounding skin develop and may lead to an ascending infection of the renal tract. Until operation can be undertaken (usually at 6 to 12 months of age) the skin should be protected by sterile ointments and barrier creams. Moist, sterile pads are applied to absorb the urine. These should be changed at frequent intervals. Alternatively Mercurochrome solution 2 per cent is applied. This may prevent infection and stimulate the formation of an epithelial cover.

After performing an osteotomy to approximate the pubic bones it is usually possible to suture the skin and bladder wall but it is often necessary to leave the repair of muscle to a later date. If there is a normally functioning urethra, repair is comparatively successful but often urethra and sphincter control are defective or absent and transplantation of the ureters into the sigmoid colon, ileum or rectum is necessary. The abnormal bladder is then removed at the same time. Alternatively the surgeon may divert the urine through a loop of bowel isolated from the ileum and brought on to the abdominal surface. A stick-on ileostomy bag catches the urine. It can be emptied or changed as required (see page 348).

Hydrocele

A hydrocele is a swelling of the scrotum caused by fluid which accumulates in the scrotal sac. It may be unilateral or bilateral. The hydrocele may close spontaneously in the first year of life. Because of this, operation is usually delayed unless the swelling causes discomfort or embarrassment. Aspiration of the fluid is obviously useless. If operation becomes necessary, the sac is incised and the opening closed by tying off the remnant of the processus vaginalis which is present and emptying the sac.

The operation is a simple one which causes little discomfort

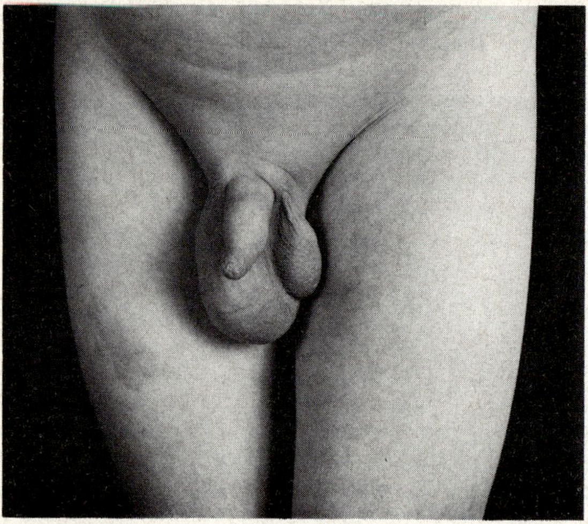

FIG. 55. A child with right hydrocele.

and few problems in the after care. The child may be treated as an outpatient or as a day case (Fig. 55).

Transplantation of Ureters

The operation of transplantation of ureters may have to be considered in cases in which there is either an abnormal or diseased bladder or an absence of sphincter control. This is frequently associated with malformation of the vagina, such as recto-vaginal fistula.

The operation is a difficult one and as a result is often disappointing. For this reason it is more usual to create an ileal loop bladder.

The ureters are brought out on to the abdominal wall and each ureter allowed to drain into a collecting bag (see page 348). Alternatively a loop of ileum is cut off from the alimentary canal and utilized as a reservoir, an opening made on to the surface and urine drained into a colostomy bag. This method lessens the risk of infection.

Nephrostomy

Drainage of the pelvis of the kidney is called nephrostomy. It is performed when some obstruction in the urinary tract has caused long-standing back pressure and dilatation of the ureters and renal pelvis (hydro-ureter and hydronephrosis) or when oedema following operation on the ureters obstructs the normal urinary flow. A Malecot catheter with a rigid tail to splint the suture line is introduced into the pelvis of the kidney and stitched in position, while a piece of corrugated rubber serves to drain the tissues around the kidney. The nephrostomy tube is kept in situ until all urinary leakage has stopped and the ureters regain their normal function. The skin around the wound should be carefully cleansed and protected against excoriation by the application of a barrier cream. Extra lengths of drainage tube are often used to allow for free movement without pulling on the tube, when this kind of drainage is used in children.

Nephrectomy

The removal of a kidney is never considered unless full investigations have shown that the other kidney is healthy and capable of taking over the total renal function. The tests carried out include intravenous pyelography, retrograde pyelography and excretion tests. It is also usual to ensure that the remaining kidney will not be at risk from the presence of infection elsewhere in the body.

Reasons for undertaking nephrectomy include congenital abnormalities of the ureters or kidney, hydronephrosis and Wilms's tumour. Tuberculosis of the kidney is rare in childhood. The child is usually admitted several days prior to operation to allow him to get used to the ward. Fluid intake and output are carefully measured for comparison with the post-operative fluid balance. A urinary antiseptic such as a course of sulphonamides may be ordered. In the case of Wilms's tumour, operation may be considered urgent and no time may be allowed for any special preparation unless a course of deep X-ray therapy is given.

Pre-Operative Preparation. This includes blood grouping, haemoglobin estimation and urine culture. Some surgeons like an aperient to be given two nights before operation. Skin preparation varies according to the wishes of the surgeon but a bath or a thorough wash with soap and water, paying special attention to axillae, groins and umbilicus should be given shortly before operation.

The Operation. The incision is usually a long one running roughly parallel with the margin of the ribs. After the kidney has been wholly or partly removed, the ureter is tied off and the wound closed. A corrugated rubber drain or small rubber tube is stitched in position to drain the kidney bed. Post-operative primary and secondary bleeding is a fairly common complication and the drain serves the dual purpose of showing any such bleeding and draining the renal cavity of serum and blood. The pad of cotton wool which covers the area should be frequently inspected. The drain is usually shortened after 24 hours and removed after 48 hours.

Nursing Care. As soon as consciousness is regained the patient is made comfortable with several pillows. He is tilted slightly towards the affected side to allow for better drainage and should be moved from side to side at intervals, as this reduces abdominal distension and further assists with drainage and prevents chest complications. The pillows should be protected by plastic covers and so arranged as to allow a hollow for the drainage tube. A small pillow placed between the knees avoids pressure and gives added comfort.

Adequate fluid intake is important and the nurse may have to spend a good deal of time persuading the reluctant patient to drink. A variety of fruit juices, tea and proprietary drinks should be given to make drinking more interesting and the young patient can be encouraged by keeping up his own fluid chart, collecting stars or making little drawings (see page 110). Pain may prevent deep breathing and so predispose to chest complications. The patient is nursed on the affected side or in the supine position to allow for good ventilation of both lungs. Breathing exercises and games which encourage deep breathing should be started as soon as possible. Regular bowel action is important.

The urinary output may at first be low and the urine blood-stained, but output should be normal and the urine regain its normal colour approximately 24 hours after operation.

In the majority of cases, nephrectomy should not present many problems. Occasionally uraemia develops, either because fluid intake has been inadequate or because the remaining kidney has not proved equal to the additional work (for uraemia see page 344). The patient is usually allowed up on the second or third day and discharged on the tenth or twelfth day. Nephrectomy should not disable the patient markedly and should not be a bar to vigorous activities or pregnancy later in life.

Wilms's Tumour (Nephroblastoma)

Wilms's tumour, which arises from the kidney, is the most commonly occurring malignant growth of childhood. Although the outlook is serious, up to 47 per cent of young children are cured after surgery followed by a course of deep X-ray therapy.

Signs and Symptoms. Frequently the first signs noticed are an enlargement of the abdomen. Pain, haematuria and suppression of urine together with general malaise, anaemia and failure to thrive occur rather later and these children do in fact remain surprisingly well for a long time despite the great malignancy of the condition and its tendency to form metastases in other parts of the body, particularly the lungs. The tumour is as a rule unilateral.

Treatment. This should be started without delay. A minimum of palpation for diagnostic purposes is allowed as there is a danger of dispersing the tumour cells into the renal vein and so encouraging spread. An intravenous pyelogram will reveal distortion of the renal pelvis and displacement of the kidney. A radiograph of the chest should be taken to ensure that there is no secondary spread of the tumour to the lungs. Operation is performed as soon as possible, blood transfusion is usually required during operation. Deep X-ray therapy, combined with cytotoxic drugs is ordered post-operatively, once the wound is healed, reducing the risk of metastases.

Nursing Care of Patients on Radium or Deep X-Ray Therapy

Patients on radiotherapy are usually given a card with instructions telling them about the treatment of local or generalized reaction or signs of intolerance to its treatment. In the case of children the mother will be given these instructions before the child is discharged home. Points of particular importance are:

Care of the Skin. Very occasionally the skin which has been exposed to radiation shows a reaction. If erythema is present the area must not be washed up to a month after treatment has been stopped. If reddened or sore a good talcum powder should be dusted over the area and if there is any reddening of the skin lanolin or Hibitane cream may be applied and is usually very soothing. The skin should not be exposed to any heat or to the sun and clothing should be very light, loose and of a smooth texture.

Generalized Reactions. These include general malaise, weariness and vomiting. Sympathy, gentleness and nursing care to give maximum rest and comfort are all that can be done for the first two reactions. Vomiting may be reduced by the administration of drugs such as chlorpromazine (Largactil). Some surgeons order pyridoxine and iron as a routine. Fluids should be given in small, frequent amounts to prevent dehydration but occasionally an intravenous infusion is necessary. The diet should be light and predigested. Milk drinks such as Bengers are often well tolerated. Extra glucose should be given with all drinks and many children enjoy sucking barley sugar and plain boiled sweets.

Points of Interest. Actinomycin D is given intravenously in doses of 15 μg/kg body weight/day for 5 days only. A dose of 75 μg/kg/day must never be exceeded as it is very toxic and may cause stomatitis, depression of bone marrow and loss of hair.

The care of patients following operation for Wilms's Tumour

and of terminal, malignant illnesses is discussed elsewhere and all that has been said applies to these unfortunate children. It is often possible to discharge the patient home after the course of deep X-ray has been completed even though readmission after some months must be expected. In that case every effort is made to admit the child to the same ward so that he is familiar with the surroundings and at least some members of the staff.

Further Reading

BLACK, D. A. K. (1968) *Essentials of Fluid Balance*, 4th ed. Oxford: Blackwell Scientific.

INNES-WILLIAMS, D. (1969) *Paediatric Urology*. London: Butterworths.

JOLLY, H. (1973) *Diseases of Children*, 3rd ed. Oxford: Blackwell Scientific.

17
The nervous system

BASICALLY, examination of a child's nervous system is the same as for an adult and it requires the same equipment. A child, however, is unable to describe his symptoms accurately and he will often be irritable and unco-operative. It will always help if a nurse whom the child knows and trusts can be present to assist the physician. It is important to allow plenty of time for the child to settle in the unfamiliar surroundings.

Most of the history will be obtained from the mother and it is taken back to include information about pregnancy and delivery. It is important to know whether there were signs of cyanosis or asphyxia at birth and whether the baby was premature or born at term. The doctor will also want to know whether there is any family history of epilepsy, mental subnormality or any other illness, which might have a bearing on the present condition.

Examination

The physician will note any abnormality of the skull such as bossing, asymmetry and the size of the fontanelle. In certain cases, such as suspected cerebral lesions or intracranial tumours, it may be important to notice the way in which the child holds his head. Facial palsy may cause him to dribble saliva from one corner of the mouth or cause only the unaffected side of the mouth to be drawn up when laughing or smiling.

The child may be unable to reach accurately for objects held out to him or he may have tremor of the hand. In certain diseases, the way in which the child raises himself from the floor to the standing position is in itself diagnostic. Sometimes the absence or presence of normal skills gives the best guide towards assessment and diagnosis.

The reflexes, as tested with the aid of a jerk hammer, are

important. Reflexes in the very young infant are unusually brisk and the plantar reflex is still extensor and only becomes flexor, as in the adult, when the child starts to walk.

Measuring the Head Circumference. The rate of growth of a child's head is often significant. In order to get accurate and comparable readings, the same person should always take the measurements if possible. The tape measure is taken round the head over the middle of the forehead and the most prominent part of the occiput.

Shaving the Child's Head. Very often the surgeon will agree, in order to avoid undue distress for the child, that the head is shaved in the anaesthetic room after the anaesthetic has been administered. The hair should be shampooed the day before operation and any scalp infection should be treated.

Signs of Raised Intracranial Pressure

While diagnosis must always be the doctor's province, early observations and accurate reporting on the part of the nurse may be invaluable in securing early and effective treatment. The signs to watch for include:

Vomiting unrelated to meals and without previous warning.
Headache, which is sometimes eased when the head is raised.
A tense, bulging anterior fontanelle.*
Distension of the scalp veins.*
Separation of sutures.*
Increase in the circumference of the head.*
Papilloedema.
Slowing of pulse rate.
Convulsions.
Meningeal cry.
Head retraction.
Arching of the back.
Internal strabismus.
Irritability.
Resentment at being touched.
Drowsiness.

* *Apply to infants only.*

Some Neurological Procedures

Lumbar Puncture

Lumbar puncture is the same for children as for adults and is done for the same reasons. It is, however, important to have complete control of the child when holding him and only an experienced person should attempt to do this. Very young children are often best lifted on to a table or a well-padded locker. Really adequate control is as a rule best achieved by the following means. The child is made comfortable on the pillow or mattress and the back flexed as much as possible in order to separate the spinous processes of the vertebrae. The nurse then hooks one arm round the neck, the other round the crook of the flexed knees and allows her hands to meet in front of the patient, so forming a complete circle with her hands and arms and the child's body (Fig. 56). Although safely restrained the child can breathe adequately and the nurse does not tire easily as the pull on her own hands gives her strength and support.

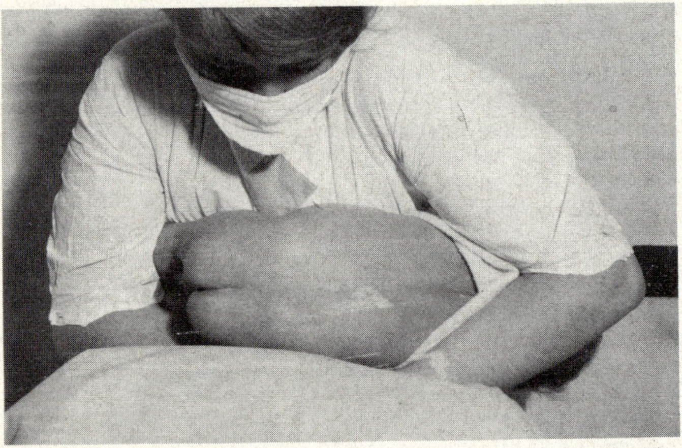

FIG. 56. Position for lumbar puncture. Note the way the neck and flexure of the knees of this young child are made to fit into the crook of the nurse's elbows.

The child should be absolutely still, neither struggling nor crying while the pressure is being read, lest false readings be obtained.

Whenever it is thought that lumbar puncture may have to be done repeatedly, a sedative should be given so as to minimize possible fear and psychological trauma.

In children headaches rarely follow lumbar puncture and the routine of keeping the patient flat and the foot of the bed raised is not necessary unless air has been injected as for the purpose of an air encephalogram.

Cisternal Puncture

When a block between the *cisterna magna* and the distal end of the spinal canal obstructs the free circulation of cerebro spinal fluid, cisternal puncture may be done instead of a lumbar puncture. A small area of hair is shaved at the nape of the neck and a special cisternal puncture needle is used. This is inserted at a point where an imaginary line, drawn from one tip of the mastoid process to the other, crosses the spine, while the head is held in complete flexion. In all other respects the procedure is the same as for lumbar puncture.

Other, more extensive procedures may be both frightening and very uncomfortable and they are therefore done under a light general, or a basal anaesthetic. It is also easier to obtain the necessary positions with the anaesthetized patient than with an unco-operative one.

In conditions in which congenital abnormalities or hydrocephalus are suspected it may be necessary to outline the ventricles of the brain. This can be done by filling them with air or pure oxygen before taking radiographs. Irregular outline, displacement or defects in filling may show up and these findings are valuable in coming to a diagnosis and in deciding on treatment. There are two methods in common use.

Pneumo-Encephalogram. A lumbar puncture is performed in the usual way and several millilitres of cerebrospinal fluid are withdrawn. The fluid is replaced by filtered air or pure oxygen, injected through a syringe attached to the lumbar puncture needle. This process is repeated several times until about 40 ml have been exchanged. When the child is sat up, the air rises within the cerebrospinal canal, like an air bubble rising in water. If there is no abnormality present the ventricles of the brain will fill with air and their outline and position can be clearly seen on a radiograph. Air encephalogram is never carried out in cases of suspected space occupying lesions as these cause raised intracranial pressure and the withdrawal of cerebrospinal fluid may lead to 'coning' of the brain-stem through the foramen magnum into the spinal canal, resulting in sudden death from pressure on this vital part of the nervous system.

Ventriculography. For ventriculography the head has to be shaved, as the blunt cannula is introduced through the scalp, directly into the ventricles. In young infants this can be done through the still-open fontanelle or the still-ununited sutures. In older patients it is necessary to make burr holes in the skull. Approximately 40 ml of filtered air or pure oxygen are then injected after withdrawing a similar quantity of cerebrospinal fluid.

In either case, radiographs are taken immediately after the air has been injected. By placing the patient in different positions the movement of the air through the ventricular system and the shape, size and position of the ventricles can be clearly seen. Alternatively a filling defect of any part of the cerebrospinal or ventricular system will be a valuable aid to diagnosis. Ventriculography is used when a brain abscess or intracranial tumour is suspected.

Radio-Opaque Methods

Angiography is used when it is desirable to outline blood vessels of the brain. An injection of a radio-opaque dye is made into the main carotid artery in the neck. As the dye circulates through the arteries their outline can be seen on the X-ray screen or film. Pictures are taken in rapid succession. In this way abnormalities such as angiomata of the brain can be clearly seen and accurately located. Angiography is a valuable diagnostic aid, particularly prior to certain operations on the brain (see Sturge-Weber Syndrome, page 375).

In cases of suspected non-communicating hydrocephalus

(see page 382) radio-opaque media may be injected into the ventricle through the anterior fontanelle or through burr holes, and the site of a hold-up may be seen in the radiograph. Radio-opaque substances may also be injected into the spinal cord to discover the site of a spinal tumour.

The procedures described above are not without hazard and shock may be considerable. Children do not complain of headache but on return to the ward their colour may be poor and they may be restless or irritable. As soon as their condition permits, extra fluids should be given as this seems to ease their discomfort and helps in their recovery.

Electro-Encephalogram

It is known that rhythmical electric charges of a certain pattern and frequency are exhibited in the human brain and that both pattern and frequency change in disease. Recordings can be made by means of electrical leads placed on the patient's scalp. The graphs obtained are typical of certain diseases or abnormalities such as cerebral abscess or degenerative diseases, and are a valuable aid to diagnosis. It is desirable to have a fully co-operative patient, capable of obeying instructions (for example to open or close his eyes) and this is often achieved by arranging for the mother or for the child's own nurse to be present. Frequently, however, a sedative has to be given.

Convulsions

Convulsions are very common in childhood and should be considered as a symptom of disease rather than as a disease in themselves. Some young children have a convulsion with every pyrexial illness and they can be expected to grow out of this tendency as they grow older. Other causes of convulsions include: dehydration, lead poisoning, hypoglycaemia, a low serum calcium level causing tetany, vitamin B deficiency, brain damage and meningitis.

Treatment and prognosis will obviously depend on the cause of the convulsions. Intellectually, many of these children develop quite normally though sometimes interrupted schooling or misguided over-protection by the parents makes them compare unfavourably with their contemporaries. By and large however, the outlook in adequately treated patients is a hopeful one.

Epilepsy

Petit Mal

Attacks of minor epilepsy may be so mild that they are only noticed by those who are in constant contact with the patient. The loss of consciousness is so fleeting that, after a momentary pause, the patient immediately resumes his activities as if nothing had happened. The eyes may take on a momentary dazed look or there may be a feeling of giddiness or a loss of postural control. In hospital it is at times necessary for a nurse to 'special' a patient in order to see one of these attacks.

Major Epilepsy

The stages of a major epileptic attack are the same in children as in adults, but children frequently become irritable or cling to their mothers as if seeking comfort during the period of aura. Occasionally there is no loss of consciousness nor are there true convulsive movements but the child shows considerable behaviour disturbances or temporary loss of memory and, in some cases, unexplained headaches or abdominal pain are thought to be of epileptic origin.

Except where children admitted during a convulsion are known to be epileptics of long standing, investigations including lumbar puncture are carried out to exclude any acute illness. Later a full neurological examination and an electroencephalogram are usually undertaken.

A variety of drugs are used to control convulsions. These include phenobarbitone, Mysolin, Epanutin or various combinations of anticonvulsant drugs. Some of these drugs have serious side-effects and the nurse should be well informed about them, and make careful observations.

In dealing with a child in a convulsion, the principal concern is to keep him from harming himself. If he has been up and about the nurse should lay him on a bed or on the floor away from any harmful object. The child's head should be turned to the side to allow saliva to drain freely and so prevent inhalation. Tight clothing should be loosened and the patient kept warm. If the attack occurs in bed, pillows are best removed and, if possible, a waterproof sheet and anaesthetic cloth should be placed underneath the head to protect the bed. A soft wedge or bandage may be inserted between the teeth to prevent the patient from biting his tongue. Restraint is best avoided. If the attack occurs in the ward, screens should be placed around him and he should be kept as quiet as possible.

As the patient regains consciousness he is likely to be bewildered and reassurance and comfort should be given. A warm drink may help to send him into a restful sleep.

In hospital, a tray containing recovery instruments and swabs is usually kept near the beds of known epileptic children but this should be covered and out of sight of both child and visitors. Occasionally oxygen has to be given and diazepam 0.3 mg/kg intravenously may be ordered.

While looking after the patient the nurse should make careful observations and chart these as soon as she is free. The points to watch for are suggested in the following list.

Observations. How did the fit start? Was there an aura, noise in the ears, flash of light? Were there any movements? Where did they begin? Where did they spread to? Were the movements tonic or clonic? Was there a tremor and eye movements?

Did the patient lose consciousness? Were the eyes open or closed? If closed, could they be opened? Towards which side were they turned? If lightly touched, did the eyes blink? Was there incontinence, cyanosis, and/or breath holding? Did the patient bite his tongue? What was the duration of the fit? Was the patient drowsy after the fit or was he confused? Did the patient show abnormal or unusual behaviour after the fit? What could the patient remember about the fit?

Temperature, pulse and respirations should be taken and recorded as soon as the convulsion is over.

General Care of Children Suffering from Epilepsy. Children whose fits are due to true epilepsy with frequent attacks need special protective measures and may have to attend special schools, but their chances of employment and their psychological adjustment can be greatly improved by attendance at ordinary schools, and understanding teachers often make this possible without any detriment to the other pupils. Unfortunately about a quarter of all epileptic children also suffer from cerebral palsy, 10 per cent have speech defects and almost half are emotionally disturbed or socially handicapped (i.e. overprotected or rejected). This accounts for the fact that more than 600 children with epilepsy in the United Kingdom are in special residential schools. As normal a life as possible should be encouraged, though regular routine with regard to meals, sleep, work and recreation can often help to keep attacks down to a minimum. About 50 per cent of children who suffer from epilepsy have an aura (warning) before an attack and can learn to protect themselves from danger before the fit starts. Convulsions seem to occur less frequently in the well-occupied child who has plenty to interest him than in those who never know what to do with themselves. Occasionally, risks have to be taken and are likely to be less serious than the effects of over-protection and constant restrictions, though commonsense precautions such as fireguards and adequate cot-sides should be provided. The parents may well be deeply affected by their child's misfortune and nurses should never forget that they deserve both sympathy and understanding.

Points of Interest. Although intelligence in epileptics is average in most instances and may even be above average mental subnormality occurs more commonly in epileptics than in other children, and the inevitable use of drugs often slows the mental processes in these children.

Pink Disease (Erythroedema, Acrodynia, Polyneuritis)

Pink disease affects very young children of either sex. The cause is thought to be hypersensitivity to mercury and with the strict control measures now in force in most countries, the disease has become less common than it once was.

The affected child presents a picture of almost complete misery and improvement may not occur for a matter of months, taxing the mother trying to nurse and comfort her child, to the utmost.

Signs and Symptoms. Children suffering from Pink Disease are extremely irritable, the skin is moist and pink and inclined to peel. Older children complain of itching and a burning sensation, the limbs may be swollen. Stomatitis causes the patient to dribble saliva, to lose teeth, to let the lips hang loosely so as to give a 'duck bill' appearance and to refuse food. All muscle tone is poor and rectal prolapse common. Loss of sleep, restlessness and refusal of food cause wasting and loss of weight. Treatment is symptomatic. Any source of infection should be eliminated and if admitted to hospital, cubicle nursing is essential. If nursed at home, it should be remembered that the mother needs relief from the exhausting day and night care of a very demanding and miserable patient. In cases where sweating is severe and much salt is lost, extra salt is given and belladonna preparations may be ordered to help dry up secretions. Penicillamine or Calcium Disodium Versenate given intravenously are used in the same way as for lead poisoning. Experiments with vasodilator and ganglion blocking agents have given occasional encouragement to research workers. Sedatives such as chloral hydrate and phenobarbitone are given to secure rest and sleep.

Nurses should remember and use every nursing trick they have at their command to make these children comfortable and to encourage them to eat (bed cradles to cool them, soothing skin applications, cool clean linen, curtains to exclude bright light, pretty crockery and coloured, varied food and occupation, all come to mind).

Mentally these children remain normal and alert but often regression in training habits is marked.

Great patience and understanding and only the best nursing attention, will manage to keep these entirely negative little patients from abysmal distress and no amount of nursing and comforting should be considered as spoiling or as a waste of time.

Meningitis
(inflammation of the covering membranes of the brain)

Meningitis is more common in children than in adults but the causative organisms are the same as in adults with the exception of *Escherichia* (*Bacterium*) *coli* which usually causes meningitis in newborn infants. Generally speaking, the acute types present a common picture and basically investigations, treatment and nursing care are the same. Infections which present special problems are mentioned under the appropriate headings; for example, tuberculous meningitis under the heading tuberculosis.

Signs and Symptoms. Most commonly the onset is sudden, with headaches, vomiting, high fever, neck stiffness and photophobia. The pulse varies and may be either increased or slower

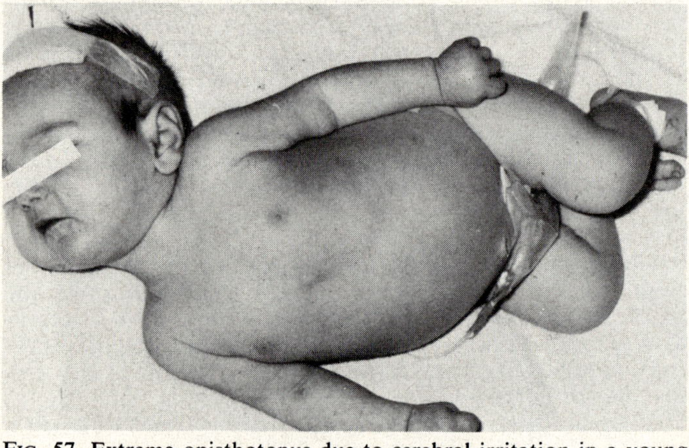

FIG. 57. Extreme opisthotonus due to cerebral irritation in a young baby.

than usual. From time to time the child gives a shrill, high-pitched scream known as the meningeal cry. He is irritable at first and resents being touched. Soon, however, he becomes drowsy, the eyes take on a staring expression and the pupils may be unequal and sluggish in their reaction to light. A squint may also develop. Occasionally convulsions occur and as a rule these must be regarded as a serious sign. As the irritation of the spinal meninges increases and the muscles of the neck become involved, head retraction and backward arching of the back result: this is known as *opisthotonos* (Fig. 57). Cheyne-Stokes type of breathing may develop and delirium, stupor and coma supervene.

As the illness progresses, generalized septicaemia may set in and in these cases the skin takes on a grey colour, and feels cold and clammy. The pulse rate rises and the volume becomes poor. The blood pressure falls. Constipation and retention of urine are common.

Examination. Examination shows the infant to have a tense, bulging fontanelle and older children will have papilloedema, sure signs of increased intracranial pressure. Lumbar puncture will confirm the diagnosis and determine the causative organism and its sensitivity to drugs.

Treatment. Treatment consists in giving the appropriate drug by intravenous or intramuscular injection. Occasionally a block forms in the channel of the cerebrospinal fluid with the result that the drugs do not reach the focus of the infection. In such cases lumbar puncture may be replaced by cisternal or ventricular puncture and surgical intervention may become necessary to assist drainage and prevent permanent damage. Sometimes fluid collects in the subdural space, causing the fever to persist and the head circumference to increase.

Prognosis. In most instances complete recovery may be expected, but much depends on early diagnosis and prompt, effective treatment. The outlook is most serious in very young infants and the prognosis should always be somewhat guarded.

Complications. Complications include neurological disturbances, hydrocephalus, mental deficiency, paralysis, deafness and convulsions. A special point worth remembering is that, in young infants, meningitis may occur in a *sub-acute form*. There may be little or no fever; diarrhoea and vomiting may lead to dehydration and sunken eyes and fontanelle. Together with these misleading symptoms neurological examination is difficult and often atypical in babies and only lumbar puncture can confirm the diagnosis of meningitis.

Meningococcal Meningitis

Meningococcal meningitis presents some special features which are particularly important as this type of meningitis is often seen in children's wards. The patient often comes from overcrowded surroundings, and the infection which is spread by droplets invades the nasopharynx and blood stream. The course of the illness may be fulminant and, if coupled with septicaemia, may rapidly lead to collapse and death. Complications such as petechial haemorrhages, temporary blindness, opisthotonos, peripheral circulatory failure, *taches cérébrales* and convulsions are common if treatment is delayed. In cases where there are signs of haemorrhage into the skin, cortisone or prednisone are given, either by intravenous or intramuscular injection.

A great danger is that an exudate may form at the base of the brain. Surgery can sometimes be carried out to remove the fibrous membrane formed but if it is not successful, blocking of the fourth ventricle, hydrocephalus, spasticity, loss of vision and hearing and mental defect may develop. With modern diagnostic methods and drug therapy, these severe cases and complications are fortunately rare in this country.

It should be remembered that meningococcal meningitis is a notifiable disease. The incubation period is 4 to 5 days only and carriers are common.

'*Haemophilus influenzae*' Meningitis

Haemophilus infection causing meningitis occurs mostly during the pre-school age. Once invariably fatal, the outlook is now much more hopeful due to treatment with drugs such as ampicilin. There remains a danger of nerve damage, causing complications such as deafness or paralysis.

Nursing Care in All Cases of Meningitis

A quiet, well-ventilated room should be chosen, and certain types of meningitis will have to be nursed with full barrier precautions. Careful observations, coupled with sound knowledge of the possible complications, are of prime importance and the observations should be carried out continuously and conscientiously.

The child's position in bed may point to increasing intracranial pressure, for example turning away from the light or hiding under the bedclothes.

Pressure areas need careful attention on account of the severe wasting which is often present, and because of restlessness and incontinence. Ripple beds are a great help. The skin should be kept healthy by careful sponging and this may at the same time serve to reduce the hyperpyrexia and help in the elimination of toxins. In all cases of bacterial meningitis broad spectrum antibiotics such as chloramphenicol are prescribed and must be given conscientiously, although the child may be very unco-operative about taking these drugs.

The bowels and bladder need watching as constipation and retention of urine are common. The urine should be tested for abnormal constituents, such as albumin, blood or acetone bodies.

Good ventilation and an electric fan may help in reducing high fever, and nursing aids such as bed cradles, ring pads for the heels and head, and soft bandages for the knees, should be used whenever necessary. Mouth toilet should be done frequently and the lips kept soft by applying petroleum jelly to prevent sores, particularly if the child is unconscious and unable to take fluids by mouth.

In the acute stages temperature, pulse and respirations are taken and charted 4-hourly and blood pressure readings may have to be taken frequently. Fluid intake and output should be measured and the charts kept up to date.

Diet. The diet should be light and nutritious, and fluids should be given in adequate amounts. Artificial feeding by nasal tube may become necessary. The problem of feeding may be aggravated by persistent vomiting. It often pays to allow the mother to bring a favourite dish from home and to give in to the child's whims where the diet is concerned, in order to maintain adequate nutrition.

Continuous and expert nursing care, using every available nursing aid and enlisting the help of occupational therapist, physiotherapist and teacher or play leader may help to bring these seriously ill children back to normal health, once they have passed the acute stage of the illness.

Cerebral Abscess

Cerebral abscess is often difficult to diagnose as the onset is insidious and neurological investigations in children a difficult task. For this reason such cases are often seen in medical wards, though the condition is essentially a surgical one.

Causes. These, in children, are the same as in adults, except that children with congenital heart disease are commonly the victims of cerebral abscess caused when a small embolus reaches the brain and becomes infected.

In the early stage of the illness the symptoms resemble those of meningitis but, as the infection becomes localized, convulsions, visual disturbances, toxaemia, drowsiness and facial palsy may develop. At this point the temperature may be only slightly raised. The diagnosis is confirmed by ventriculography, immediately prior to surgical intervention.

Treatment. Antibiotics are given in large doses and, as soon as the abscess is sufficiently localized, an operation for drainage is carried out. A small catheter may be left draining the abscess bed, and can be used to give antibiotics. The subsequent treatment is purely surgical.

The prognosis is good though children who have recovered in all other respects may be left with convulsions.

The *nursing care* includes all points observed when looking after seriously ill or even unconscious patients suffering from a prolonged illness, as well as the care for the underlying condition, for example endocarditis or otitis media. These patients may become restless and difficult to manage, and need careful and constant nursing attention.

Intracranial Tumour

Intracranial, space-occupying lesions are fairly common, particularly in children of five to ten years old. Treatment is surgical or by deep X-ray therapy. Both boys and girls are, as a rule, very sensitive to the loss of hair caused by deep X-ray therapy. They can be made happier by arranging for them to wear a temporary wig and by assuring them that their hair will eventually grow again. According to their situation the lesions cause complications by pressure, for instance pressure on the pituitary gland, causing *diabetes insipidus.* Some of these tumours are malignant and inoperable but in many cases there is reasonable hope of successful treatment. The commonest site is the cerebellum and the pressure here causes the patient to suffer from vomiting which is difficult to control. Papilloedema is usually present and the child is grossly ataxic.

During the period in which investigations are carried out it is important to keep these children happy and generally fit. Whenever possible they should be up and about and gentle physiotherapy helps to keep their muscles in trim. But as these patients are often unstable on their feet this places extra responsibility on the nursing staff to avoid accidents. When deep X-ray therapy is given, vomiting and anorexia may become a problem and ingenuity is needed in keeping up the patient's nutrition. Avomine and other drugs may be prescribed to stop vomiting.

Sturge-Weber Syndrome

Some children have a facial naevus and a naevus of the meninges on one side, associated with hemiplegia of the opposite side and fits which may affect only the opposite side or be general. This is known as Sturge-Weber syndrome. The naevus on the meninges consists of dilated capillaries of a web-like appearance (telangiectasis) which calcify after a time. The associated convulsions may be so severe as ultimately to affect the child's mental development.

Treatment consists in trying to control the convulsions by drugs but frequently surgical treatment becomes necessary. In this case either the affected area or the entire hemisphere has to be removed (hemispherectomy).

Acute Encephalitis

Acute encephalitis may be caused by virus or bacterial infection, specific fevers or influenza and rarely by immunization.

Signs and symptoms. The onset of the disease is very acute with high fever, severe headache, vomiting, visual disturbances and sometimes convulsions and loss of consciousness. Patients may be so confused as to become irrational and violent to an extent which necessitates restraint.

A high lymphocyte count in the cerebrospinal fluid often confirms the diagnosis. The illness is a short one and has a high mortality rate. Brain damage may be permanent in those children who recover from the acute illness.

Treatment. This is symptomatic and principally aims at reducing the intracranial pressure by repeated lumbar punctures. The nursing care is exacting as the patient cannot be expected to co-operate. Restlessness creates problems regarding pressure areas. Artificial feeding may become necessary during the confused stage and constant vigilance is essential to keep up a high standard of care and prevent accidents. Steroid therapy may have dramatic results.

Rare types of encephalitis include encephalitis lethargica, which is now hardly ever seen in this country, post-vaccination encephalitis and toxoplasmosis.

Toxoplasmosis

Toxoplasmosis is a form of infection caused by a protozoon.

If the child is affected in utero the symptoms are present at birth. The infant fails to thrive, vomiting and diarrhoea, convulsions and changes in the retina develop and, as the lesions rapidly become calcified, they cause blindness, mental deficiency and hydrocephalus. The outlook is bad but not hopeless.

The presence of the disease is confirmed by serological tests. Early treatment with pyrimethamine (Daraprim) and sulphadimidine has been found to result in some improvement, but prolonged use of the drug may cause megaloblastic anaemia, due to folic acid deficiency.

Lead Encephalopathy

Lead encephalopathy is mentioned mainly because it should be possible to avoid its occurrence altogether. It is usually due to the use of paint containing lead which, in one way or another, has come within reach of young children. Toddlers, who carry everything to their mouths or who rub their sore gums on the cool bars of their cots when teething, are particularly exposed to this danger. By law, lead paint may not be used where such risks arise, but sometimes father may brighten up the child's furniture or toys with a little paint left over from an outside painting job, and so become the unwitting cause of the illness. Poisoning may also result from the chewing of lead soldiers, or yellow and orange crayons which contain lead chromate. By health teaching nurses can do much to prevent such accidents.

The symptoms include pallor, irritability, vomiting, colic, constipation, anaemia, neuritis, convulsions, symptoms of intracranial pressure, coma and death.

Penicillamine or calcium versenate (EDTA) are used to treat lead poisoning.

There is a serious risk of mental handicap if the child survives. These children should be followed up for at least one year to ensure that the blood lead level returns to normal, and to detect any further exposure. Siblings at risk should also be screened for evidence of exposure to lead.

Cerebral Palsy

Cerebral palsy is caused by defect or disease of the brain affecting the upper motor neurones and liable to occur any time before, during or after birth. The disease is not progressive. Muscular control may be so little impaired that it is barely noticeable, or all muscle groups of the body may be involved, completely incapacitating the victim. About six out of every 1000 live births suffer from a degree of cerebral palsy.

Some of the sufferers appear mentally handicapped as they are unable to control their facial expressions, but in reality half are mentally normal or of superior intelligence. Inability to enunciate may add to the impression that there is mental impairment.

Low birth weight babies in particular seem likely to be affected, but there are many other causes, including ill health during pregnancy and an abnormal delivery.

The earlier these children can be treated, the greater the hope of teaching them sufficient muscular relaxation and control to make their lives tolerable to themselves, their parents and the community in general.

Nurses have special opportunities for spotting these cerebral palsy babies who are sometimes admitted to the children's ward under another diagnosis. These may include babies who suck and swallow badly, babies who are abnormally quiet or always restless, babies who start up with a jerk at a sudden noise, babies who never cry and those who let their heads drop back when they are picked up or always hold them turned towards one side. Babies who suffer from haemolytic disease of the newborn (see page 68) are potential cerebral palsy sufferers and should be kept under careful supervision, so that treatment, if necessary, may be started at the earliest moment.

These babies should be brought to the notice of a doctor without delay so that they can be watched, and physiotherapy started as soon as practicable, as this will reduce spasticity as much as possible and prevent an abnormal pattern of movement from developing. Where there is doubt, the nurse should compare her patient's progress with the milestones set out in Chapter 1 and try to judge whether her young charge's achievements fall within the normal limits of development. Mothers are often reluctant to admit, even to themselves, that their own child's progress compares unfavourably with others, and tact and careful observation may be needed if treatment is to be started at the best time.

Children suffering from cerebral palsy have difficulty in carrying out co-ordinated movements. The adductor muscles of the thigh in particular go into spasm (the scissor attitude). The gait is unsteady or clumsy, and is often reminiscent of a drunken man, charging forward, dragging a foot and stumbling about (Fig. 58), or the movements may be slow and writhing. The inco-ordination of the respiratory muscles leads to frequent chest infections. Speech is difficult if the lip, tongue and laryngeal muscles are affected and the child may grimace in an attempt at forming words. What speech is possible is often explosive and the abnormal functioning of the respiratory muscles causes the child to make uncontrolled, animal-like noises. This may intensify the impression that the child is mentally abnormal. In addition he has difficulty in swallowing and he may have a constant dribble of saliva down his chin. Poor mastication causes dental decay, anaemia and malnutrition.

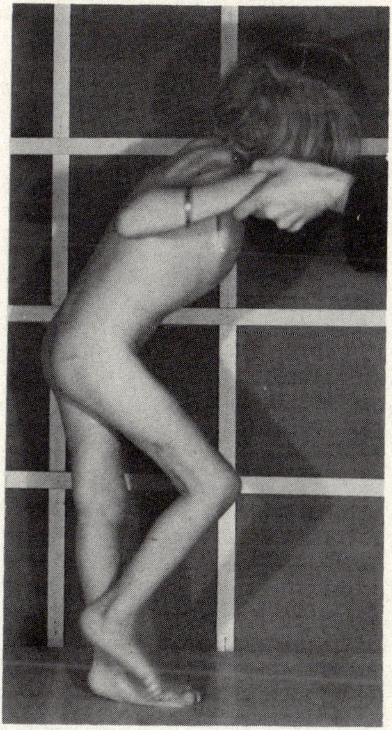

FIG. 58. Cerebral palsy. Note the typical stumbling gait.

Many spastic children have a squint caused by muscle spasm, and visual disturbances such as double vision are common. Hearing defects are often associated with cerebral palsy, and these and the visual defects are often partly responsible for the delay in acquiring speech and learning to read.

Some of these children have particularly lovable ways, but others suffer from temper tantrums brought on by frustration and by a tendency to convulsions. Doctors and nurses can help to enlighten the general public about cerebral palsy sufferers and thus get them accepted with constructive sympathy.

Investigations are carried out by a specialist and should be very extensive. The aim is to make a full assessment and then set to work on those muscle groups and abilities which give hope of response and seem capable of development. Teamwork is the essence in the treatment of cerebral palsy. An educational psychologist is asked to assess the child's mental ability, a very difficult task as poor muscular control and sensory defects, such as deafness or double vision, may make the use of the usual testing material impossible.

It is often possible to correct or alleviate some of the associated defects, by giving the child glasses, a hearing aid and walking calipers. The general health should be regularly supervised. As these children have difficulty in masticating due to bad muscular co-ordination, malnutrition is common and the teeth may be bad or ill developed. Septic tonsils are frequently another cause of general ill health. Deformities of various kinds may develop, caused by the unequal pull of muscles on the bony structures. The paediatrician will therefore often enlist the help of orthopaedic, dental, ear, nose and throat and ophthalmic surgeons who may be able to correct or ameliorate existing defects.

From the earliest moment the use of splints, small pillows, specially constructed chairs, gentle, passive movements and massage should be encouraged and teaching of conscious relaxation started.

The brunt of treatment will fall on the parents, teachers and physiotherapist. These children can attend nursery schools and schools for the physically handicapped, where physiotherapy is available and where they can be shown how the powers left to them can be used to the best advantage. Often this means tedious exercises in relaxation and only when this has been mastered will it be possible to teach voluntary movements with success. Progress will be slow and such aids as mirrors, walking skis and rails at suitable levels may give the much-needed encouragement. Tape recorders, on which progress in speech can be followed, are an invaluable stimulus both to the children and to their parents and teachers.

Films or video recordings taken of the patient at various stages may also be used to remind all concerned of the initial difficulties and so make them appreciate better what has been achieved. Building up the handles of eating utensils, adjusting lavatory seats and other ingenious adaptations may be learnt at special centres and schools or thought of by intelligent, enterprising parents.

Parents of spastic children have in fact come together and founded a society through which they work for better treatment and education for their children as well as encouraging each other and exchanging useful ideas on their children's upbringing.

Later in life no trouble should be spared to integrate these young people into the life of the community, and it will be found that given suitable help and employment a large majority can earn their living and fend for themselves.

The problem, though great, is one where there is no need for despair, and the reader will be rewarded if she makes a more thorough study of this condition.

Friedreich's Ataxia

Friedreich's ataxia is a fairly uncommon condition and the reader is referred to larger textbooks for greater detail. The disease is familial, and usually becomes established at the age of 5 to 10 years; it is caused by degenerative changes in the spinal cord and cerebellum. The child develops unco-ordinated movements, ataxia, pes cavus (hollow instep and retraction of the toes), difficulty with speech and swallowing, generalized weakness and mental deterioration

There is no known cure for this disease and nursing and medical care are confined to symptomatic treatment and prevention of deformities.

Progressive Spinal Muscular Atrophy

In this condition the motor cells in the spinal cord fail to develop properly and in consequence the muscles of the limbs and trunk are very feeble and flaccid. In one form, *amyotonia congenita*, most of the damage occurs before birth and the infant can merely lie flat. Some slight improvement may occur and permits life to continue for years, but sooner or later respiratory infection causes death, for the child is unable to clear the respiratory passages by coughing.

In another form, *Werdnig-Hoffman's disease*, the condition is less severe at birth but weakness increases and death occurs at an early age. Nursing care concentrates on preventing inhalation of food and infection and in moving the child and changing his position and caring for the skin. Diagnosis in both instances is confirmed by electromyogram, muscular biopsy, and rectal biopsy. Once this condition has been diagnosed the parents should be given genetic counselling as this disease is hereditary and future siblings may be affected.

Hydrocephalus

Hydrocephalus is the name given to an excessive accumulation of cerebrospinal fluid within the skull. The resulting pressure causes the skull bones to separate, the skull circumference to increase, the ventricles to becomes distended and the substance of the brain to be compressed.

The excess accumulation is produced by obstruction of the flow or absorption of the fluid, due to congenital malformation, birth injury, inflammatory processes or pressure from a tumour.

Nurses will hear the doctors mention a communicating and a non-communicating type of hydrocephalus and investigations will aim at establishing which of the two varieties affects the child.

In the *communicating type* there is a block within the subarachnoid space although there is free communication between the ventricular system and the spinal theca.

In the *non-communicating type*, the outflow from within the brain to the subarachnoid space is blocked; in either case various methods of drainage have been tried with some success. Lately the use of the *Spitz-Holter* (Fig. 60) and the *Pudenz valve* has given good results in a proportion of cases.

The Care of Children with Spitz-Holter Valves. In many

instances it is now possible to prevent hydrocephalus from developing. If it is seen that the head circumference is increasing, a device which enables the cerebrospinal fluid to drain from the ventricles into the general circulation, can be inserted. A

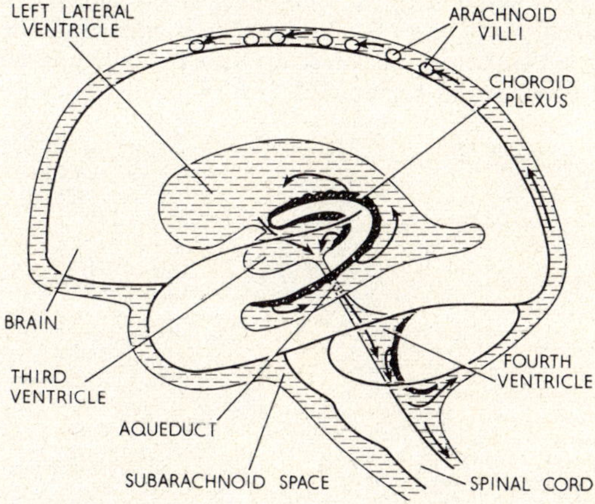

FIG. 59. Diagram of the skull and brain, showing the ventricles and the circulation of cerebrospinal fluid.

thin tube is fixed in the ventricle and brought out behind the ear to lie in a groove in the skull and from there led into the jugular vein and on to the vena cava. A valve, which prevents reflux is incorporated. It is possible to 'milk' the tube in order to prevent blocking and the mother may be taught to do this once or twice a day.

In some cases the abnormality is slight and may arrest spontaneously. If this happens and the brain has not been damaged, the child may be able to lead a near-normal life attending ordinary schools and attaining average standards of education.

Unfortunately there remains a proportion of cases in which hydrocephalus can neither be prevented nor arrested. The nursing problem is then a considerable one. These infants should be given as much attention as possible to keep them happy and to help them to develop in spite of their limitations.

The *nursing care* of hydrocephalic children is chiefly concerned with the prevention of pressure sores and of hypostatic pneumonia and giving love and attention to a chronically sick child. Owing to the considerable weight of the head, these patients are unable to move themselves freely and they have to be turned carefully every few hours. The weight of the head also causes great pressure on the scalp and ingenuity is needed if pressure sores are to be avoided. Soft pillows are unsuitable for

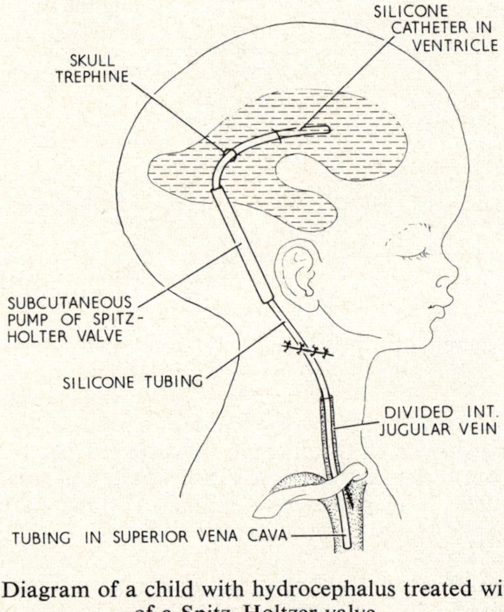

FIG. 60. Diagram of a child with hydrocephalus treated with the aid of a Spitz–Holtzer valve.

young children but polyurethane pads covered with some washable material give the necessary softness. Sometimes a ring of polyurethene can be used to give added protection to any prominence on the skull.

When lifting the infant from his cot the head must be picked up first and given adequate support before the rest of the baby is lifted out. It is unnecessary and unkind to deprive these infants of the usual 'cuddle' for fear of 'breaking the neck' and skill and the help of a soft pillow, on which to support the head while feeding, makes it perfectly possible to pick them up in the usual way.

Babies with hydrocephalus often have pretty faces which seem doubly dainty compared with the large vault of the skull. The forehead is usually drawn up tightly and it is not always possible for these infants to close their eyelids. Castor oil or 1 per cent Albucid drops should be instilled every 4 hrs to keep the cornea moist and free from infection and injury.

Some hydrocephalic babies are troubled by persistent vomiting. In these cases the feeds should be small and frequent, and diluted or Bengerized milk is sometimes well tolerated even though the vomiting is of cerebral and not of digestive origin. Special care must be taken to avoid inhalation of vomitus. Convulsions and screaming attacks are common, and should be dealt with in the usual way.

In some instances the condition is not amenable to treatment and the infant survives for a year or more and may present a grave problem within a family. Many are alert and intelligent in spite of their deformity. They should never be allowed to vegetate, but their cots should be raised so that they can look around, and they should be given extra attention whenever possible to keep them happy and help them to develop.

If these children are nursed in general paediatric wards, nurses should always remember that they may seem frightening or repulsive to other children and to lay personnel. Their beds should therefore be appropriately placed and their heads covered by a shawl or a pretty bonnet. This also helps to prevent undue loss of heat from the large expanse of skin on the head.

Spina Bifida

Spina bifida is a congenital abnormality due to a defect in the formation of the skeletal arch enclosing the spinal cord. It occurs most frequently in the lumbar region but may be present anywhere along the spinal column or even on the skull.

There are various degrees of this abnormality. In the mildest there is nothing beyond the bony defect. At other times a patch of hair or naevus over the spinal defect should lead the nurse to suspect the presence of spina bifida. Next in severity is the *meningocele* in which case the spinal meninges herniate and the sac contains cerebrospinal fluid. If the sac contains nerve tissue as well as fluid the lesion is called *meningomyelocele* (Fig. 61).

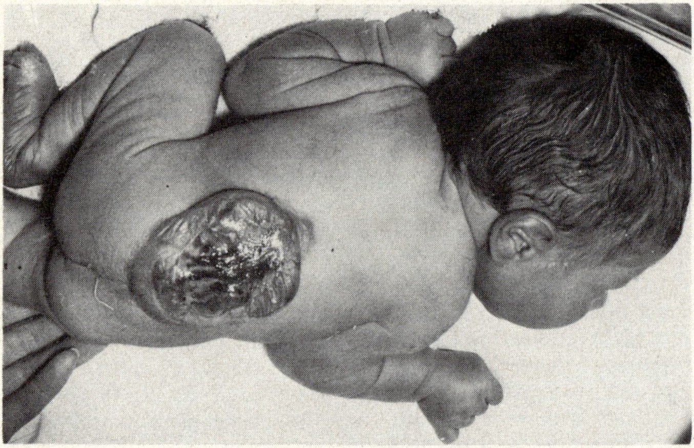

FIG. 61. A newly born infant with meningomyelocele.

In the case of babies who show signs of leg movement, immediate treatment, which should include expert physiotherapy, is of paramount importance. Early operation may lessen the danger of the motor and sensory lesions associated with this type of deformity. In many cases other abnormalities, such as talipes equinovarus, congenital dislocation of the hip joint and abnormalities of the urinary tract are also present. The most severe type is not compatible with life, as the central canal is exposed on the surface of the body and the sac is filled with nerve tissue.

When a baby with a meningocele is born, immediate steps should be taken to assess the problem and prepare for possible surgery, the lesion must be kept moist with saline soaks or with a bland non-adherent, non-greasy dressing such as Nusan B, as any damage at this stage may aggravate the neurological damage, already present. Paediatric surgeons now generally feel that early surgery should be restricted to those with mild or moderate neurological involvement.

The operation, which should ideally take place within hours of birth, aims at giving the lesion a good cover of skin. The skin is undermined, often right round to the umbilicus, and drawn together over the meningocele. Direct suture is usually possible after the underlying sac of meninges has been excised. The skin cover gives good protection, prevents infection (e.g. meningitis), helps to reduce paralysis and makes the care of the baby easier for all concerned.

When surgery is delayed or even impossible, nurses should then use their ingenuity in the way they protect the protruding lesion. Polyurethane rings are most satisfactory but even such primitive adaptations as half a rubber ball, perforated to allow for ventilation or a small kitchen strainer can serve a useful purpose.

Nursing care. This mainly aims at keeping the area dry and clean, not always an easy task with a young baby. The suture line must also be kept free of friction, and injury and abrasions prevented. The skin is best covered with a soft sterile dressing or tulle gras and a protective barrier should be devised between the buttocks and the operation site. It is often important to nurse these infants in the prone position with felt kneepads to avoid flexion contractive of the hips. This is best done by means of building up the mattress with pillows and sand bags. The chief difficulty is to leave the face free and to give an adequate air way. Special care should be taken to prevent trophic ulceration and to keep these babies warm, bearing in mind the fact that many are paralysed and lack sensory appreciation. Measurements of the head circumference should be made daily. Early signs of developing hydrocephalus include a tense fontanelle which remains wider than normal for the age, and in some cases vomiting. If a progressive enlargement is observed, surgery will be indicated. Although, a period of further observation will be required as, for reasons unknown, spontaneous arrest occurs in 40 per cent of all cases.

Where possible the mother should be admitted to be with her

child. The shock of having a deformed child should never be underestimated by the nursing staff, who by nature of their work become 'matter of fact' about this condition. Much time will be needed in sympathetic discussion with the parents who will need the support of the whole paediatric team, doctors, social workers, physiotherapists, health visitors and nurses. The Association for Spina Bifida and Hydrocephalus (address on p. 461) founded by parents of children with this handicap, will be able to give comfort as well as practical advice and support. It is important that the aim of care should be to send the mother and baby home as soon as possible in order that the natural bonds of affection can develop within the family setting. Parents who have one child with spina bifida have an increased chance that any subsequent baby may have a malformation of the central nervous system also, hence the importance that they should be offered genetic counselling.

Long-Term Care. The degree of handicap varies from one child to another, and each poses a different set of problems. Whilst each must be considered individually, the main areas of concern can be considered under the following headings.

Urinary problems may range from stress incontinence to complete loss of sphincter control. Some children develop over-distended bladders with the consequent risk of infection which will require intensive treatment with antibiotics. Where the bladder becomes over-distended, a method of manual expression of urine can be taught to the mother and later the child. Girls, particularly, present difficult problems; if incontinence pads and protective plastic pants do not provide the answer a urinary diversion may become necessary. The usual technique is to divert the ureters into an isolated segment of the ileum, of which one end is closed and the other brought out on to the anterior abdominal wall. A disposable bag can then be fitted to collect the urine. Boys can use a penile clamp or a fitted penile urinal. It is important to ensure that these children take plenty of fluids by mouth.

Bowel Control. Most of these children can achieve bowel continence with good management. This involves giving a low residue diet together with an enema once or twice a week.

Voluntary defecation can also be achieved in some children, by straining at stool after a meal or hot drink. Care must be taken that the rectum does not become impacted with faeces thus causing overflow incontinence.

Orthopaedic handicaps. Intensive physiotherapy, training and splinting will all help in the management of any limb deformities. Most of these children can be taught to walk using calipers although great care must be taken in view of the skin anaesthesia which makes them very vulnerable to trophic sores and ulceration. Some children will need to use a wheelchair and a surprising agility can often be achieved, sometimes to the envy of their friends!

Hydrocephalus. Although hydrocephalus will usually have been treated with the insertion of a shunt system, the treatment itself may lead to difficulties and complications. The tubes may need to be lengthened as the child grows or the shunt may become blocked and needs to be replaced urgently. Occasionally, the tubes themselves may become disconnected, and need surgical correction. Low grade, persistent septicaemia, most commonly due to *Staphylococcus albus* may occur and this is difficult to control until the valve is removed and it may be difficult to insert another.

Social and psychological problems. Children with physical handicaps are not necessarily also emotionally disturbed, but research findings do suggest that these children tend to be less mature and more disturbed than those without any handicap. Mental handicap too may present a problem, although the intelligence level varies and is usually related to the type of defect. Many of these children attend normal schools, but the majority attend special schools for the physically handicapped.

Some Behaviour Problems

Enuresis

A child who repeatedly passes urine involuntarily at an age when he can normally be expected to be toilet-trained is said to be suffering from enuresis. He may either never have been dry, or may have relapsed after a period of normal control of micturition. Wetting may occur several times a night, very occasionally, or perhaps once or twice per month.

Causes include renal infections, nephrosis, diabetes, psychological disturbances, congenital abnormalities of the urinary tract, spina bifida, neurological lesions, mental subnormality, chronic constipation, and intestinal worms. A frequent cause is behaviour disturbance following the birth of a new baby, a change to a new school, a severe illness or other experience causing a loss of security.

A thorough physical examination, urinalysis and full investigations of the renal tract must be done to exclude organic disease, and if these are negative, psychological treatment may be advised. This will include full enquiry into home background, and the parents will be interviewed as well as the child. They may be advised to restrict fluid intake during the evening, to rouse the child and offer a pot before they themselves go to bed and to leave a small light burning. Punishment and scolding are as a rule out of place, although an overworked exasperated mother may well be forgiven if she loses patience with the child. Constant wet sheets may be a great trial in a small town flat and the criticism of neighbours is not easy to bear.

Every small improvement should be hailed as a hopeful sign and encouragement and praise given whenever possible. Sometimes drugs are used such as the tri-cyclic antidepressants. A 'conditioned reflex' can be created in older children by using a specially designed buzzer which goes off and rouses the child as he starts to void urine. Properly used these may score successes in 75 per cent of cases treated.

Faecal Incontinence (Encopresis)

Faecal incontinence, i.e. soiling at an age when a child may reasonably be expected to be toilet-trained, may be due to a number of reasons. A common cause is constipation with overflow, and reasons for this situation range from 'pot refusal' due to painful anal fissure in toddlers, to emotional disturbances, congenital abnormalities and bad housing conditions. Another example is the child who notes his mother's distress if he does not have his bowels open regularly and uses bowel function to attract attention, 'please' or 'punish'. Sometimes the lavatory itself is to blame: it may be situated on a dark landing in an old tenement building or in the garden, or it may be so high that the child dreads using it for fear of falling in.

The cause of faecal incontinence should therefore be investigated very carefully and patiently. Good teamwork between parents, paediatrician, child guidance clinic and health visitor will usually cure the condition, but sometimes repeated enemata or such medicines as Senokot may be prescribed.

Although chronic constipation very frequently has a psychological background, it is also a common complication in mentally subnormal children and in those suffering from such conditions as spina bifida and neuromuscular diseases. If due to psychological reasons, the condition usually starts after the child has been successfully toilet-trained. Strange habits such as passing a stool 'secretly' and 'hiding' it in strange places may develop. Only skilled psychiatric treatment can successfully cure such children.

Mental Handicap

Mental handicap or mental defect can be defined as inadequate mental development resulting in incapacity for independent social and intellectual adaptation in everyday life. There are many causes for this handicap which can be classified into the following groups:

(1) Genetically determined, e.g. Down's syndrome.
(2) Ante-natal infection, e.g. rubella or syphilis.
(3) Birth injury.
(4) Post-natal, e.g. encephalitis, cerebral infection, trauma.

Mental handicap may also be associated with other handicaps, e.g. cerebral palsy or the child with hydrocephalus and myelomeningocele.

Only a few types of mental handicap are obvious at birth, such as Down's syndrome or microcephaly, whilst with others the condition may be unsuspected for several months. The first indication of this handicap in the young child is usually noticed in a delay by the child to reach the normal milestones in sitting, standing and walking; speech too is delayed. The child often appears placid and 'good' or conversely may appear hyperactive, restless and difficult to feed. Occasionally the handicap is only recognized when the child starts school and has difficulty in learning the three 'Rs'.

Whatever the cause and whenever it is diagnosed the news will cause much anxiety and distress for the parents and the family. The parents may vacillate between extreme feelings of total rejection of their child to overwhelming possessiveness which may lead to neglect of their other children. The parents often try to find a cause for the handicap and may blame themselves. The nurse must recognize that these feelings are very real to the parents who will need much support and help in adopting a positive acceptance of their child's handicap. Many parents benefit from having contact with parents in a similar situation and help both practical and emotional is provided by voluntary agencies for the handicapped child.

The parents will have many questions to ask, wanting to know what their child's potential will be, how best to help him and what type of schooling will be needed? In order to answer these questions a complete assessment will be made by the multidisciplinary team concerned with the care for the child. Measurements of the intelligence quotient will be made by the clinical psychologist and compared with the chronological age; physical ability will be assessed by the physiotherapist, social behaviour by the nurse and the child's medical history thoroughly investigated by the paediatrician. Even with this initial assessment it is difficult to forecast how the child will develop and progress. Assessment therefore should be carried out periodically in order that appropriate stimulation and training is given at the right stage of development.

Parents will need to know that their mentally handicapped child requires more and not less of the normal childhood pleasures and activities. It is through play, nursery rhymes, songs and stories that the young child learns. He should be cuddled, praised and made a fuss of so that he feels secure and will want to do his best. As far as possible the parents should treat the child normally whilst recognizing that because of this handicap he will be slower and less able than other children of the same age.

All children whatever their disability are able to go to school. Special schooling with small groups of children and specially qualified teachers provide education and training that is geared to the individual child's needs and potential.

In the past many mentally handicapped children were placed in large institutions for care and protection where they were often forgotten by their families. It is now recognized that with training and care many more mentally handicapped people can take their place in society where they may work in sheltered workshops and live in a hostel if there is no family home.

However it is important to recognize that many children because of their handicap or social background may require admission into a specialist hospital; here doctors and nurses with special expertise will provide an environment which will give the child the opportunity to learn social skills and to be cared for. Even though care must be planned in the long term; parents are encouraged to maintain family links joining in hospital and ward activities and where possible taking their child home for week-ends and holidays.

As with all children the mentally handicapped child may need admission into the paediatric unit with a superimposed medical or surgical condition. The nurse should especially remember how distressing this situation will be for the child. In order to avoid too much bewilderment and distress the child should whenever possible be looked after by 'his nurse'. Every effort should be made to follow the child's home routine whilst he is in hospital in order to maintain the progress he is making. Facilities for mother or father to be resident should be provided.

Further Reading

ANDERSON, E. M. & SPAIN, B. (1977) *Your Child with Spina Bifida*. London: Methuen.

CARLSON, B. W. & GINGLEND, D. R. (1962) *Play Activities for the Retarded Child*. London: Ballière, Tindall & Cox.

FIELD, A. (1970) *The Challenge of Spina Bifida*. London: Heinemann.

KIRMAN, B. H. (1972) *The Mentally Handicapped Child*, London: Nelson.

LORBER, J. (1975) *Your Child with Spina Bifida*. London: Association for Spina Bifida and Hydrocephalus.

MORRIS, P. (1969) *Put Away*. London: Routledge & Kegan Paul.

OSWIN, M. (1967) *Behaviour Problems Amongst Children with Cerebral Palsy*. Bristol: John Wright.

STONE, J. & CHURCH, J. (1968) *Childhood and Adolescence*. New York: Random House.

TILL, K. (1975) *Paediatric Neuro-Surgery*. Oxford: Blackwell Scientific.

18

Diseases of the skin

Infantile Eczema

Infantile eczema is an allergic skin condition seen in varying degrees of severity. In mild cases only the flexor surfaces of the legs and arms are affected, in severe cases the rash may cover most of the body including the cheeks, forehead and scalp.

Infantile eczema mostly affects very young children. It is rarely seen before the age of 3 months and with the exception of localized patches may be expected to clear up by the age of 2 to 3 years. A definite family history of eczema, asthma or hay fever is typical and some children who suffer from eczema in infancy develop asthma later in life.

Boys are more frequently affected than girls and the babies are often blue-eyed, fair-haired and frequently delightful patients to look after. Allergy to certain foods such as eggs, fish, cow's milk and certain pollen or household dust can sometimes be found, either by taking a careful history or by performing intradermal tests.

Signs and Symptoms. The rash is commonly first noticed over the forehead, cheeks and scalp but the areas around the mouth stay clear. As the eczema spreads the flexures of the elbows and knees and the folds behind the ears become affected and patchy areas may occur in any part of the body. Initially the skin is red, hot and scaly but soon papules and vesicles appear and as they break down clear serum exudes from the lesion. This is known as weeping eczema and at this stage the skin easily becomes infected. Irritation is intense and it may be almost impossible to stop the infant from scratching. As the exudate dries up thick crusts are formed. In spite of the extensive lesions, eczema leaves no scars.

Treatment. Treatment often includes a full investigation of the possible exciting causes. Intradermal tests with specific proteins, pollen or dust may show a positive reaction to a certain agent which can then be eliminated from the diet or the child's environment. Psychological disturbances may be present and both parents and patient need guidance and psychotherapy. Dietary idiosyncrasies must be corrected and certain foods may have to be excluded from the diet. Starchy foods should be given in moderation, but extra protein in the form of Casilan or Complan are useful during the acute, weeping stage. Occasionally there is an intolerance of cow's milk and this can be substituted by soya-bean 'milk'. Special dried milks such as Allergilac (Cow & Gate) are on the market.

Local Treatment. This includes the use of coal tar preparations, calamine lotion with or without an oily base and the addition of a mild antiseptic. More recently creams containing hydrocortisone have been used with good effect though improvement is often not maintained when treatment is discontinued. It is also important to realize that absorption of cortisone can lead to dangerous complications, e.g. if an operation has to be performed. Irritation may be allayed by giving baths to which Ung. Emulsificans has been added. The preparation is soothing and assists with the separation of crusts while replacing soap. Children enjoy these baths and they give mothers an opportunity to make a special fuss of their children. A soft towel should be used for drying and the skin gently dabbed and never rubbed.

The Applications. These vary according to the stage of the rash. When dry and scaly, creams or liniments may be ordered. They are either applied direct to the skin and left exposed or thinly spread on to old linen and bandaged to the affected area. Infected areas may be treated with some kind of antiseptic lotion or cream such as, for instance, proflavine or an antibiotic. Bandages should always be of the open woven type as they are cooler and more economical than other types. Tubular gauze is very useful as it is easy to keep in position, porous and light. The skin of convalescent children can be suitably protected by tubular gauze 'sleeves, stockings and mittens'. When elbow splints are applied, they should be made of spatulas or cardboard (see page 117) and a minimum of padding used to avoid over-heating the skin. Any knots should be tied on the posterior aspect of the splint so that the child cannot rub his face on them. Inventive nurses can make good use of tubular gauze for the purpose of restraining, in lieu of using splinting.

Nursing Care. The brunt of the treatment will fall on the mother or nursing staff. Irritation is intense and the infant manages to scratch by every possible means. Even when the extremities are effectively restrained he manages to wriggle his little body and rolls his head and if inadvertently released, a newly healed area may be scratched to bleeding point in next to no time. Mittens made of tubular gauze (see page 61) may have to be left on during a bath to prevent scratching and the hands always dried first and clean mittens applied after a bath.

The infant should be kept cool and well occupied. During the acute stages it is necessary in many cases to secure rest and sleep by sedation. Special smooth sheets should be used. With small children it has been found useful to nurse them on a large sheet of X-ray film or acetate sheets which are smooth and cool and can easily be cleaned. Tied to the mattress this can be a most effective means to comfort. Clothes must be light and cool and should be of thin cotton or silk. Mittens and socks can be used to keep the extremities warm but they should be of cool light cotton or tubular gauze. The patients are often happiest if left entirely without clothes. Clothing is best done up in the front, as buttons or tapes down the back give the baby an opportunity for scratching by moving his body. The bedclothes are best cradled and an electric fan may be used to keep the air circulating and cool. Sedatives such as chloral hydrate in large doses, Benadryl, Phenergan, Trimeprazine elixir and Disprin may be ordered. It is usual to admit these infants into cubicles to minimize the danger of cross-infection but this consideration must be carefully weighed against the need for company and diversion. Extra visiting and attention from the mother are desirable not only because she can divert the infant but also because she can learn to handle her child and assist with the care of his skin while under expert supervision. Thus she will gain confidence and the child will learn to accept treatment from her. A good ward sister may also be able to observe any psychological conflicts which may exist between mother and child.

Children suffering from eczema are prone to asthma and gastro-intestinal upsets. The latter may cause alarming losses of weight and apparent wasting due to the loss of abnormal fluid present in the tissues. Both these complications may prove serious and babies with infantile eczema should be nursed with special care. Exposure to infection is minimized by admission to a cubicle or a 'clean' ward. Barrier gowns are worn and anyone suffering from a cold should keep away from these babies. Exacerbations during teething are common.

Care has to be taken to avoid indiscretions in the diet where an allergy is known to exist. Not infrequently there is a definite psychological background, as in many allergic conditions. This point must never be ignored and a child guidance expert may be able to help and advise. A happy emotional background is of great importance. The mother-child relationship should always be carefully examined, but even if the mother is entirely adequate, exhaustion from nursing the child and constant disturbed nights may be so great that a period of rest is imperative and the infant's admission to hospital unavoidable. A calm but non-restrictive atmosphere in the home is of prime importance.

Immunization and Vaccination. Children with eczema can be treated as any others with regard to immunization. Vaccination against smallpox may, however, be highly dangerous and the child should never be allowed to go near another child recently vaccinated. There is a great risk of generalized vaccinia coupled with severe toxic symptoms. This very serious condition is known as Kaposi's vericelliform dermatitis. Kaposi's dermatitis is however, more often due to infection by the virus of herpes simplex.

Acne Vulgaris

This very common and distressing condition occurs at puberty. It is due to an excessive output and overgrowth of sebaceous glands particularly on the face, chest and shoulders. Blockage of sebum occurs and a comedo or 'black head' is produced.

Treatment. It is of utmost importance to reduce the greasiness of the skin. The face should be washed in hot water as often as possible and the comedos removed with a comedo extractor. Calamine lotion with 3 per cent sulphur is then applied and rubbed in well. The hair must be shampooed regularly. Ultraviolet light increases the amount of desquamation and may be used in the home providing the eyes are protected with dark glasses. Long-term tetracycline therapy has been found to be of value in severe cases. Diet does not appear to make any difference. The patient is always very self-conscious about these spots and will need constant reassurance that once puberty is over these lesions will disappear, but that squeezing of the spots produces scars and should be avoided.

Impetigo Contagiosa

Impetigo is a skin infection caused by the streptococcus or staphylococcus. It is very common in children of school age and spreads easily, particularly in overcrowded homes with poor hygiene. The organism enters the skin through a crack or a scratch and for that reason is often associated with an infested head.

At first small vesicles appear and as they break the lesion becomes red and weeping and as the exudate dries up thick crusts form. Typical sites are on the scalp, the chin and around the lips. The crusts have the appearance of being 'stuck on' (Fig. 62).

Local Treatment. Local treatment consists in softening the crusts with warm saline bathings or a solution of potassium permanganate 1:4000. The skin may be painted with an antiseptic preparation such as boracic cream or an antibiotic cream. Occasionally antibiotics may be ordered by mouth if the infection is severe or fails to respond to local treatment. If the hair is crusted, a small area may have to be shaved after obtaining medical and parental consent. Once the crusts are removed a 1 per cent cetrimide solution may be used for cleansing the skin.

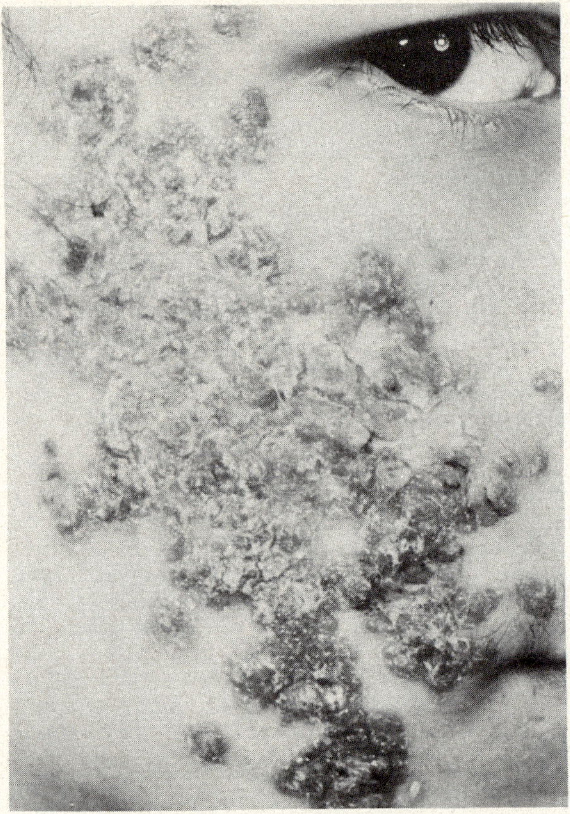

FIG. 62. A typical case of severe impetigo.

Systemic treatment with penicillin should be given. It is important to remember that other members of the family may also be affected and need treatment.

Prophylactic treatment consists of using medicated soap and antiseptic creams. The cream is introduced into the vestibule of the nose of all the family until the infection on the affected child has been completely eliminated.

The child suffering from impetigo is likely to infect others and if admitted to hospital should be nursed with barrier precautions. Crockery and cutlery should be sterilized until the last lesion has healed. Scratching is prevented by splinting in the same way as in the case of infantile eczema (see page 117).

The condition may clear within a few days and rarely leaves any scars. Recurrence should be prevented by giving the mother guidance with regard to personal hygiene and building up the child's general resistance, by good diet, exercise in the fresh air and an adequate vitamin intake.

Scabies

Scabies is a skin infection caused by a minute parasite. The female mite burrows into the skin where she lays her eggs, and it is usually possible to see the burrows with the help of a magnifying glass. As the eggs hatch, the larvae move to the hair follicles. Intense iritation results and this is particularly marked when the skin becomes warm at night. In young babies the soft skin allows for access in any part and lesions are found anywhere on the body. In babies who have not started walking, lesions may even occur on the soft skin of the soles of the feet. Secondary infections are common as a result of scratching.

Treatment. This aims at softening the skin and opening the burrows prior to the application of benzyl benzoate (25 per cent solution). The patient is given a warm bath after which the skin is dabbed dry and the whole body painted with benzyl benzoate and allowed to dry. On the second day the body is again painted all over and on the third day a final bath is given. After that, both personal clothing and bed linen are changed. The infected clothing and linen are sterilized by boiling or by pressing with a hot iron.

Benzyl benzoate may sting on application, particularly if there are open scratch-wounds. Care must be taken not to apply the lotion too near the eyes. Alternatively monosulfiram (Tetmosol) may be used and is less irritating for some children. For small infants Eurax 10 per cent ointment may be used instead of the benzyl benzoate. This is applied in the same manner as benzyl benzoate.

Ringworm

A fungus infection caused by a micro-sporon is responsible for this skin condition. Ringworm usually affects the scalp or nails of school children and is highly contagious.

Since the advent of the oral antibiotic drug Griseofulvin the former, routine treatment with X-rays has been abandoned. The diagnosis is confirmed by examination under a Wood's glass filter which shows the hair with a characteristic fluorescent green colour.

Athlete's Foot (*Tinea interdigitalis*)

This very common condition, due to an epidermophyton, is highly contagious. The disease is spread through towels, bath mats and communal baths, becoming a particular problem in boarding schools. Areas of sodden skin with cracks and fissures appear between the toes spreading to the sole of the foot which may become quite sore.

Treatment. The sodden skin should be removed each day and zinc undecylenate ointment applied. This substance is also available as a dusting powder to be used in socks and shoes. Treatment should be continued for at least a week after the last sign of infection has disappeared to prevent a relapse. Meticulous attention to hygiene is essential to prevent the spread of this infection to others. Where a pupil is reported with this condition attention must be paid by the authorities to the bath-room and swimming pool floors to avoid an outbreak throughout the school.

Head Lice (*Pediculosis capitis*)

The incidence of infestation with head lice rises each year. It is estimated that at least one million people are affected in the United Kingdom. Schoolchildren especially in junior schools are the most commonly infested. Head lice may be found in the hair of children who may have become infected, perhaps by sitting next to an already infected child at school, or from an infected member of the family. Infestation of the hair by

Pediculosis capitis should be suspected if the child is noticed to be scratching the scalp frequently, particularly at the back, as the head lice tend to inhabit the occipital region rather than the front part of the scalp. Secondary infection of the scratches on the scalp may produce a coincident impetigo. In some children where infestation is severe, cervical adenitis, associated with malaise and pyrexia may occur as a result of septic absorption from these areas of secondary infection.

The louse reproduces by means of hatching eggs which are attached to hair follicles by means of a 'cement-like' substance. This makes removal of the eggs or 'nits' difficult.

Treatment. The treatment of choice is to use an insecticide lotion containing malathion 0.5 per cent, e.g. Prioderm. The lotion kills both the lice and the eggs, 30 minutes after application, the hair is washed with a bland shampoo. Alternatively, an insecticidal shampoo containing either DDT or Gamma BHC which will destroy the lice rapidly but is ineffective against the nits, may be used. As the nits will hatch out after treatment with these shampoos, the hair should be washed with the shampoo again after 8 days. Failure to shampoo a second time allows for a resurgence of the infestation. Following treatment, the hair must be carefully and repeatedly combed with a fine-toothed metal comb such as the Sacker comb.

The basis for successful treatment is both educational and practical. It is essential that the whole family be treated and this should include all the adults as well as any pre-school children who are also at risk. When infestation occurs in a school-aged child the school authorities should be notified.

Further Reading

WILKINSON, D. S. (1970) *The Nursing and Management of Skin Diseases*, 3rd ed., Part 4. London: Faber & Faber.

19

Diseases of muscle, bones and joints

Muscular Dystrophies (Myopathies)

A number of variants of the myopathies exist which all have the characteristics of progressive, degenerative changes in the muscle fibres, leading to wasting and weakness. The nerves are not affected in this group and there are neither sensory changes nor paralysis. The diseases are often hereditary and familial and usually lead to early death due to intercurrent infections such as pneumonia. A proportion of children with muscular dystrophy are mentally handicapped but the majority are of normal intelligence.

The various types of myopathies affect different muscle groups in particular, causing degenerative changes in the muscle fibres and their replacement by connective tissue and fat. Whole groups of muscles may thus be weakened and although the process may be a very slow one, it is always progressive and the patient eventually becomes completely incapacitated and crippled.

Diagnosis. Diagnosis is confirmed by electromyography by which means the changes can be differentiated from those in other diseases of muscles. The destruction of muscle causes excretion of creatinine in the urine.

Pseudo-Hypertrophic Muscular Dystrophy

The most common of the myopathies in childhood is pseudo-hypertrophic muscular dystrophy so called because of the enlargement of certain muscles in this condition.

Signs and Symptoms. The child may be normal up to school age but gradually it is noticed that he tires easily, that he prefers to sit about rather than play with other children, and finds it difficult to walk up stairs without the help of the banister. The gait becomes unstable and he is easily pushed over in play. The muscles of the shoulder girdle may become so weak that the child cannot raise his arms above his head and when the doctor places his hands underneath the arms to lift the patient, the child literally slips through his hands.

Weakness of the muscles of the pelvic girdle and the spine lead to kyphosis and lordosis. The gait is waddling at first and later walking becomes impossible. When the child tries to raise himself from the lying position, he first has to roll on to his front and then raise himself on to his hands and knees; by gradually moving one hand after the other up his legs and above his knees he eventually succeeds in raising himself to the upright position. This manoeuvre is very characteristic of the disease.

As the muscular weakness progresses the child becomes bed-ridden and deformities through contractions develop.

Treatment. Treatment aims at preventing crippling and wasting by massage and exercises. Movement should be encouraged as disuse leads to more rapid wasting. Pneumonia usually causes death after a few years.

Other Types of the Myopathies. These affect specific muscle groups in particular. The rate of progress may vary greatly and in spite of crippling the patient may survive into middle age. The more common varieties are the facio-scapulo-humeral type and myotonia-congenita. As the name implies, the muscles affected in the facio-scapulo-humeral type, are those of the face, arms and shoulder girdle. The first signs may be difficulty in sucking and in closing the eyes completely. The handicap is as a rule slight and a fairly normal existence is possible. Myotonia congenita causes voluntary muscles to go into protracted contractions followed by slow relaxation. Muscle biopsy shows enlargement and thickening of muscle fibres. Muscle biopsy and electromyography are usually carried out to confirm diagnosis as the changes in the electrical activity in the muscle and those in the structure of the muscles are characteristic of the various types of the disease.

Genetic counselling should be offered to all parents considering enlarging their family.

Torticollis (Wry Neck)

Torticollis may be present from birth or arise later in life caused by diseases such as inflamed glands of the neck, tuberculosis of the cervical spine and paralysis. Occasionally the cause is psychological.

The postural changes are characteristic and include rotation of the head to one side with head flexion and a raising of the shoulder on the other. If allowed to persist, the angle at which the head is constantly held causes visual disturbances.

Treatment. This depends on the child's age and on the underlying cause. In infants stretching and passive exercises should be carried out several times daily and correct posture maintained by means of sandbags and possibly a cap and light harness made of 12 mm webbing. Collars made of corrugated paper covered with a piece of soft material, Perspex splints and supports and collars made from polystyrene are used to keep the head in an over-corrected position. In resistant cases, subcutaneous or open tenotomy may have to be carried out to lengthen the sternomastoid muscle. Post-operative overcorrection is maintained for some time by one of the methods given above.

Sternomastoid Tumour

Difficult labour associated with excessive rotation and lateral extension of the neck and head are occasionally the cause of a sternomastoid tumour. The tumour is rarely noticed before the baby is about 2 weeks old. It is painless and firm and the size varies from a small lump the size of a pea to that of a walnut. The condition is harmless and resolves spontaneously after some weeks. Passive movement and massage are given to help recovery and minimize any risk of permanent torticollis from habitually wrong posture.

Klippel-Feil Syndrome

In this skeletal abnormality the patient has a short neck, fused cervical vertebrae, a low hair line and a curious tilting of the head. Sometimes the condition is seen in conjunction with spina bifida, spastic paralysis and other abnormalities.

Perthe's Disease

Osteochondritis is a fairly common abnormality of growth and development of the epiphyses in children. The most common of the diseases in this group is Perthe's disease. This disease affects boys more frequently than girls and develops between the ages of 5 to 10 years. It is usually unilateral.

The cause is a disturbance in the blood supply to the epiphysis, which leads to deformity of the epiphysial plate and in the later stages, if untreated, to collapse of the head of the femur and arrest of the development of the epiphysis.

Examination reveals that the range of movement is limited in all directions. Changes may not show up on radiographs for some time; after a while there may be wasting of the leg and in some cases shortening. The latter is due to collapse of the head and later premature epiphysial arrest. The disease takes a long course, the average time from onset to final healing is 4 years.

Treatment. There are two distinct approaches to the treatment of Perthe's disease. Some surgeons consider that prolonged immobilization with traction is required to prevent osteoarthritis in later life. Others believe that once the early stage of muscle spasm is passed, the use of weight-bearing crutches or the Synder sling with crutches for non-weight bearing ambulation is all that is required. If the disease process affects the entire femoral head osteotomy may be necessary. To avoid the effects of prolonged hospitalization these children, where possible, should be cared for at home with the support of the community nursing services.

Nursing Care. Those children who are treated by bed-rest combined with traction and splinting and those with calipers have to be given special care of skin and pressure areas to prevent soreness. With the surgeon's permission groin and any other straps should be released twice daily and the skin washed, carefully dried and kept healthy by applying powder and zinc and castor oil cream (with or without the addition of compound of tincture of benzoin, sufficient to colour the cream light brown) and padding with a layer of lint or polyurethane.

General muscle tone should be maintained by giving daily massage and exercises. As the stay in hospital may extend over many months, schooling and occupational therapy should be made available and whenever possible little treats such as outings or a week-end visit home can be arranged.

Prognosis. The prognosis is excellent provided adequate, early treatment is given but late cases may develop severe arthritis when they grow older.

Congenital Dislocation of the Hip Joint

Children with congenital dislocation of the hip joint have an abnormally shallow acetabulum which causes the femoral head to be displaced upwards and backwards when the child begins to put weight upon the limb. The neck of the femur may be shortened and the capsule becomes stretched. Sometimes the femoral head lies outside the acetabulum at the time of birth. As the child walks she dips on the affected side or has a waddling gait if the dislocation is a bilateral one. Because the pelvis is tipped forward, lordosis develops.

Congenital dislocation of the hip joint is a fairly common condition. Successful treatment depends on an early assessment and this should not be delayed beyond the first week of life.

The abnormality occurs mostly in girls; the condition runs in families and although usually present at birth it is often not noticed until the child begins to walk. The dislocation may be unilateral or bilateral and it may be partial or complete.

Signs and Symptoms. The observant nurse may notice that one leg is shorter than the other and that the perineum is wider than usual. A telescoping movement of the leg may be possible. When the baby lies prone, the gluteal crease on the affected side is higher than that on the good side and the buttocks may be flattened.

When the baby is being medically examined she is placed on her back with the legs towards the examining doctor with hips and knees flexed to right angles. The middle finger of each hand is placed over the great trochanter while the flexed leg is contained in the palm of the hand and the thumb on the inner side of the thigh opposite the lesser trochanter. Keeping the legs flexed at 45° abduction the middle finger of each hand is pressed on the great trochanter to test whether or not the femoral head can be lifted into the acetabulum. If the test is positive, a click will be heard. This is known as the Ortolani sign.

Not in all cases in which the test is positive will treatment be necessary. An experienced orthopaedic surgeon must however be asked to see the baby without delay.

Treatment. Treatment should be started as soon as the condition has been recognized as its duration and success depend on the age of the child. In very young babies a special webbing harness may be used. Older children may be placed on a special abduction frame and skin traction is applied to bring the head of the femur into position opposite the acetabulum. The legs are gradually abducted, one leg at a time, at intervals of 2 or 3 days to allow for gradual stretching of the muscles. When both legs have been abducted to right angles to the trunk (Fig. 63), the child is taken to the theatre.

Two different methods of treatment are commonly used, depending on the age of the child, radiograph appearance and the surgeon's wishes:

1. The dislocation is reduced and the legs rotated to bring the femoral head into the acetabulum. The legs are fixed externally rotated and in full abduction with the knees flexed at right angles to the femora. A so-called '*frog plaster*' is applied, which reaches from the nipple line to the ankles.

2. The dislocation is reduced, the femora internally rotated and the legs fully abducted from the knees downward. A plaster, reaching from the groins to the ankles enables the child to move freely in the hip joint while maintaining flexion and extension. A wooden cross-bar is incorporated into the plaster from one knee across to the other: this is called a *Batchelor plaster*. After

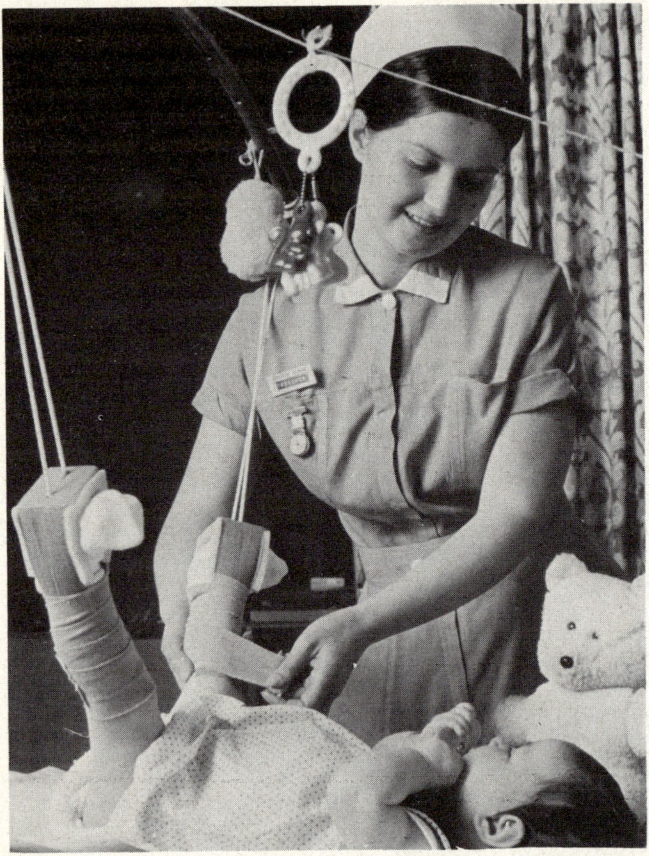

FIG. 63. Nurse renewing bandages following daily inspection of skin for child on hoop traction.

a time the child learns to move about and even to 'walk' on her knees.

In either case treatment has to be continued for a year to 18 months and during that time the child may be discharged home and brought back for changes of plaster at intervals of approximately 3 months. Occasionally neither of these methods is successful and open reduction and rotation osteotomy to correct the angle of the femur on the hip may be necessary. This would not be done until the baby is at least 1 year old. In very persistent cases shelf operation, acetabuloplasty, is performed to deepen the acetabulum, and a hip spica applied.

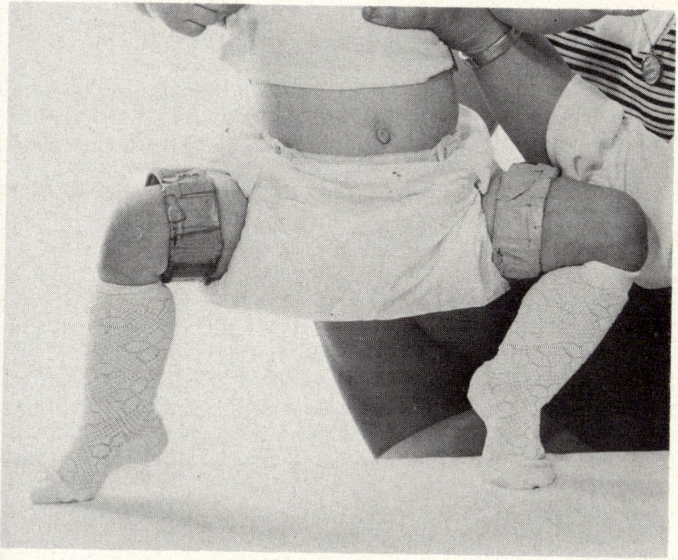

FIG. 64. Congenital dislocation of the hip. A simple splint that the mother can easily apply, comfortable to wear and which maintains the correct position.

Nursing Care. During the stage of abduction the child suffers considerable discomfort and frustration due to the immobility and her position on the frame. Firm sympathy, a great deal of individual attention and occupation and free visiting all help to comfort the child and in the initial stages sedatives should be given generously. The nurse will have to use much patience and imagination to get the child to take fluids and food in this position and to teach her to pass urine and faeces without unduly soiling the padding of the frame. The bandages are taken off the legs daily and the skin inspected for reaction to strapping. They are washed and powdered before reapplying the bandages. The frame padding or plaster can be protected by thin plastic sheeting or waterproof adhesive tape.

After manipulation and application of the plaster the new position will again cause distress for some days and sleep may be very light and disturbed. Individual small pillows to support arms, shoulders and feet should be available. Even though the plaster is left exposed to allow for drying, the chest and extremities should be covered with little blankets, bootees and mittens. The toes should be carefully watched. They should be warm and rosy and should flush quickly with blood on release of digital pressure. The patient is turned 4-hourly to ensure drying of the plaster on the back as well as the front.

As soon as the plaster has set, the child should be turned on to her side and front at intervals for change of position and to reduce abdominal distension as far as possible and give a different outlook. A special watch should be kept for possible plaster sores. The young child is unable to express her pain and discomfort but restlessness, itching, fretfulness and a slight rise in temperature should all be considered carefully as possible signs of trouble. It must always be remembered that, once the sore deepens, all pain disappears. A foul smell and staining of the plaster are later, more obvious signs that a sore has developed. As the child digs her elbows into the bed in an attempt at raising herself to look around, the elbows are particularly liable to get sore. Heels and ankles should also have attention and be kept off the bed by support with small pillows or heel rings while lying down. Various adjustable frames with a detachable tray can be used to support the child in the upright position and some children can even manage to 'walk' in a frog plaster. A 'twin push-chair' will make it possible to take the child out and a little platform on wheels on to which the child is placed in the prone position, gives the slightly older patient excellent means of mobility.

Treatment has to continue over a period of 1 to 2 years depending in part on the age of the child, as the longer the condition has been left untreated the more difficult is successful treatment. When the plaster is eventually omitted, the child is at first allowed the freedom of the bed. Daily physiotherapy is given and after about 3 weeks, if X-ray appearance is satisfactory, is allowed to start weight-bearing. In early, successful cases walking should be normal and a complete, permanent cure can be expected.

If home conditions are good, the child is usually sent home and only readmitted for change of plaster and reassessment at intervals of 2 to 3 months. The mother can be taught how to keep the plaster clean and special little supports and chairs can be made at low cost to facilitate sitting up and for toilet purposes. If the child has to remain in hospital, everything should be done to keep up contact with the home by allowing free visiting and if possible week-end visits home. Suitable occupation and little outings to the hospital grounds or even the surrounding streets are important if the young child is to be given a chance of developing the experiences appropriate to her age. If these points are neglected it may well happen that as a result of treatment the hip joint is normal at the expense of serious psychological disturbance in the young patient.

Talipes

Talipes (Fig. 65) may occur on one or both sides and is often associated with other congenital abnormalities such as spina bifida. There are variants in both severity and in the type of the deformity. Usually several joints of the foot are involved, often causing inversion of the forefoot, internal rotation of the tibia and plantar flexion of the ankle joint. There are four types, and any may be seen in varying degrees of severity.

1. *Talipes equinovarus* (*clubfoot*). The deformity consists of inversion (turning in) of the forefoot, internal rotation of the tibia and plantar flexion of the ankle joint.
2. *Congenital talipes calcaneovalgus.* The deformity consists of eversion (turning out) of the foot and dorsiflexion at the ankle joint. The tendon Achillis is lengthened. This deformity is less severe and yields more easily to treatment than the equinovarus deformity. In mild cases it may be sufficient for the mother to stretch the foot into equinus and varus position several times before each feed. She

will also have to do this in cases which require surgery.

3. *Talipes equinovalgus.* In this deformity there is eversion and plantar flexion.
4. *Talipes calcaneovarus.* In this deformity there is inversion and dorsiflexion.

The two last-mentioned deformities are usually seen in patients suffering from paralysis and/or cerebral palsy.

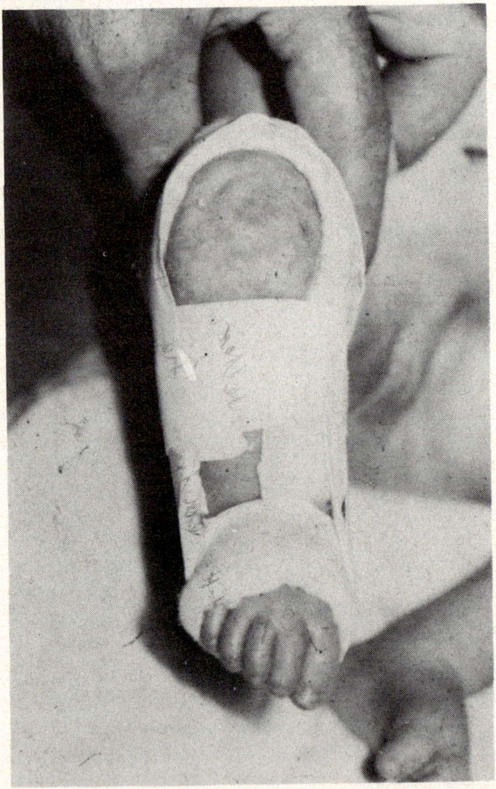

FIG. 65. Talipes equinovarus foot strapped in the correct position.

Treatment of Talipes Equinovarus. This should be commenced within 36 hours of birth and its success depends greatly on the promptness with which it is started. The foot is manipulated manually until the little toe touches the peroneal surface of the leg. The over-corrected position is maintained by adhesive strapping, splints, plaster of Paris or special Denis Browne boots. Manipulation is repeated weekly at first. Kicking and standing on the splints when the child is old enough are encouraged as this helps to develop the leg muscles.

Manipulation often causes reactionary swelling and as treatment is often given in the out-patient department full instructions to bring her baby back if there is reason for concern, should be given to the mother, in the same way as would be done in cases of fractures treated by plaster of Paris. If the baby is treated in the maternity ward, the weight of the bedclothes is taken off by using a cradle and the feet are inspected frequently to make sure that swelling is not excessive and that there is no serious constriction to the blood supply. As it would seriously interfere with treatment if the splints were to be left off, even for short periods, it is necessary to persevere regardless of strapping reactions or even blistering of the skin. If treated from birth correction may be complete by the age of 6 months or a year but a special night boot is usually worn for another year or two. Occasionally the outside of the shoe heel is raised or an inside iron with a 'T' strap fixed to the shoes when the baby starts to walk. Cases treated less promptly may need many years of treatment, and cure may not be permanent. Parents are usually very pleased with the initial improvement and it may be difficult to impress on them the importance of continuing treatment for a number of years. Sometimes manipulation, stretching and splinting fail and operation becomes necessary. This may be either open or closed tenotomy, or, as a last resort, Steindler's operation or triple arthrodesis. Supervision by the orthopaedic surgeon is as a rule maintained until growth is complete.

Osteomyelitis

Osteomyelitis is an infection causing acute inflammation beneath the periosteum resulting in an abscess and sequestrum formation (death of the bone). Osteomyelitis used to be one of the most severe illnesses of childhood usually affecting children whose general health was poor and who came from overcrowded homes. With the advent of modern drug therapy the outlook has greatly improved, but the patient may still be seriously ill and relapses are common.

The disease commonly attacks children between the ages of 2 and 12 years, although babies in the neonatal period may be affected. The femur, humerus, clavicle and maxilla are common sites of infection and there may be evidence of a recent knock or injury. There is frequently a history of infected tonsils, boils or septic spots and the causative organism is then in many cases a staphylococcus, although in recent years other organisms, e.g. *E. coli*, have caused osteomyelitis. The condition in the latter case is not so acute, but the site has to be drained more often before the infection is overcome.

Signs and Symptoms. The onset may be acute with hyperpyrexia, tachycardia, headaches, rigor, toxaemia or septicaemia, but at times it can be quite insidious. Infants appear to have little pain, but the general disturbances include vomiting and diarrhoea, causing dehydration. In older children pain can be very severe until tension subsides following the discharge or release of pus or decrease of infection following treatment with antibiotics. The limb is held immobilized in a relaxed position and occasionally the condition may be mistaken for some form of paralysis. Any handling is deeply resented. The skin over the affected area may be found to be red, shiny and hot, although it may take a day or two for the inflammation to become obvious. The white cell count is high (mainly polymorphonuclear cells) and blood culture is sometimes positive. X-ray appearance is rarely abnormal before the second or third week.

Treatment. Large doses of antibiotics together with immobilization, may bring about a cure, but sometimes the patient does not respond well. The usual antibiotics in this case are penicillin, kanamycin and cloxacillin, given by injection. Surgery may become necessary to either drain an abscess that has formed, or to remove damaged bone.

Nursing Care. As there may be exquisite pain, jarring of the bed must be avoided and for that reason the bed should be situated in a corner of the ward in the acute stage. Temperature, pulse and respirations are taken every 4 hours and fluid intake and output charts kept up to date. Abundant fluids are given and as the child is often negative and reluctant to drink, it is important to vary the drinks by using different flavours and by alternating hot and cold drinks. Savoury fluids, such as Bovril or Marmite are at times taken when sweet drinks are refused. They serve the additional purpose of causing thirst because of their high salt content. Once the fever has subsided, a nourishing, high protein diet is given to build up the child's general health. Small pillows, sand-bags and air rings should be used to ensure a comfortable position and rest for the affected part. As the illness may be a long one, the child should be wheeled into the fresh air whenever this is possible and schooling, occupational therapy and extra visiting are important if general morale and happiness are to be maintained.

Achondroplasia

Achondroplasia is a congenital abnormality which runs in families and is characterized by a shortness of the limbs and a large head with marked frontal bossing. The long bones are short, thick and curved and the overlying subcutaneous tissues and skin are in folds as if there were more of them than fits the length of the limb. The hands are broad and the child is unable to extend the elbow joint fully. The ligaments are relaxed and this produces a waddling gait. Growth is slow and this fact, together with the shortness of the long bones, causes dwarfism. The patient has a peculiar ability to rise from the sitting position on the ground to the standing position without using his hands. Adults with achondroplasia often earn their living as clowns in a circus. So far there is no known treatment.

Syndactyly

Syndactyly or webbing of the digits of the hands and feet may be partial or complete. The underlying bones and joints may be normal, or sections may be missing or fused. The plastic surgeon may be able to separate the digits and to give the hand an aesthetically good appearance, without much difficulty. Or it may be necessary to utilize one of the fingers as a thumb by transplanting muscles in such a way as to bring one digit into apposition to the others to make gripping possible. Occasionally skin grafting is undertaken to supply skin for the surfaces between the divided digits.

In looking after these patients post-operatively it is important to watch for signs of impaired circulation, sometimes a difficult task as the entire hand or foot may be covered in a tight crêpe bandage. Fine judgment may be needed in assessing any complaints of discomfort the child may make. As a rule children are very adaptable and manage to lead a normal life in spite of their handicap and up to the age of approximately 10 years they rarely seem aware of, or disturbed by their appearance.

Osteogenesis Imperfecta (Fragilitas Ossium)

As the name suggests the bones in fragilitas ossium are fragile and fractures occur on the least provocation. There are two main types of the disease. In the antenatal variety most of the bones of the fetal skull and skeleton have sustained fractures before birth. Callus formation causes the bones to be thickened

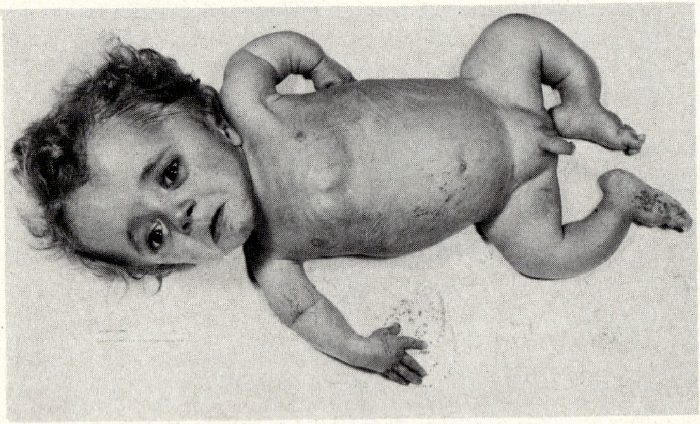

FIG. 66. Fragilitas ossium in a 2-year-old child.

and deformed. Babies with this complaint have markedly blue sclerotics. The condition is familial and severe cases become seriously handicapped, while others die at birth due to fractures occurring during labour (Fig. 66).

In the second variety the fractures occur mostly after the first year of life. The bones are porous and the teeth translucent. Although the fractures heal rapidly, deformities inevitably result and these children lead sheltered lives with schooling frequently interrupted by treatment or admissions to hospital. Occasionally the condition improves at puberty. Neither the cause nor any effective treatment are known.

Correction of Deformities caused by Paralysis

The abnormal and imbalanced pulls of certain muscle groups against others weakened by paralysis can cause severe and progressive deformities in the growing child. Surgical treatment is often necessary to prevent deformity and to stabilize joints and so to improve function. The results of infantile paralysis, congenital abnormalitics of the spine (e.g. myelomeningocele) and cerebral palsy are examples.

Corrective operations include transplantation of tendons in the leg or foot. This transplantation aims at counteracting an abnormal pull from a group of healthy muscles which would lead to deformity. Transplantation of the tendons of the hamstring muscles, for instance to the back of the femur, may enable a child with spastic paralysis to straighten his knees and to walk almost normally.

Tenotomy may be performed to lengthen certain tendons; a contracted Achilles tendon is a typical example. Paralysis of one leg only, may cause the healthy leg to grow and develop more rapidly than the affected one. The growth of the sound leg can be slowed down by inserting staples into the epiphysis and in this way both legs will be equal and the need for a surgical boot become unnecessary.

The nursing care of these patients is basically the same as for any child in plaster or extension.

Special points about children in plaster:

It is important to remember that where there is sensory loss the child would not complain of pain if a pressure sore should develop. The skin is also liable to break down easily due to poor blood supply. Urinary incontinence may present special problems and the plaster of Paris needs to be protected in order to keep it dry and avoid sores and unpleasant smells.

When the plaster is removed special care must be taken to prevent re-fracture or other damage, as the child, being without pain has no fear and takes greater risks in his newly found mobility than other children might do.

Children with cerebral palsy are liable to sudden spasm. This again will make them more liable to plaster sores than other patients. Re-assurance may help them to relax.

Further Reading

ASTON, J. N. (1972) *Short Textbook of Orthopaedics and Traumatology* 2nd ed. London: English Universities Press.

HUNT, P. (ed.) (1966) *Stigma: The Experience of Disability*. London: Geoffrey Chapman.

LLOYD-ROBERTS, G. (1971) *Orthopaedics in Infancy and Childhood.* London: Butterworth.

20

Tuberculosis in childhood

ALTHOUGH the death rate due to tuberculosis has fallen during the past 20 years it is still one of the most significant of the communicable diseases, especially in the developing countries. In Great Britain, tuberculosis is a notifiable disease, although neither treatment nor segregation of patients suffering from it is compulsory without special legal measures being taken.

Many factors predispose towards the development of tubercular disease; children under the age of two are more prone than the older child; although the condition is not hereditary, it is thought that a susceptibility to it may be. Over-crowding, poor living conditions and malnutrition all play their part in the incidence of the disease.

Definition. An infection due to the tubercle bacillus which may be acute, sub-acute or chronic, commonly affects the respiratory system, usually the lungs, but may involve other systems of the body, e.g. the genito-urinary, skeletal, nervous or gastro-intestinal tract. Pathologically it is characterized by an acute or chronic inflammatory process.

Source of infection. Most children who develop tuberculosis have acquired the disease from contact with an infected person either from within the family or at school or nursery. Whenever the diagnosis of tuberculosis is made in a child it is important that all close contacts are also investigated as there may be unsuspected infection present.

Two distinct strains of the tubercle bacillus are pathogenic to man, the human type mainly responsible for pulmonary infection and the bovine type acquired usually by drinking infected milk.

Immunity. Acquired immunity may develop through infection

by repeated small doses of tubercle bacilli. Children living in large cities can become immune in this way, even though the symptoms of infection may be so slight as to go unnoticed. Artificial immunity may be conferred by inoculation with BCG vaccine.

Bacillus Calmette-Guérin (BCG). Calmette and Guérin developed non-virulent tubercle bacilli and used them for inoculation. In some countries all children are immunized, with the result that the incidence of the disease has decreased. In Great Britain BCG is reserved for those who are exposed to special risks, e.g. for infants who have a close relative suffering from tuberculosis, for secondary school pupils who are still Mantoux negative (see below) and for nurses.

Tests. Various tests, such as the Mantoux and Heaf tests are used to check whether individuals have been exposed to tuberculous infection or are infected at the time of exposure. This is indicated by a positive or negative reaction.

Mantoux test. The Mantoux test consists of an intradermal injection of 0.1 ml of tuberculin solution into the patient's forearm. All these tests become positive within 48 hours, and should be read on the second or third day. A positive reaction consists of a slightly raised indurated patch at the site of the injection that should measure at least 10 mm across. The solution used for the injection is made in varying strengths, the strength most commonly used being 1:10 000.

Heaf test. A solution of old tuberculin is applied to the area, small punctures are made in the skin by means of a special spring injector, whose sharp points penetrate the skin. The reaction is similar to that of the Mantoux test and the results are read in the same way.

General Nursing Care of Tuberculosis. With the advent of anti-tuberculosis therapy, the majority of patients will make a complete recovery. However the illness may be a protracted one and the general nursing care will present special considerations and problems.

Observations. Primary lesions of tuberculous infection do not always remain confined to the one area and the nurse should at all times be on the alert for any change in her patient that might indicate a spread of the disease, e.g. in temperature, pulse and respiration. Changes in the patient's temperament may also be significant; an otherwise cheerful and contented child who suddenly becomes fractious or irritable may, for instance, be showing early signs of tuberculous meningitis. The onset of diarrhoea may indicate involvement of the gastro-intestinal tract. Frequency of micturition or the onset of haematuria may be early symptoms of renal tract disease. Stiffness or reluctance to move a limb must always be reported immediately as it may indicate abscess formation or tuberculous disease of the joint.

Regular weighings should be recorded as these will act as a guide to progress during the illness.

General Care. Rest, good nursing and a nourishing diet are the basic principles for the management of these patients.

The child's bed should be in a light place in the ward preferably near a door or window that can be left open. A french window leading to a garden or balcony can be a great asset. Nursing aids such as back rests, soft pillows and air rings will add to the patient's comfort and will enable him to rest more quietly.

The patient need only be nursed with strict infectious precautions if suffering from miliary tuberculosis, or if he has an infected discharge, sputum or cerebrospinal fluid. In these instances strict precautions must be observed. Any sputum or infected material should be adequately disinfected before disposal. As far as practical, disposable equipment is used in the care of these patients so that the used equipment can be incinerated.

The diet should be nourishing, appetizing and well served. The basic diet is supplemented by extra protein in the form of milk shakes and milk jellies. Special dishes prepared by the patient's own nurse or a particular treat brought in by the child's mother will help to encourage the appetite.

Adequate occupational facilities for the child during the illness are most important, toys and books should be readily accessible for the young patient. The parents should be encouraged to visit frequently, having first determined that they are free from tuberculosis. If financial difficulties are encountered in meeting fares, help may be available through the medical social worker who will also arrange a convalescent holiday, if this should be needed before the child returns home. Once discharged from hospital these children need to be under medical supervision for many years in order to ensure that any recurrence of the disease is treated immediately.

Investigations will include full blood investigations including haemoglobin estimations and total white blood cell count which may be raised during the acute stage of severe illness. Frequent estimations of the ESR are useful as an indication of progress. A return to normal value of 10 mm in 1 hour, is accepted as a good indication of the body having successfully combated the infection.

Radiographs of the affected part are taken frequently. In cases of tuberculous meningitis lumbar punctures are performed.

Young children are not usually able to co-operate in producing specimens of sputum as they frequently have an entirely unproductive cough, and it may be necessary to search for the tubercle bacillus in gastric washings.

Gastric washings. On waking and before anything is given by mouth, a gastric tube is passed and any resting juice withdrawn. This is placed in a sterile bottle and labelled. A few millilitres of sterile saline are then introduced through the tube and withdrawn. This second specimen, which often contains a fair amount of mucus, is placed in another bottle and labelled. Both specimens are sent to the laboratory. Gastric washings are usually repeated on three successive mornings. The nurse will have to use much tact and sympathy when carrying out this procedure, in order that the child may be co-operative and easily managed (see page 174 for method of holding a young patient).

Urine tests. In order to eliminate the danger of overlooking an infection of the renal tract weekly tests are carried out to exclude the presence of blood, albumin and pus cells in the patient's urine.

Drugs Used in the Treatment of Tuberculosis. The main drugs used in the treatment of tuberculosis are:

Streptomycin. May be given by intramuscular injection (40 mg/kg body weight per day) or, in tuberculous meningitis, by the intrathecal route (50 to 100 mg daily). Side effects; rashes, nausea, vomiting, giddiness and deafness.

Para-aminosalicylic acid (PAS). Given orally as tablets, syrup or enteric-coated granules (200 mg/kg body weight daily in divided doses). Side effects; nausea, vomiting, rashes and jaundice. Patients usually get used to the drug rapidly and tolerate it well after initial difficulties.

Isonicotinic acid hydrazide (INAH). Given orally either as tablets, sachets or as a mixture (20 mg/kg body weight) once or twice daily. This is usually well tolerated. Side effects; rashes, purpura, dizziness, convulsions and neuritis.

As a rule these drugs are given in combination, at least two at a time, and the combination is varied during the course of treatment which may last several months. The giving of these drugs in combination makes each more efficacious and prevents the tubercle bacilli from becoming resistant to any of them.

Amongst the newer anti-tuberculous drugs recently developed is Rifamycin often given as a syrup (20 mg/kg body weight daily). This is usually well tolerated, but nurses will observe it tends to colour the urine pink.

Other drugs. Sedatives may occasionally be necessary especially in cases of tuberculous meningitis. Aperients, iron and extra vitamins are amongst the other medications frequently prescribed as the need arises.

Primary Tuberculosis of Childhood

In childhood, infection with the tubercle bacillus follows a fairly set and typical pattern. As a rule the tubercle bacillus reaches the lungs by inhalation and produces a local lesion which is frequently so slight that it goes unnoticed. The infected area may become encapsulated by fibrous tissue and calcifies;

this lesion may only be the size of a split pea, and is called the 'Ghon focus'. As a result of tuberculous infection the glands at the roots of the lung become enlarged and the X-ray report will refer to enlarged hilar glands or mediastinal lymph nodes.

The Ghon focus and the enlarged hilar glands form what is known as the primary complex, and this may now develop in any of the following ways:

1. The primary focus becomes arrested and heals by calcification; that is to say the patient is cured.
2. The primary focus becomes arrested but is re-activated later in life.
3. The pressure of the tuberculous glands causes collapse of a part of the lung, in which case the lung may eventually re-expand spontaneously or the gland may rupture into the bronchus and cause tuberculous bronchopneumonia which will show as a wedge-shaped shadow on radiographs.
4. The infection spreads via the blood stream and may cause miliary tuberculous infection of the bones, the renal system or gastro-intestinal tract.

The Primary Complex

Signs and Symptoms. The child is usually quite well and frequently the infection is only detected when contacts of tuberculous adults are X-rayed. Occasionally, however, the child may be less interested in his normal activities and more demanding than usual, lose interest in his food and therefore fail to gain weight. There may be slight anaemia. The mother may give a history of a recent chill after which the child has failed to return to normal health.

The temperature and pulse rate may be slightly raised and there may be a mild dry cough, often paroxysmal in nature which raises the mother's concern. When an infected gland presses on a bronchus the cough may be irritating and have a brassy tone. Dyspnoea may develop and become quite alarming, especially at night.

Nursing Care. What has been written about the general care of children with tuberculosis applies also to these cases. In mild cases complete symptomatic recovery may occur in about 6 weeks. In severe cases where the primary focus is larger and caseation has occurred, recovery will take longer.

Further Reading

JOLLY, H. (1976) *Diseases of Children*, 3rd ed. Oxford: Blackwell Scientific.

21

Communicable diseases

THE TABLES on pages 432 to 436 give a summary of the acute infectious fevers which may be encountered in a children's ward. Further details of each condition can be found in specific textbooks. Brief notes on other conditions that may be met follow, but larger textbooks should also be consulted.

Coxsackie and Echovirus Group

The Coxsackie and Echoviruses cause a variety of conditions and include those listed below.

Benign lymphocytic meningitis, with fever, headache, nausea, neck stiffness and raised cell levels in the cerebrospinal fluid (predominantly lymphocytes).

Epidemic myalgia (Bornholm's Disease) (Coxsackie). Acute, severe pain of the intercostal muscles, painful, rapid shallow respirations, pleural rub, low grade fever, possibly lymphocytosis. Lasts 7 to 10 days. Symptomatic treatment.

Herpangina (Coxsackie Group A). Mild febrile illness of infancy. Vesicular and ulcerative lesions on soft palate and in fauces.

Epidemic diarrhoea (Echo).

Aseptic meningitis (Echo). Without paralysis or sequelae.

Adenovirus. Acute upper respiratory tract infection or severe influenza-like fever. Sore throat. Cough. Conjunctivitis. Painful enlargement of lymph glands. Sometimes causes pneumonic consolidation.

Catscratch fever. Probably a virus infection. Cat apparently healthy. A few days after scratch, ulcer or sore. A week or two later—regional lymph nodes very enlarged, some fever. Nodes may suppurate or adenitis persist for some months. Pus sterile, white cell count normal. Treated with broad-spectrum antibiotic to prevent suppuration.

Tetanus (Lockjaw)

Tetanus is caused by *Clostridium tetani* which is found on cultivated land. Anaerobic bacillus—danger in deep penetrating wounds which do not bleed much. Exotoxin forms, which attacks muscle, motor nerves, central nervous system. Neonatal tetanus may complicate umbilical sepsis.

The *incubation period* is variable. The shorter the time, the worse the prognosis. Non-infectious.

Signs and Symptoms. Local muscle weakness, trismus, spasm of face muscles (risus sardonicus), tonic spasmopisthotonos, rigid abdomen. Fever common. Paroxysmal state, precipitated by any disturbance such as feeding, noise, examination, painful spasm, arching back, extension of limbs, clenching teeth. Lasts seconds or minutes. If severe or increasing frequency—death from exhaustion.

Treatment. Intravenous antitoxin after subcutaneous test dose initially (need to be prepared for anaphylactic shock) followed by intramuscular injections of antitoxin daily. One hour after antitoxin—surgical débridement under light anaesthetic. Muscle relaxants to control spasm. Penicillin prophylaxis. If respirations cease—oxygen from anaesthetic machine, tracheal intubation as soon as relaxed, tracheostomy later, elevate foot of bed, sucker, intragastric feeds at first, intravenous fluids and electrolyte balance. Chlorpromazine may be given to control spasm and sedate the restless child.

Prophylaxis (Prevention). Active immunization—tetanus toxoid by triple immunization or separately (see page 14). Booster dose at 4 to 5 years, and every 5 years, and 0.5 ml if the patient has an accident involving penetrating wound or possible infection.

Passive Immunization. Anti-tetanus serum at time of accident. Not as efficient and more danger of anaphylactic reactions.

Poliomyelitis

Poliomyelitis is caused by a virus infection of the nasopharynx or alimentary tract.

The *incubation period* is 7 to 14 days or 21 days depending on the type. Isolate for 6 weeks.

Signs and Symptoms. Coryza, fever, malaise, headache, vomiting, neck and back stiffness or rigidity, drowsiness or irritability; pain in limbs when patient sits up—back rigid and hands placed behind 'tripod sign', to support the body; Kernig's sign may be positive. Cerebrospinal fluid under increased pressure, 10 to 200 cells/mm^3, at first polymorphonuclear, later lymphocytes, protein sometimes increased; this increases with paralysis; raised globulin; sugar and chlorides normal.

Virus affects anterior horn cells and motor nuclei of brain stem. The poliomyelitis may be abortive, or progress to a flaccid paralysis of legs, arms, trunk, tongue, pharynx, larynx, face, diaphragm and intercostal muscles, or respiratory centre in the medulla. There is no sensory loss and the paralysis develops rapidly, but may advance for 3 to 5 days, during which time fever subsides. There may be retention of faeces and urine, and reflexes are absent or decreased, although in pre-paralytic stage they may be increased.

Treatment. Treatment is symptomatic. In *pre-paralytic stage* —rest, analgesics (exertion increases likelihood of paralysis and respiratory difficulty). Isolation. Reassurance.

If paralysed—gentle, frequent passive movements to weak limbs, hot packs to painful muscles, cradle, footrest, prevent shortening, expression of bladder to prevent retention of urine, enemata, adequate airway and oxygen, tracheostomy if necessary, probably with cuff and intermittent positive pressure or artificial respirator.

After acute stage—early and vigorous activity, schooling, rehabilitation, active physiotherapy. Paralysis usually diminishes over 2 or more weeks, or improvement may continue for several months; deformity can be minimized by adequate splinting where indicated, and if necessary tenotomy or arthrodesis can be introduced at a later date.

Bulbar Involvement. Early difficulty in swallowing and speaking. Patient nursed in respirator to prevent mucus and vomit

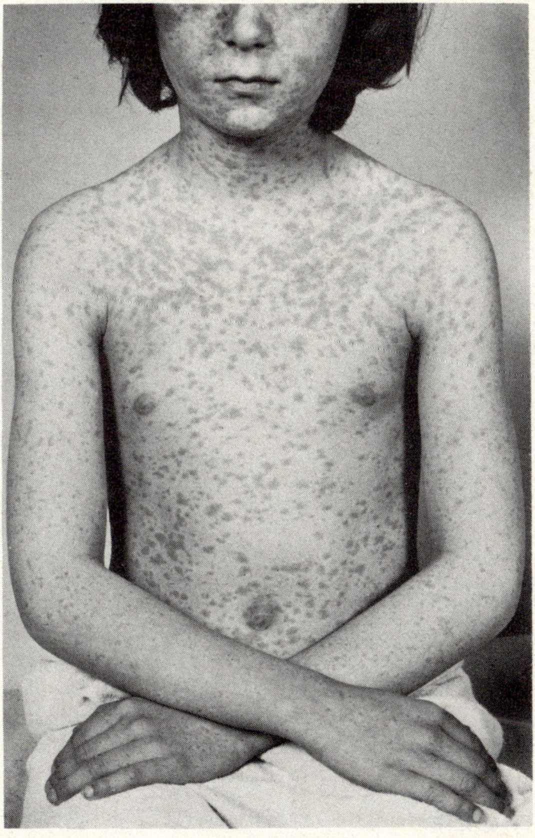

FIG. 67. Measles.

PRINCIPAL COMMUNICABLE DISEASES

Disease	*Incubation period*	*Organism and mode of spread*	*Signs and symptoms*	*Treatment and complications*	*Other remarks*
Measles (morbilli Fig. 71)	10–14 days	Virus Droplet	Running eyes and nose. Dry, irritating cough. Conjunctivitis. Photophobia. Pyrexia. Transient prodromal rash. Koplik spots—white on red base on buccal mucous membrane. 3rd day: temperature subsides. 4th day: rash appears—dusky red macular rash behind ears → face, trunk, limbs. Temperature again elevated. Rash becomes large irregular blotchy areas of darker red.	Bed. Symptomatic. Antibiotic for secondary infections. Otitis media. Blepharitis. Corneal ulcerations. Bronchopneumonia. Collapsed lobe of lung. Bronchiectasis and lung abscess (if collapse insufficiently treated). Tuberculosis. Encephalitis and encephalomyelitis (gastro-enteritis in infancy.)	Notifiable. Segregate until rash fades. Passive immunity for 3 months after birth (if mother has had measles). Older or sick children are given convalescent serum 5–10 ml or adult serum or gamma-globulin for protection. *Gamma-globulin* 250 mg prevent attack under 1 year, attenuates attack at all ages. Later 750 mg should prevent attack. Second dose after 6 weeks.
German measles (rubella)	14–21 days	Virus Droplet	Mild malaise and pyrexia day before rash. Generalized tender lymphadenitis especially posterior cervical and occipital. Rash: pink macules and papules at first discrete then confluent.	Very little necessary—symptomatic. Occasionally: Encephalitis. Arthritis.	Danger to fetus during first 14 weeks in utero if mother affected. Baby may be born deaf, with cataract, glaucoma, or heart disease (also risk of abortion). Mother should be given gamma-globulin.
Scarlet fever (scarlatina)	1–7 days	Haemolytic streptococci (Lancefield Group A) Droplet, fomites, milk	Headache, vomiting, pyrexia. Sore throat—soft yellow exudate. 'Strawberry tongue'. Polymorphonuclear leucocytosis. Raised antistreptolysin titre. Cervical lymphadenitis. Rash-punctuate erythema, bright scarlet, behind ears and sides of neck →whole body except circumoral pallor. Desquamation after 1 week.	(Septic and toxic forms very rare.) Bed. Penicillin and sulphonamides. Fluids. Mouth care. Pneumonia. Septicaemia. Otitis media. Acute nephritis and rheumatism. Anaphylactoid purpura. Sinusitis. Encephalitis. Quinsy. Retropharyngeal abscess. Cervical adenitis and abscess.	Notifiable. Dick test for diagnosis—rarely used. Possibility of cardiac lesions from acute rheumatism. Scarlet fever antitoxin sometimes given.

Whooping cough (pertussis)	7–14 days	*Bordetella (Haemophilus) pertussis* Droplet	Cold → chest infection → cough which becomes paroxysmal with vomiting and may end with a whoop. Ulcer on fraenum. Lymphocytosis. Low erythrocyte sedimentation rate. Baby vomits, cyanosed, limp, no paroxysms.	Feed after vomiting. Sedation. Broad-spectrum antibiotics for secondary infections. Deal with debility—long convalescence, high-calorie diet. Otitis media. Bronchopneumonia. Pulmonary collapse. Bronchiectasis. Tuberculosis. Subconjunctival haemorrhage. Cerebral anoxia or haemor rhage. Convulsions. Rectal prolapse. Hernia. Spontaneous pneumothorax.	Notifiable. No passive immunity in babies Mild abortive case in immunized child, but equally infectious. Child often 'whoops' for months after attack—not infectious. Routine immunization—not to child with epilepsy or prone to convulsions—he may develop encephalopathy if immunized. Resuscitation equipment and oxygen available in case a severe apnoeic attack should occur.
Chickenpox (varicella)	14–21 days	Virus Contact and droplet	Minimal malaise and headache. Fever. Transient prodromal rash. Main rash appears in crops—mainly on face, head and trunk, (centripetal) oval, unilocular papules → vesicles → pustules → crusts. Irritating rash. Lymphocytosis.	Prevent from scratching to avoid scarring. Baths. Calamine. Keep cool. Short nails. Elbow splints if necessary. Antihistamines. Antibiotics for secondary infections—impetigo, boils, cellulitis, conjunctivitis, polyneuritis, encephalitis, transverse myelitis.	Notifiable only in smallpox epidemic. Herpes zoster closely allied. Severe or fatal if child has leukaemia or is on steroid therapy. Segregate until scabs dry.
Smallpox (variola)	8–18 usually 10–12 days	Virus Contact and droplet	*Variola major* Sudden onset—headache, fever, shivering, severe pain in back and aching of limbs. Toxaemia. Prodromal rash—purpuric. True rash, 3rd day, 1 crop only. Thickest on peripheral parts of limbs (centrifugal) round, multilocular → confluent. Macule → papule → vesicle → pustule → crust → scab → scar.	Strict isolation until all scabs off. Care of mouth, eyes, skin, otherwise symptomatic. Antibiotics against secondary infection. Otitis media, conjunctivitis, corneal ulceration, nephritis, cardiac failure, septicaemia, bronchopneumonia, encephalitis.	Notifiable. *Variola major*—high mortality. Quarantine 16 days. Routine vaccination advised—except for children with eczema. Vaccination of contacts effective to modify the attack. Very high infectivity.

Disease	Incubation period	Organism and mode of spread	Signs and symptoms	Treatment and complications	Other remarks
Smallpox (cont.)			Toxic, septicaemic, confusion state with pyrexia when pustules form. Slower developing rash than chickenpox. *Variola minor* Relatively trivial and difficult to distinguish from chickenpox.		
Mumps	14–28 days	Virus Droplet	Fever, malaise, stiff jaw, swelling of salivary gland—parotid and submandibular. Unilateral or bilateral. Trismus. Pain on eating—especially sugars. Furred tongue, mouth dry—diminution of saliva. Moderate lymphocytosis.	Symptomatic. Mouth care—drink with straw. Avoid foods which are sweet and stimulate salivary glands. Mastitis, oophoritis, prostatitis, pancreatitis (all rare), meningitis, encephalitis (may lead to permanent deafness), facial paralysis. Orchitis at or after puberty (steroids given to lessen symptoms).	Complement fixation test reaction to confirm diagnosis—rarely necessary.
Influenza	1–2 days	Virus—A, B, and C strains Droplet	Sudden onset—fever, shivering headache, upper respiratory tract infection. Profound malaise, severe aching in back and limbs. Remittent fever for up to 1 week—falls by lysis.	Analgesics when necessary. Antibiotics for secondary infections—pneumonia, post-influenzal debility and depression.	Vaccines A and B strain—partial immunity for 6 months—used in epidemics.
Roseola infantum (exanthema subitum, sixth disease, pseudo-rubella)	8–15 days	Virus Droplets	Fever, macular rash—appears immediately temperature fallen, fades on pressure. On trunk, neck, proximal part of limbs; *not* face. Lasts 1–3 days. Little malaise. Catarrhal pharyngitis, cervical lymphadenopathy. Neutrophil leucopenia with rela-[illegible]	Nil	Practically confined to first 3 years of life.

Glandular fever (infectious mono-nucleosis)	6–14 days	*Epstein-Barr virus (EBV)* Droplet. Low infectivity.	Lassitude, anorexia, general malaise, pyrexia, headache, sore throat with tonsillar exudate which separates easily without bleeding. May be petechiae on palate. Enlarged lymph nodes and spleen. Transient macular rash—chest trunk, limbs and particularly dorsum of hands and feet. Leucocytosis with raised monocytes (atypical). Paul Bunnell test may be positive.	Symptomatic. Treat general debility and depression—prolonged convalescence. Treat secondary infections—hepatitis, meningitis, encephalitis. Nephritis.	Relapses common, but complete recovery eventually.
Diphtheria	2–7 days	*Corynebacterium diphtheriae* Droplet	Malaise, headache, rapid, feeble pulse, some rise in temperature, toxic. Albuminuria, exhaustion. *Faucial:* Slight sore throat, continuous greyish membrane spreading to soft palate and pharynx, which bleeds when attempt made to remove. Glands of neck very enlarged.—'Bull neck', myocarditis. *Nasal:* Thin bloodstained nasal discharge with offensive smell. Crusting of external nares. *Laryngeal:* Croupy cough, laryngeal stridor, loss of voice, asphyxia.	Diphtheria antitoxin if any question of infection possible. Absolute bed rest, mouth care, tube feed if necessary. Steam tent for mild cases of respiratory obstruction. Tracheotomy may become necessary. Penicillin to treat secondary infection. Respirator will be necessary if diaphragm paralysed. Physiotherapy after acute stage. Myocarditis, paralysis of limbs, palate, diaphragm, ciliary muscles and external rectus muscles, nephritis, peripheral neuritis.	Notifiable. Follow up contacts and possible carriers. Treat carriers with antibiotic and possibly tonsillectomy. Immunization advisable to prevent infection and epidemics. Schick test to assess immunity—negative if immune.
Enteric fever	2 weeks	Typhoid (*Salmonella typhi*). Paratyphoid A, B and C (*S. paratyphi* A, B and C) (non-lactose fermenters).	Headache, tiredness, aching limbs, cough, fever rising in 'step-ladder' fashion, relative bradycardia, palpable spleen, abdominal discomfort, 'rose spots' on abdomen or chest—constipated—later 'pea soup' stools.	Symptomatic. High calorie, low roughage, diet. Care of mouth and skin. Watch for haemorrhage from perforated Peyer's patches. Transfusion if necessary.	Notifiable. Isolate until 2 negative stool cultures (consecutive). Immunize contacts. Treat carriers—if necessary with cholecystectomy.

Disease	Incubation period	Organism and mode of spread	Signs and symptoms	Treatment and complications	Other remarks
Enteric fever (cont.)		Contamination of food or water by excreta from carriers or patients with the disease. Fomites, flies.	Leucopenia if no secondary infection. Typhoid state—drowsy, confused, muttering, plucking at bedclothes, 'coma vigil'. Blood culture positive in first few days. Widal test—rising titre.	Venous thrombosis, acute arthritis, cholecystitis, bone abscess and periostitis, peritonitis. Parotitis if inadequate mouth care. Chloramphenicol.	
Brucellosis (undulant fever)	1–3 weeks	*Brucella abortus* (cattle). *Brucella melitensis* (goats). *Brucella suis* (pigs). Infected, unpasteurized milk, meat, dairy products. Infected hides and carcases.	Headache, malaise, anorexia, constipation, fever—settles by lysis in 10 days, but recurs. Cough, backache, profuse sweating, palpable spleen. Transient arthritis. *Abortus fever* (chronic brucellosis). Insidious, milder and more prolonged. Recurrent night sweats without serious general ill health. (*In both*) Blood culture may be positive. Rising agglutination titre. Leucopenia, mild anaemia.	Tetracycline, streptomycin, vitamin B. Symptomatic—treat debility with long convalescence. Disinfect excreta—especially urine.	Notifiable. Recurring at short intervals for many months. Pasteurization of milk, clean water and destroying infected animals prevents disease.
Psittacosis (ornithosis)	1–2 weeks	Virus from infected birds (who may not be ill). Most virulent strain from parrots. Droplet and contact with infected birds.	Gradual onset, cough, fever, relative bradycardia, headache, backache, general malaise, splenomegaly. Pneumonia spreading from hilum. White cell count low or normal. Diagnosis—complement fixation test.	Symptomatic. Tetracycline for 1 week. Convalescence slow and prolonged. Fulminating—high fever delirium, rising pulse and respiration rate, poor prognosis.	

going into lungs, with head tilted down for drainage. Alternatively respirator with tracheostomy and suction or positive pressure respirator with tracheostomy and suction. *Never* put patient with bulbar paralysis in ordinary respirator without prior tipping, or secretions are immediately sucked into lungs.

Prophylaxis. Prevents disease and epidemics (see page 14). Gamma-globulin can be given for passive immunity to close contacts who have not been immunized.

NOTE. Immunization against diphtheria and pertussis should be avoided if there is a poliomyelitis epidemic, as the injected limb is more liable to paralysis if the child develops poliomyelitis. A child who develops poliomyelitis after a recent tonsillectomy is prone to develop bulbar paralysis.

Further Reading

BRIMBLECOMBE, F. & BARLTROP, D. (1978) *Children in Health and Disease*. London: Baillière Tindall.

KRUGMAN, S. & WARD, R. (1968) *Infectious Diseases of Children*, 4th ed. St Louis: Mosby.

MEREDITH-DAVIS, J. B. (1965) *Preventative Medicine for Nurses and Social Workers*. London: English Universities Press.

WARIN, J. & IRONSIDE, A. (1969) *Lecture Notes on Infectious Diseases* Oxford: Blackwell Scientific.

22

Burns, scalds and accidents

BURNS and scalds are among the most frequently occurring accidents in childhood (some thousand patients are admitted annually to the hospitals in the London area alone) and they are the more tragic, because so many of them are preventable.

Common Causes

The causes of such accidents are not only failure to use fire guards for open fires. In many households electric fires still remain unguarded, mirrors or pretty pictures hung above fireplaces attract children, saucepan handles are left within reach of toddlers, scalding hot water is left standing about in readiness for a bath, the weekly wash or for scrubbing the floor. Toddlers have been known to sit on top of draining boards from where they have slipped into scalding-hot water or they have been scalded by detaching the hose-pipe from washing machines.

Tablecloths should not be used in homes where there is a danger of a toddler getting hold of the cloth and so pulling the teapot over himself. Older children run particular risks when playing with fireworks, partly empty oil or paint drums, bonfires on demolition sites or rubbish dumps and when playing with matches. Baths should never be filled with hot water before running in some cold, otherwise a small child may step into water which is hot enough to scald him, or the bottom of the bath may become hot enough to burn the soles of his feet. Special precautions are necessary in the homes of mentally handicapped children or those suffering from epileptic fits, as not even the most devoted mother can be expected to be with her child all the time.

Children admitted with burns (Fig. 68) are frequently little girls whose nightdresses have caught fire or who have stood in

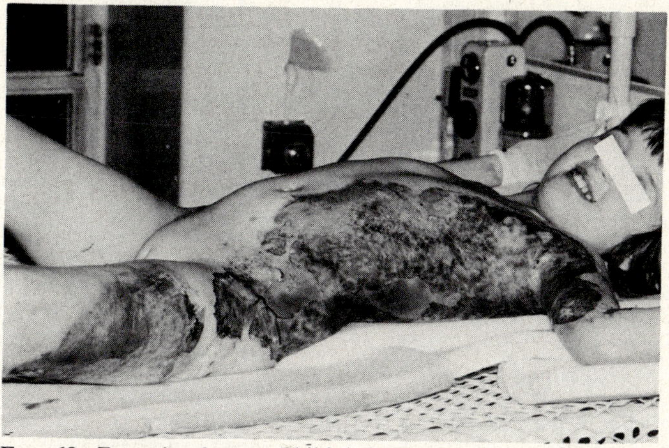

FIG. 68. Extensive burns. Child being nursed using the exposed method on foam pads which are changed frequently.

front of fires in flimsy party clothes in an attempt to keep warm. Young children of either sex should wear pyjamas or at least nightdresses made of flame-proof materials such as Proban.

First-Aid Treatment

Very slight burns and scalds are best treated by running cold water over the area (this reduces pain) and then covering it with a loosely applied, clean cloth to exclude air. Anthisan cream is sometimes preferred and may reduce pain as well as blistering.

More severe burns should be covered with clean linen to exclude air. Burnt clothing (sterilized by the heat) should be left untouched, but any wet clothing should be gently removed before covering the wound. Regardless of the possibility of an anaesthetic within a few hours, bland fluids such as sugar water or very weak tea should be given at once, as with children promptness in this respect may be the most important factor in saving life by reducing shock.

Classification of Burns and Scalds

Modern surgery refers to only two degrees of burns and scalds: superficial burns, and full thickness or deep burns. As a rule *superficial burns* may be expected to heal with little scarring, while *full thickness burns* are slow to heal and may cause scarring, crippling contractions and loss of function, and usually require skin grafting and prolonged and repeated treatment in hospital.

The extent of the burn is as important as the depth. For purposes of classification the 'Waller Method' is frequently used. The body surface is divided into sections of 9 per cent of the total and thus, with reference to a chart, it is easy to estimate the extent of the burn as being a multiple of 9 per cent. The seriousness of the burn or scald is often far more dependent on the extent of the affected area, than on the thickness. A child may lose his life with an 18 per cent superficial burn but an older patient may be expected to survive deep burns covering 50 per cent of the body surface.

The Lund & Browder method of estimating the extent of burns is shown in Fig. 69. As in Waller's 'Rule of Nines'

FIG. 69. The Lund and Browder method of measuring burns (from Lund, C. C. & Browder, N. N., *Surg. Gynec. Obstet.*).

Areas affected by growth	Age				
	1 month	1 year	5 years	10 years	15 years
A=half of head	9½	8½	6½	5½	4½
B=half of one thigh	2¾	3¼	4	4¼	4½
C=half of one lower leg	2½	2½	2¾	3	3¼

method, the body is divided into areas each of which is given a percentage value, but the values of certain areas alter with age as the proportions of the child's body are changed by normal growth.

Treatment for Shock

No time should be lost in treating shock, even if the usual symptoms may at first not be evident because shock is delayed. Shock is always directly proportionate to the area involved, as the loss of salts, protein and fluids into the tissue spaces and on to the body surface reduces the volume of circulating blood. The body reacts to this by a drop in blood pressure, subnormal temperature, pallor, thirst, restlessness and failure to secrete urine.

Intravenous Therapy

This should be started immediately in all cases in which the area involved exceeds 9 per cent of the body surface. It is usual to take blood for grouping and haemoglobin estimation before starting the infusion.

Plasma or the modern dextrans are the fluids of choice although fresh blood may be given according to the level of the haemoglobin which should never be allowed to fall below 70 per cent.

The rate of fluid loss is estimated by repeated haematocrit readings, the haemoconcentration and the amount of urinary output. On the first day approximately two-thirds of the fluid loss is replaced in the first 8 hours after admission. After that, chemical tests of both blood and urine are done at least daily and the findings are taken as a guide for further intravenous therapy.

Oxygen Therapy

Shock and the loss of red blood cells from the burnt surface may cause sufficient reduction in the oxygenating power of the blood to make oxygen therapy necessary. This is usually best given by nasal catheters as oxygen given by means of a tent interferes with local treatment and also influences bacterial growth.

Cubicle Nursing

Whenever possible the patient is admitted into a special cubicle which is kept as free from infection as possible by daily cleaning with plenty of soap and water, disinfectant solution, aerosol spray and special ventilation, and by employing barrier technique. The humidity is regulated according to need. At first a dry atmosphere (approximately 35 to 40 per cent humidity) is maintained to allow for crust formation and to discourage bacterial growth, but humidity may be raised gradually to 50 or 60 per cent particularly if chest complications are feared. The temperature of the cubicle is kept to 21° or 24°C (70° or 75°F), sufficient to keep the patient comfortable but not enough to encourage bacterial growth. For small babies who have not yet developed a 'shivering reflex' higher temperatures may be necessary.

Local Treatment

Treatment of the burnt area may vary from one hospital to another and according to the wishes of the surgeon, and the nursing and laboratory facilities available. Prevention of infection and early grafting are accepted standards of treatment at the present time. Limbs are usually dressed and covered irrespective of age, but patients are often best nursed by the exposure method, which has the advantage of inhibiting bacterial growth by keeping the area cool, dry and exposed to light, and eliminating painful dressings while promoting healing with a minimum of scarring. The patient can move around freely and observation of the progress is possible; both these considerations are of psychological and clinical importance. Few dressings under anaesthetic are necessary and this means, among other things, that nutrition is not constantly being interrupted.

The affected area and surrounding skin are usually cleansed with a solution of 1 per cent cetrimide or of Hibitane 1:2000. Large, heavy blisters may be punctured and drained but small ones are left and dead skin is not removed unless it is very dirty.

A hard, dry crust of plasma exudate usually forms within 24 to 36 hours and provides a sterile covering for the underlying surface. Air is allowed to circulate freely to aid the drying process and for that purpose special beds, polyurethane pads, extensions and slings may be used and the patient's position changed according to need. Using an aerosol spray topical antibiotics can be applied, e.g. polymyxin and bacitracin. Pressure on the affected part must be avoided as a good blood supply is essential to healing.

Immediately on admission, and before cleansing the area, swabs are taken from various parts of the burnt area, the nose and throat and of one or two areas of normal skin. The swabs are dipped into sterile broth before use and they are sent to the laboratory for culture and sensitivity tests. A dose of tetanus toxoid is usually given. In some centres human plasma is used to accelerate crust formation but in the majority of cases this is not considered necessary. In favourable cases the crusts begin to peel off after approximately 3 weeks when new epidermis has formed. Very thick crusts may be loosened by liquid paraffin soaks (gauze swabs saturated with paraffin) which are renewed every 4 hours. After approximately 12 hours much of the crust can be lifted off with the aid of sterile forceps. This should only be done if the treatment is entirely painless, i.e. adequate healing underneath the crust has taken place.

Full thickness burns are treated in the same way initially, but after 1 to 2 weeks the patient is taken to the theatre for thorough examination and wound toilet. By now it is possible to decide how much of the tissue is dead and consequently incapable of primary healing. As a rule partial thickness burns may be expected to heal in 3 to 4 weeks, but full thickness burns will require grafting and usually are associated with some degree of deformity. Any sloughs are removed and skin grafting is undertaken. This operation is called *escharectomy* (eschar = slough). Loss of blood may be considerable but by now the patient's general condition should be so much better that he can stand up to operation even though further blood transfusion may be necessary.

In ideal conditions the grafted areas may be left exposed following operation. If the areas have been covered with dressings and bandages, it is important that the nurse should watch any exposed and pendant parts, the extremities particularly, for oedema and for bleeding. Either must be reported at once. The bandaging requires great skill as considerable pressure is required in order to prevent blood or exudate from lifting the graft off its bed. At the same time it is obviously dangerous to apply the crêpe bandages too tightly. Oedema may be severe and may cause the bandage to become tight and impede circulation with consequent death of the skin graft. Nursing methods, such as elevating the part, are attempted to reduce the swelling before interfering with the bandage as this is often applied with the intention of correcting deformities and contractions, as well as covering the operation area.

General Treatment

Drug Therapy

A broad spectrum antibiotic or a combination of one of these with penicillin is given prophylactically for the first 24 hours. The drug may then be changed according to the sensitivity report. Some surgeons change the drug routinely every time the patient has to be taken to the theatre in order to guard against his becoming resistant to any one drug.

Morphine (0.05 mg/kg body weight) is a suitable sedative and analgesic to give to the child who will be frightened as well as in pain. This should always be relieved, as pain does exacerbate shock. The nurse should remember that this drug should not be given subcutaneously for the first day or so, as in the presence of shock it may not be adequately absorbed until later, with dangerous results. Initially the intravenous route is safest. Alternatively Nepenthe (0.06 ml per year of age) may be given orally.

Usually by 48 hours pain subsides and drugs such as codeine or phenobarbitone are sufficient. Elixir Phenergan has a sedative effect and at the same time reduces tissue swelling. It may have to be continued for some time and should never be withheld merely for fear of forming a habit. Iron in the form of Colliron 1 to 2 ml three times a day is usually ordered.

Diet

Oral fluids should be commenced as soon as possible after admission to the ward and are best given at this stage as 5 per cent glucose 40 ml/kg/24 hours. It may be necessary to pass a nasogastric tube in order to avoid disturbing the child too much. Once the shock associated with the injury has passed, usually in about 2 to 3 days the child should be given a diet high in protein and calories. It may be necessary for this to be continued for several weeks, for much protein is lost from the burns and healing is delayed by malnutrition. Initially the child may be given a fortified milk preparation if necessary through a naso-gastric tube. A suitable mixture that can be used is:

Milk	1000 ml (35 oz)
Casilan	40 g ($1\frac{1}{3}$ oz)

which supplies 70 g of protein and a total of approximately 810 calories.

As soon as the patient can tolerate it, a full diet is given which is augmented by eggs, milk, vitamins and foods which are rich in iron. Such foods are red meat, liver, kidney, sardines, black treacle, whole meal and rye bread and Bovril and Marmite. As most of these foods are both palatable and colourful, there should be little difficulty in arranging attractive meals. The food intake must be measured accurately and the amounts taken should be known and supplemented by tube feeding if necessary. Much patience and ingenuity may be needed to achieve the necessary fluid and calorie (joule) intake but as so much of the patient's treatment and progress depends on this factor, success brings its own reward.

Point of Interest. Burns cause rapid muscle wasting and survival may depend on nutritional replacement. The rapid tissue breakdown may have a serious effect on the kidneys and serious renal complications are common in patients suffering from burns and scalds.

Nursing Observations

Observations of the child's appearance, pulse rate and blood pressure should be made frequently, as they are of considerable importance in assessing the child's general progress. In addition any girl with extensive burns (more than 10 per cent surface area) should have an in-dwelling catheter in the bladder, and any boy should have Paul's tubing attached to the penis, so that urine output can be measured and recorded hourly. A rising pulse rate, hypotension and oliguria are all indications that the infusion rate should be increased to meet the body's fluid requirements. The nurse should realize that shivering and vomiting in these children are more likely to be due to inadequate fluid replacement or infection than to their being cold. The child should be weighed on admission and at intervals during treatment in order that fluid replacement and drug therapy can be safely calculated.

Nursing Care

If the foot end of the bed is at first raised to counteract shock it is necessary to watch for oedema of face and neck which may in turn spread to the brain and cause cerebral congestion. In this case the bed must be lowered at once and in more extreme cases the head end of the bed is elevated. Local oedema of the limbs and excess fluid loss from exudate is prevented by raising the affected extremity by means of extension. Sterilized polyurethane foam slings attached to a balkan beam or an intravenous stand and positioning with the help of foam pillows is possible in most cases. Toddlers with burns of buttocks can sometimes be kept dry by using a gallows extension. Burns of the trunk may be nursed on a 'Bradford frame' padded with sterilized polyurethane foam pads, which are changed twice daily. The supporting nylon net is divided into sections and this facilitates the giving of bedpans without disturbance to the patient who lies, as it were, suspended over the gap. Intermittent pressure mattresses which move automatically in waves at about 10-minute intervals are suitable for older children. Foam pieces can be sterilized in the same way as rubber gloves and it is a good idea to use pads of different colours for the amusement of the child and so make a bit more tolerable the frequent change which may be a disturbing procedure to the patient.

Complications

Damage of liver and kidneys, pneumonia, reactions to blood transfusion, sepsis, uraemia and psychological disturbances are common. Treatment of any of these at the earliest stage is essential and in many cases these complications can be avoided by adequate medical and nursing care. Local complications may arise from sloughs and crusts which by their position or extent may restrict chest movement or the blood supply to extremities, causing chest complications or thrombosis and gangrene of the parts. Burns and scalds of the eyelids are likely to cause contractions followed by exposure of the cornea, resulting in keratitis. Careful swabbing and the use of chloramphenicol Applicaps may prevent complications but in some cases it is deemed best temporarily to stitch the upper and lower lid margins together or to excise the contracted lids and graft them.

Burns of the hands and external genitalia present further problems which have to be dealt with as the individual case demands. Warm baths will help the child to 'kick out' any contractures although splinting with Kramer wire or plaster of Paris may still be necessary. The application of lanolin or Anthisan cream will help to soften healed areas and grafts.

Lesions of groins, neck and armpits should be prevented from contracting by separating them or extending them fully with the aid of pillows or rolls of polyurethane foam. Steam scalds of face, neck and tongue may require tracheostomy and so add to the already difficult nursing problem.

Mental Welfare

However exacting the routine nursing care, no nurse must ever forget the mental welfare of these children. They are usually severely shocked and numbed in the first hours but after this initial stage they need a great deal of assurance, company and occupation. They are frightened by the accident and the sudden admission to hospital and often haunted by memories of the burst of flames and by feelings of guilt. Flame burns in particular cause severe nightmares after 2 or 3 days, and the children easily develop feelings of resentment and a bad relationship towards their parents.

Patient assignment nursing and the presence of the mother for as much time as possible is of great psychological value. Any relatives or neighbours involved in the accident should be allowed to visit and speak to the child in order to reassure him. Sometimes it is possible to admit the mother with the child, provided she can spare the time from her other commitments. She can help to feed her child and play with him and sometimes may get him to sleep when he is wakeful or frightened. The idea that the mother can only be admitted or frequent visiting be arranged after the first days when the child is better, is completely mistaken. *It is in the first, initial stages that comfort from the mother is so important.* It is useless to cure a child physically while allowing psychological damage to persist or to develop. The greatest danger in this respect exists in units where children are nursed side by side with adults and where nursing staff are unaware of the special psychological needs of young children, notwithstanding their devoted and expert care of the injuries which are the cause of the admission. Although a physiotherapist will carry out daily treatment to prevent and correct contractions and bad posture, mothers can often be taught to assist, e.g. when games are played which encourage deep breathing and so help to prevent chest infections. As soon as possible full occupation is needed to keep these patients happy.

Boredom encourages scratching and picking at the crusts, both factors which may lead to infection, delayed healing and unnecessary scarring. Adequate occupation and company are far better means of preventing this than sedation or restraint. Toys and occupational material must at first be of the sterilizable kind. In situations of stress such as this, the child should not be deprived of a loved toy and if this cannot be sterilized even a teddy bear can be covered by a clean polythene bag.

It is interesting to note that children who sustain burns or scalds often appear to be of rather low intelligence and that they often come from homes with several other young brothers and sisters, so that the mother is overworked and unable to give much supervision. This also seems to be one of the reasons why many of these patients are still used to drinking from the bottle, well after the usual age. This possibility should always be kept in mind if there is difficulty in getting a young child to drink.

Children nursed by the exposure method often miss their usual coverings at first and if cold, can be covered by sterile towels and wear sterilized bootees and mittens. Little girls enjoy wearing pretty hair ribbons even if this is the only 'clothing' they are allowed. The young patients soon get used to their nakedness and although they may at first feel cold when transferred to the open ward they then often dislike being dressed.

Consideration for the mental welfare of the parents is as important as for the child. Parents often blame themselves in some way for the accident and some time may have to be spent with anxious parents outlining the treatment, the probable outcome of the illness and the degree of scarring and length of hospitalization to be expected. Parents of newly admitted children should be encouraged to speak to those of convalescent patients as they may be able to give them comfort from their own experiences.

Convalescence

Convalescence may be prolonged in many cases and go on for months after the accident, until healing and repeated skin grafting are complete. Occupational therapy or schooling are essential during this period and short outings or week-ends at home should be arranged when possible. The skin is often kept supple by massaging with lanolin; this treatment together with exercising, helps to stretch newly forming skin and prevents contractions and should be carried out several times daily and not merely when the physiotherapist visits the ward.

ACCIDENTS

Dangers	*How to guard against them*
	FIRES
Electric fires, gas fires, coal fires	Efficient guards fixed to fire surround. Fix on wall whenever possible. Wire netting fixed to fire.
	ELECTRICITY
Sockets	Locked sockets prevent children from poking fingers or pointed articles into the holes. 'Baby Guards' can be obtained to fit over all 5, 13 and 15 amp British plugs.
Flexes	Short flexes prevent accidents from tripping over them. Long flexes tempt children to pull on them, e.g. flex from electric iron.
	HOT WATER
Water taps	Fix out of reach if possible. Detachable in bathroom.
Baths	Run cold water in before the hot to prevent floor of bath from getting too hot.
Bath water	Mix well, use thermometer, do not rely on sense of touch.
Hot-water bottles	Use tap (not boiling) water. Cover completely with two protective layers. Never give hot water bottles to unconscious or paralysed patients.
	SCALDS
Teapots, kettles	Point spout away from table or stove edge. Drinking from the spouts of teapots and kettles seems attractive to the very young child. Oedema of the mouth, larynx and oesophagus may necessitate tracheostomy. Keep well out of the way.
Tablecloths	Tablecloths should not be used or should at leas not exceed the size of the table surface. If allowec to hang over table edge the toddler may tug o them when wanting to reach something on th table. Serious scalds may result, if there is a teapo on the table.
Saucepans	Saucepan handles should always be directed back wards or inwards. Safety rails for stoves ar available. The child may reach for the handle in a attempt at 'peeping inside' to see what is cooking
Scrubbing buckets	Buckets filled with scalding water should never b left standing on the floor unguarded. The youn child may fall or plunge his hands into it.

ACCIDENTS—*contd.*

Dangers	*How to guard against them*
	SWALLOWING AND INHALING
Toys	Toys should be large enough to make it impossible for younger children to swallow or inhale them. Beads, nails and small marbles should not be given to very young toddlers. Toys should not have sharp edges—danger of cuts and abrasions. They should be coloured with vegetable (not lead) paint.
	SUFFOCATION
Pillows	Should not be used in cots before the age of 1 year or until the child can safely move himself. They are particularly dangerous if they are soft.
Plastic bibs	Avoid. They may fall over the baby's face and interfere with breathing.
Plastic bags	Children should never be allowed to play with these.
	GANGRENE
Mittens	These are best avoided. A thread of cotton or strand of wool hanging off the inside edge of the mitten has been known to wrap itself round the tip of a finger causing constriction and gangrene.
	FOREIGN BODIES
Small objects	All body orifices offer opportunities for young children to push beads, peas, ball of paper, etc., into them. Sepsis and foul-smelling discharge will result. The observant and watchful mother or nurse should spot the toddler doing this sort of thing before the harm is done.
	SHARP THINGS
Knives, saws, axes, scissors	All these should be kept out of harm's way. If left lying around they are likely to be misused and dangerous. Playing with them should be forbidden, while very young. When a little older their use should be supervised. The 'first' scissors should have rounded ends and they should not be too sharp. A child who has 'his own' will not want adult ones.

ACCIDENTS—*contd.*

Dangers	*How to guard against them*
Safety pins	If left lying around they should be fastened. If in use they should be inaccessible to the child. On napkins they should be pinned horizontally.
Pin boxes and needle books	Should be kept well out of reach.
	FIRE AND BURNING
Matches	Children should be taught to respect matches as dangerous when used by very young people or indiscriminately.
Matchboxes	Should not be left lying around the house.
Lighters	The same applies to them as to matches.
Fire-works and bonfires	Children should know that both may be enjoyed only while supervised by adults.
Clothing	Pyjamas are preferable for girls as well as boys as their closer fit diminishes the danger of catching fire. Flame-proofed materials are obtainable, their advantages greatly outweigh the extra cost.
Mirrors	Should not be fixed over fireplaces. Clothes easily catch fire as one leans over the fireplace to look in the mirror.
	WINDOWS
Guards	Safety guards should be fixed on windows of any rooms in which young children may have to be left alone.
Chairs and step ladders	May invite the child to climb on to them and lean out of the window. If unguarded this may have serious results.
	STAIRS
Safety gates	Where there is a toddler in the house stairs should be made safe by placing safety gates at the top and bottom of flights of stairs.
	POISONING
Marking ink	Until it has been fixed by boiling, the aniline dye in marking ink (e.g. on baby napkins) may be absorbed via the skin and cause methaemoglobinaemia, a serious condition.

ACCIDENTS—*contd.*

Dangers	*How to guard against them*
	LOTIONS
Disinfectants	Should be kept locked away or out of reach even if the toddler climbs to get at them. They should always be clearly labelled, but it must also be remembered that the child may not be able to read. Disinfectants should not be stored in old fruit-juice bottles which still have the original label on.
	EATING HARMFUL THINGS
Pills	Pills should, if possible, be distinct in shape and colour. As the young child loves putting things in his mouth, pills should be inaccessible to him. They should preferably be wrapped separately in foil or wax paper and put out of the child's reach. Pills often resemble familiar sweets and may be almost indistinguishable from them. New regulations require that aspirin and paracetamol must be sold in child-resistant containers. The Medicines Commission has recommended that these containers should in the future be used for other medicines as well.
Berries	A firm warning against picking and eating berries must be given in early days.
Cosmetics	Cosmetics should be kept out of reach of toddlers as some are harmful when taken internally.
	WATER SAFETY
Paddling and swimming	Young children should be taught to swim early in life. The child should be shown danger spots such as sudden drops in depth, dangerous currents and outlets from drains. When on holiday by lake, sea or river children should wear safety belts or jackets. Parents should insist on children paddling or swimming where other people are about.
	ROAD SAFETY
Road deaths and injuries (1974)	The Safety Code should be taught untiringly by parents and in schools. Deaths: 719 Injuries: 53 560

ACCIDENTS—*contd.*

Dangers	*How to guard against them*
Deaths from other accidents (1974)	Burns and scalds: 147 Asphyxia, drowning and choking: 199 Poisoning: 29 *N.B.* These figures apply to children under the age of 15 years
	GENERAL POINTS Many children were seriously injured and are scarred or incapacitated for life. In addition to the more obvious results of accidents, psychological trauma resulting from shock, hospitalization handicaps and disfigurement must be of the greatest possible concern to all.

Further Reading

BARCLAY, T. & MUIR, I. (1964) *Burns and Their Treatment*. London: Lloyd-Luke.

ELLIS, M. (1967) *Accidents to Children*. London: Evans.

ELLSWORTH LAING, J. & HARVEY, JOYCE, (1967) *Management and Nursing of Burns*. London: English Universities Press.

MILLER, M. & MILLER, J. (1972) *Orthopaedics and Accidents*. London: English Universities Press.

23

Terminal illness and death in the children's ward

THE CARE of children suffering from a hopeless disease calls for some of the nurse's finest qualities and there is probably no situation that taxes her emotions more severely, nor any other group of illnesses in which she would more sincerely wish to give of her best, both in the care of her patient and by offering mental and spiritual help to the parents.

Sometimes it is the nurse who is looking after the child, who, because she herself has a live faith and religious outlook, can give just the right kind of comfort by word or attitude. Even the parent who has not thought of religion and has got out of the habit of prayer may find solace in a prayer said together by the child's bedside. Some nurses feel that this aspect should be left to others more experienced in dealing with deep sorrow. But it is often in the unplanned and unexpected moment that the right word or action, however simple, brings greatest relief and assures the parents of the sympathetic sharing of their burden. The nurse closest to the child should at this time also be closest to the parents.

Once a hopeless diagnosis has been made, the parents will want to ask innumerable questions of every possible person, in the hope of getting some information which might give a ray of hope. It is best to allow only the smallest possible number of people to discuss prognosis and treatment, as doubts may arise even if merely different words are used to describe the same thing. Any information given should be consistent and it is often possible to lead up to the subject of a hopeless outcome in several separate conversations. Parents often sense what will have to be said and some will ask a direct question. An honest answer is probably the only right one in such a case but at the same time the parent can be assured that everything possible will be done to relieve pain and keep suffering to a minimum. The child too will need to know something of his illness, although a great deal will depend on his age and understanding. In order to help him maintain his trust in the medical and nursing staff it is important that information is not withheld from the child. Children rarely ask outright, 'Am I going to die?' but, if the nurse finds herself in this situation she should first ascertain what does the child mean by dying? Children at different stages of development have different ideas, fantasies and experience. One way of handling this sort of situation is to convey gradually the idea of the long-term nature of his illness. That it is not a disorder that can be treated straightaway and finished with, but that it has an up and down course and cannot be measured in a day or a week. This will relieve his anxiety and enable him to anticipate and understand when he has bad days. Children should also be told whenever there are changes in their medication or treatment. Pain should never be denied, and the nurse should never say, 'It won't hurt' when it will, or, 'Don't be a cry baby' when an older child has recourse to tears. But, rather when a child asks, 'Will it hurt?' the nurse should say—'It does hurt a bit, but I'll be very quick and it will hurt as little as I can make it.' Encourage the child to count as the injection or treatment is carried out, one . . . two . . . three, which will help to allay his fear and anxiety.

Parents should be allowed to be with their hopelessly sick children as much as they wish, and should be allowed and encouraged to do those little things for the child which only a mother would know how to do. Both parents and child should be kept occupied and entertained as far as possible. As a rule it is kinder to keep the child in a general ward rather than in a side ward, unless the final weariness becomes too much for him.

Little treats, such as food brought from home, an unusual visit to another part of the hospital, or a week-end at home should be allowed without fear of 'spoiling the child'. The visit of a granny, a beloved teacher or the family vicar should always be permitted.

Children with malignant or terminal illnesses often develop curious fancies; one typical one is the desire to have 'a special meal in the middle of the night'. No nurse should be too busy or too rigid in her routine to grant such a request. There is always time to see to these children. There is little doubt that dying children sometimes realize what is about to happen. A compassionate nurse will be aware of this and often a little verse or story about Jesus who loves little children, or of happy children in God's blue heaven, is not mawkish and sentimental, but kindly and deeply comforting. No child should be allowed to die alone. Anticipation of impending death is one of a nurse's primary duties. If they desire it, parents should be allowed to sleep in the hospital and they should be called when the end approaches. When all is over, those nearest to the child should be left alone for a few moments by the bedside and then led away with quiet, sympathetic firmness. It is common-sense kindness to ensure some rest by giving the parents, with the permission of the attending house officer, one dose of sleeping tablets to be taken when they reach home.

Many hospitals have the services of a chaplain available. Whether normally religious or not, most people find it helpful to talk to him at this time and he should always be called. A sympathetic nurse will soon sense what kind of comfort will best help each individual parent. Often the parents have been so preoccupied with their dying child and their impending loss that they have for the time being hardly given a thought to their other children at home. The nurse can then remind them of the other children's needs and of their good fortune in having others who need their love. This is positive comfort and may be very helpful as it reminds the parents that their responsibilities have not come to an end and that there is much purpose left for them in life. The reminder that death is releasing their beloved little one from suffering or from an invalid life is comfort which may help in other cases. In all cases it is possible to remind parents that children probably lack the apprehension and fear an adult may feel and that their passing is thus made a great deal easier.

The parents' wishes as regards religious observances and orthodox rites should be ascertained and the necessary arrangements made in good time. It is every nurse's duty to be familiar with the practices of other denominations as well as her own, and all children should be christened, confirmed or given the last rites, as the case may be.

The Cot Death Syndrome

Most cot deaths occur in the early hours of the morning, between midnight and 6 a.m. The tragic silent nature of this event is testified to by many parents who have not been awoken even when sleeping in the same room as the child. The death of a child is extremely difficult for parents to accept under any circumstances, but this is particularly so when there is no apparent cause. A great deal of supportive counselling is required for the whole family. The parents need to be reassured that the death could not have been foreseen, nor that anything they did contributed to the child's death.

Relationships within the family often become disturbed, older siblings may have severe guilt feelings, or the parents blame one another. The health visitor has an especially important role to play in this situation, as an informed listener able to reassure and help to alleviate any guilt feelings and anxiety. These tragedies are always sudden and unexpected, and the cause remains unknown. Certain factors however have been implicated. It seems that cot deaths most frequently occur in bottle-fed babies and seems also to be common in those with a mild respiratory infection. These deaths are commoner in males and those infants of low birth weight and where the mother is a smoker with a history of poor prenatal health and diet. The sudden cot death remains the main cause of death in all infants between the age of one week to one year.

Prevention is important, and the health visitor and nurse should be aware of high-risk families in low socio-economic groups. The active encouragement of breast-feeding is of value, but if the infant is artificially fed· one of the modified milks should be used. Mothers should also be advised to place the baby in his cot lying on either side but not face down. The mother should also be aware of the need to seek early medical attention for all illnesses and minor ailments in the young baby. The Foundation for the Study of Infant Deaths publish a very helpful booklet for bereaved parents. It is also helpful for the parents to know, through the Foundation, that many other parents have been faced with the same situation and that they are not alone in their distress.

Last Offices

The general procedure of carrying out the last offices differs little from that customary for adults. Detail may, however, be adapted to suit the special cases. Unless the relatives have brought a little gown and socks, a plain white cotton gown or shroud is supplied by the hospital. This should be sufficiently long to cover the feet. If the jaw is inclined to drop, 2.5- to 3-cm bandage, still rolled up as supplied, can be used as a prop between chin and sternum and camouflaged by the gown. This is particularly easily done with infants whose necks are short. With young infants the knees may be drawn up, and they should be straightened by bandaging, some cotton wool being placed between the prominences of the knees to avoid marking the skin. The child's hands are placed together with the fingers interlaced, holding a little white flower. If the arms tend to sag, a roll of cotton wool or a rolled-up napkin can be placed underneath the elbows beside the body to support their weight. The face is covered with a square of gauze or an embroidered handkerchief reserved for the purpose. After securing the body in a sheet, a pall is placed over it and it is carried to the mortuary. Fresh flowers should be placed in the chapel and a light is left burning until the body is removed for burial.

Personal belongings or toys are parcelled up in the usual way but occasionally the parents appreciate the suggestion that a beloved toy should be left with the child.

Answering the questions of other children in the ward about the sudden disappearance of a patient or the inevitable disturbance caused by a death may not be easy. Psychologists are not yet agreed as to what is the best way of dealing with the problem and no two children are likely to react in the same manner, though they will all sense that something unusual has taken place. In the majority of cases it is probably best to state the truth simply, as for instance 'Johnny was so weak he fell asleep and will not wake up again because God has taken him to heaven'. But the nurse should also add immediately—'this will not happen to you—you are not weak, are you?', or words to that effect. As a rule children will be satisfied with this straightforward, honest statement. The few who may ponder or seem disturbed will soon be picked out by the ward sister, who can have a more personal talk with the individual child. The interest and variety of ward life will soon restore the usual, happy atmosphere.

Further Reading

Kubler-Ross, E. (1976) *On Death and Dying*. New York: Macmillan.

Martinson, I. M. (1978) *Home Care of the Dying Child*. Hemel Hempstead: Prentice-Hall.

Toynbee, A. (ed.) (1968) *Man's Concern with Death*, Chapter 4. London: Hodder & Stoughton.

Appendix 1

List of useful addresses

Association of British Paediatric Nurses,
c/o The President, Children's Hospital, Western Bank, Sheffield S10 2TH, England

Association of Spina Bifida and Hydrocephalus,
Devonshire Street House, Devonshire Street, London W1

British Association of Early Childhood Education,
Montgomery Hall, Kennington, Oval, London SE11

British Epilepsy Association,
Crowthorne House, New Wokingham Road, Wokingham, Berks

British Heart Foundation,
57 Gloucester Place, London W1

Children's Chest Circle,
Tavistock House North, Tavistock Square, London WC1

Coeliac Society,
P.O. Box 181, London NW2

Colostomy Welfare Group,
38 Eccleston Square, London SW1

Compassionate Friends (these deal with bereaved relatives),
50 Woodwaye, Watford, Herts (who will supply local Branch address)

Cystic Fibrosis Research Foundation Trust,
59 Holborn Viaduct, London EC1

Diabetic Association,
3–6 Alfred Place, London WC1

Disabled Living Foundation,
346 Kensington High Street, London W1

Down's Babies Association,
Queenbournc Community Centre, Ridgacre Road, Quinton, Birmingham

Family Fund (Joseph Rowntree Social Service Trust Ltd),
9 Poland Street, London W1 or Beverley House, Skipton, Yorks.

Family Planning Association,
27 Mortimer Street, London W1

Family Welfare Association Ltd,
501 Kingsland Road, London E8

Foundation for the Study of Infant Deaths,
23 St Peter's Square, London W6

Genetic Counselling: every General Practitioner should hold a list issued by the Department of Health and Social Security

Haemophilia Society,
16 Trinity Street, London SE1

Handicapped children, supplies and equipment:
E. J. Arnold & Son Ltd,
Buttersley Street, Leeds
James Galt & Co Ltd,
Brookfield Road, Cheadle, Cheshire
Task Master Ltd,
Morris Road, Clarendon Park, Leicester

Hospital Centre (King Edward 7th),
126 Albert Street, Camden Town, London NW1

Ileostomy Association of Great Britain,
149 Harley Street, London W1

Invalid Children's Aid Association,
126 Buckingham Palace Road, London SW1

Leukaemia Society,
186 Torbay Road, Rayners Lane, Harrow, Middlesex

Muscular Dystrophy Group,
Macauley Road, London SW4

National Advisory Centre for Battered Children,
Denver House, Bound's Green Road, London N11

National Association for Deaf/Blind and Rubella Children,
164 Cromwell Lane, Coventry CV4 8AP

National Association for Gifted Children,
1 South Audley Street, London W1

National Association for Maternity and Child Welfare,
1 South Audley Street, London W1

National Association for the Welfare of Children in Hospital,
7 Exton Street, London SE1

National Birthday Trust,
57 Lower Belgrave Street, London SW1

National Children's Adoption Association,
71 Knightsbridge, London SW1

National Children's Bureau,
8 Wakeley Street, London EC1

National Children's Homes,
85 Highbury Park, London N5

National Council for One-Parent Families,
255 Kentish Town Road, London NW5

National Council for Social Service,
26 Bedford Square, London WC1

National Council of Voluntary Child Care,
Cheriton Barton, Cheriton Fitzpaine, Devon

National Deaf Children's Society,
31 Gloucester Place, London W1

National Kidney Centre,
1 Fairholm Gardens, London N3

National Society for Autistic Children,
1a Golders Green Road, London NW11

National Society for Brain Damaged Children,
Honorary Secretary: 35 Larchmere Drive, Hall Green, Birmingham

NSPCC,
1 Riding House Street, London W1

Royal Association for Disability and Rehabilitation (*RADAR*),
25 Mortimer Street, London W1

Royal National Institute for the Blind,
224 Great Portland Street, London W1

Royal National Institute for the Deaf,
105 Gower Street, London WC1

ROSPA (Royal Society for the Prevention of Accidents),
1 Grosvenor Crescent, London SW1

Society of Compassionate Friends (these deal with bereaved relatives),
Honorary Secretary:
8 Westfield Road, Rugby, Warwickshire (who will supply local Branch addresses)

The Spastics Society,
12 Park Crescent, London WI

Variety Club of Great Britain,
5th floor, 1–4 Argyll Street, London W1 (gives financial aid to varied charities)

Appendix 2

Normal values and conversion tables

Normal Values

Haemoglobin	
Newborn	16·6 g/dl
Age 12 years	13·8 g/dl girls 14·0 g/dl boys
Red Blood Cells	
Newborn	4·5 to 5·0 $\times$ 10^6/mm^3
Age 12 years	4·2 to 5·4 $\times$ 10^6/mm^3
White Blood Cells	
Newborn	16 to 20 $\times$ 10^3/mm^3
Age 12 years	4 to 12 $\times$ 10^3/mm^3

Platelets
200 to 500 $\times$ 10^3/mm^3

Sedimentation Rate (Westergren)
2 to 10 mm/hour

Total Protein	5·2 to 7·8 g/dl
Albumin	3·5 to 5·0 g/dl
Globulin	1·7 to 2·8 g/dl
Fibrinogen	0·2 to 0·4 g/dl
Bilirubin	0·1 to 0·5 mg/dl
Serum Electrolyte	
Sodium	136 to 143 mmol/l
Potassium	4·1 to 5·6 mmol/l
Chloride	98 to 106 mmol/l
Bicarbonate	21 to 25 mmol/l
Urea	2·5 to 6·7 mmol/l

Blood Sugar

Serum glucose (fasting)	3·4 to 5·6 mmol/l

Cerebrospinal Fluid

Pressure	50 to 150 mm H_2O (7·5 to 20 kPa)
Sugar	3·9 to 4·8 mmol/l
Total protein	10 to 30 mg/dl
Cells	< 5 lymphocytes/mm^3

Faeces

After the age of one year 90 per cent dietary fat is absorbed and only 10 per cent excreted in the stools of healthy children.

Total fat	15 to 30% by weight of dried stool
Free fatty acids	5 to 15% by weight of dried stool
Soaps	5 to 15% by weight of dried stool
Neutral fat	1 to 2% by weight of dried stool

Urine (24-hr content)

Protein (total)	30 to 50 mg
Urea	200 to 500 mg/kg body weight/day

Average Blood Pressures

Age	*Systolic*		*Diastolic*	
	(mmHg)	(kPa)	(mmHg)	(kPa)
Birth	65–95	8·5–13	30–60	4–8
5 years	80–110	11–15	45–65	6–8·5
10 years	90–120	12–16	50–70	7–9

Weight Conversion Table

1 ounce = 30 grams (approx.)
2·2 pounds = 1 kilogram (approx.)

Pounds	*Kilograms*
1	0·45
2·2	1 kg or 1000 g
3	1·36
4	1·81
5	2·27
6	2·72
7	3·18
8	3·63
9	4·09
10	4·50
15	6·81
20	9·09
25	11·34
30	13·63
35	15·90
40	18·18
45	20·45
50	22·72

Fluid Conversion Table

Fl ounces	*Millilitres*
½	15
1	30
2	60
4	115
6	170
8	230
Pint	
1	568
Gallon	*Litres*
1	4·55

Thermometric Equivalents

Fahrenheit to Centigrade (within clinical range only)

°F	°C
93	33·9
94	34·42
95	35
96	35·56
97	36·11
98	36·66
99	37·22
100	37·78
101	38·33
102	38·89
103	39·44
104	40
105	40·56
106	41·11
107	41·67
108	42·22

Height Conversion Table

1 inch = 2·54 centimetres
100 centimetres = 1 metre

Inches	*Centimetres*
18	45·72
20	50·80
22	55·88
24	60·96
26	66·04
28	71·12
30	76·20
32	81·28
34	86·36
36	91·44
38	96·52
40	101·60

Index

Principal references in **bold type**

abdominal
  colic 295
  distension 265, 276, 302, 303, 307, 356
  pain 222, 229, 246, 276, 290, 303, 318, 366
abnormalities in babies **59**–85
abscess
  cerebral **374**
  pelvic **271**
absorption, disorders of 272–311
accidents 8
  in hospital 118
  to children **450–4**
acetabuloplasty **411**
acetest tablets 318
acetone 318, 319
acetylcysteine 162, 310
acholuric jaundice **229**, 275
achondroplasia 75, **417**
acidosis 154, 246, 260, 343
acne 316, **398**
acrodynia (Pink disease) **368**
acute rheumatic fever **210**
Addison's disease **315**
adenitis 301
adenoidectomy **167**
adenovirus 428
adrenal gland **315**
  failure 341
adrenocorticotrophic hormone (ACTH) **315**
adrenogenital syndrome **316**
admission
  booklet 105, **129**
  of mothers **102**
  questionnaire **99**
  routine **98**, 228, 232
agenesis of the kidney **347**
agranulocytosis 211
air (pneumo) encephalogram **363**
albuminuria 222
alkalosis 261
allergy **152**
alopecia 232, 234
ammonia dermatitis 353
amyotonia congenita **382**
anaemia 211, 221, 223, 224, 225, 260, 271, 296, 304, 313, 357, 377, 426, 441
  acute haemolytic **228**
  aplastic 228
  congenital **69**
  Cooley's **229**, 230
  haemorrhagic 225
  hypoplastic **228**
  iron deficiency **226**
  megaloblastic 376
  sickle cell **230**
anal
  fissure **254**
  stenosis **82**
  stricture 254
anaphylactic shock 343
anaphylactoid purpura 210, **222**, 267
anastomosis 265
  bile duct 84
  intestinal tract **82**, 83, 84
anencephaly 74
aneurism 223
angiography **207**
  nervous system **364**
ankylosis, fibrous 220
anorexia 190, 230, 255, 268, 281, 295, 332, 343, 375
ano-rectal manometry **284**
antenatal development **2**
anterior poliomyelitis 160, **430**
antigen-antibody reaction 315
anti-haemophylic globulin **238**
anti-spasmodic drugs (asthma) **152**
anti-streptolysin titre 336
antrum washout 139
anuria 338
anus
  ectopic **289**, **290**
  imperforate **82**
  stricture of 254
aorta, overriding 197
aortic
  regurgitation 213
  stenosis **196**
  valve incompetence 214
apex beat **186**, 192, 202

aphthous stomatitis **240**
apnoea 52, 317
  alarm mattress 52
appendicitis, acute 165, 246, **267**, 290, 333
appendix
  pelvic 268
  perforated 269
Arabon 306
arteritis, temporal 223
artificial
  feeding **19**, 376
  respirations **114**
  ventilation **114**
arthrodesis 415
ascites 278, **339**
aseptic meningitis 428
asphyxia 237
aspiration pneumonia 242
asthma **150**, 315, 316, 395
asthmatic bronchitis 154
ataxia 375
  Friedreich's **381**
atelectasis **52**
athlete's foot **402**
atresia
  bile duct **83**
  of bowel **44**
  of duodenum **81**
  of oesophagus **78**
atrial
  fibrillation **186**
  septal defect 196
atrio-ventricular node 181
audiometry 171
aura **368**
auto-immune reaction **210**, 222, 240
average standards **1**

babies, infectious **48**, 72
Babysitta 145
balanitis **349**
barium
  enema 266, 284
  meal 78, 249, 302
  X-ray 78
barrier nursing **46**, 242, 277, 332, 373, 401
basal metabolic rate 313
Batchelor plaster **409**
bat ears 74
bathing the sick baby **39**–43
BCG (Bacille Calmette-Guérin) vaccination 15, **422**
bed
  sores 216
  wetting 255, 279
behaviour problems 273
Bengers food 78, 148, 247, 385
benign lymphocytic meningitis **428**
bile pigment 274, 276
biliary atresia 275
bilirubin 69
  serum levels 52
biopsy
  jejunal 305
  muscle 223
  rectal 284
  renal 223
birth injury 62, 315, 382
bladder
  drainage 351
  eversion 353
  lavage 351
  neck sclerosis 348
  neuro-muscular incoordination **348**
Blalock–Hanlon operation **198**
Blalock–Taussig operation **197**
bleeding, subperiosteal **296**
bleeding time 200
blindness 372, 376
blood
  calcium 317
  chemistry 249
  cholesterol 313
  diseases **225**–38
  nitrogen 249
  picture 340
  plasma transfusion 237
  potassium 306
  pressure **187**, 202, 336, 337, 344, 371, 441
  sedimentation rate 139, 151
  shunting 196
  sodium levels 260, 340
  sugar estimation 318
  transfusion **86**, 221, 227, 228, 229, 230, 233, 235, 237, 260, 267, 270, 304, 329, 341, 344, 357, 441, 447
    dangers **89**
    exchange **70**
    management **86**
    packed cells **228**
blurred vision 225
Boehringer meconium strip 307
boils 419
  meatal 170
bone
  congenital abnormalities **75**
  marrow puncture **231**
borborygmi **283**
Bornholm disease 428
bossing (skull) 293, 360, 417
bowel sounds **270**, 271, 285, 286
Bradford frame 446
bradycardia **185**
brain
  abscess 176

brain—*contd.*
  damage **63**, 183, 365, **376**
breast
  enlarged in babies 62
  feeding **17**, 18, 187, 250
  milk 191, 250
  mothers' 19
breath
  holding 187
  typical odours **240**
breathing exercises **139**, 153, 190, 200, 356
bronchial spasm 151
bronchiectasis **138**, 147, 167
bronchitis
  acute **136**
    spasmodic 154
  allergic 136
  asthmatic 154
bronchography **133**, 139
bronchopneumonia **146**, 147, 426
bronchoscopy **133**, 137, 160
brucellosis **436**
buffalo hump, 316
bulbar paralysis **437**
buphthalmos 74
burns and scalds **438**–49
burns 329, 343
  causes of 438
  classification 440
  complications 447
  diet 445
  drug therapy 444
  first-aid 439
  full thickness 440, 443
  general treatment 444
  intravenous therapy 441
  Lundt and Browder method 440
  mental welfare 448
  oxygen therapy 442
  partial thickness 443
  rule of nines 440
  shock treatment 441
  superficial 440
  Waller method 440
burr holes 364
butterfly rash 224

calciferol (vitamin D) 317
calcium
  deficiency 303
  disodium versenate **369**, 377
  gluconate 70
  levels 317
  metabolism 292
caloric requirements **20**
calculi, renal 329
caput succedaneum **63**
carbohydrate metabolism 304, 315
cardiac
  arrythmia 204
  by-pass machine 198
  catheterization 198, **207**, 346
  failure 188, 214, 223, 229, 300, 329, 338
    common causes 188
    drugs in 191
    infant feeds in **191**
  incompetence 211
  massage 115
  murmur 226, 300
  surgery **200–7**
    complications 204
    equipment post-operation 201
    nursing care **201**
  valve vegetation 213
cardiograph 219
cardio-vascular system **185**–209
carditis 211
  rheumatic 209
carpo-pedal spasm 293
cataract 299
  congenital **74**
catarrh 156, **164**
catarrhal jaundice 276
catheter, in-dwelling urinary 326, 346
catheterization **326**, 330, 346
catheter specimens of urine **326**, 330, 332, 334
catscratch fever **429**
central venous pressure **202**
cephalhaematoma 62
cerebral
  abscess **374**
  haemorrhage 223, 237, 296
  lesions 360, 365
  palsy 63, 170, 368, **377**, 378, 380, 391, 414
    spasm 420
  thrombosis 204
  tumour 315
  vomiting 385
cervical adenitis 117, **403**, 432
changing stools **44**, 256
chaplain 457
charcoal biscuits 328
cerebrospinal fluid 382, 428, 430
chest
  aspiration **134**, 149
  examination **132**
  infections **281**–309
Cheyne–Stokes type breathing **371**
chicken pox (varicella) **433**
chilblains 329
child guidance clinics 14, 391
children at birth 2
  contact with home **106**
  emotional reactions **111**

children—*contd.*
  in hospital **96**–123
  questionnaire 99
  sick at home **125**
  resident mothers **102**
chiron bag 258
choanal atresia 74, **157**
chlorophyll tablets 306
cholecystography **84**
choledochus cyst **275**
chorea **215**
christening 252
Christmas disease **238**
chromosome studies 316
  in Down's syndrome **73**
chronic
  constipation **390**
  heart failure 188
  hepatitis **278**
circulatory failure 263
circumcision **349**, 350
circumoral pallor 223
cirrhosis of the liver 84, **278**, 299
cisternal puncture **363**, 371
clean specimen of urine 268
cleft
  lip 74, 177, **178**, 179
  palate 74, 177, **181**
clinistix 300
Clostridium tetani 429
clotting time 200
clubbing of fingers 138
coarctation of aorta **195**
cod liver oil 295
coeliac
  crises 306
  disease 293
  syndrome 301, **303**
cold baby syndrome **71**
colic 266, 333, 346, 377
collagen diseases **222**
collapse of lung 133, 426
collateral circulation **195**
Colliron 182
colonic lavage 257
colostomy 282, **284**
  bag 354
  psychological aspect **286**
  washout **286**
coma 278, 317, 371
common cold **156**, 171, 259
communicable diseases **428**–37
complementary feeds **31**
complete rest 212
composition of milk **21**
confusion, post-operation 204
congenital
  abnormalities **302**
  anatomical abnormalities **74**
  atresia of bile duct 83
congenital—*contd.*
  dislocation of hip joint 74, 388, **408**
  heart disease 74, 166, 188, **193**, 374
  hypertrophic pyloric stenosis **247**, 254
  largyngeal stridor **158**
  malformation, heart and great vessels **194**
  obliteration of bile duct 62, 74, 75, **83**, 275, 329
  congestion of lungs 213
coning of the brain stem **364**
conjunctivitis 428
constipation 145, 190, 210, 231, 232, 234, 249, **253**, 276, 281, 283, 295, 313, 314, 318, 334, 377
  causes **254**
  chronic 375, 390, 391
  complications **255**
  in cretins **312**
  intestinal obstruction 264
  with overflow **255**, 390
  total 265
contact with home **106**
convulsions 52, 63, 73, 147, 166, 170, 197, 259–60, 280, 300, 317, 333, 343, 361, 365, **366**, 368, 371–2, 374, 375–6, 380, 385
  in gastro-enteritis 259
  in the newborn 64
  in otitis media 171
  post-natal 62
  in tonsillitis 166
  observations **366**
contact with home **106**
Cooley's haemolytic anaemia **229**
cortisone **315**, 317, 320
coryza 430
cough reflex 168
cow's milk modification **22**
cot death syndrome **458**
cot sides 116
Coxsackie virus 428
craniotabes **293**
creatinine
  iodine levels 313
  urinary levels 223
cretinism 240, 254, **312**
Crosby capsule **305**
cross infection 45
croup **158**
Croupaire 135, 159
cubicle nursing **46**, **262**, 442
Cushing syndrome 232, **316**
cyanosis 63, 154, 160, **187**, 197, 235, 239, 367
cyanotic attacks 53, 183, 317
cyanotic heart lesions 197

cyclical vomiting **245**
cystic
  fibrosis of pancreas (mucoviscidosis) 276, **307**, 311
  Fibrosis Society 311
  spina bifida 74, **385**, 390, 391, 407, 413
cystitis 329, **334**
cystogram, micturating 329
cystography 330
cystoscopy **330**
cytotoxic drugs 231, 234, 358

deafness 73, **170**, 371, 372
  in cerebral palsy 379
death in the children's ward 110, **455**
defecation, pain in 254
deep X-ray therapy 234, 355, 357, **358**, 375
dehydration 239, 246, 249, 259, 260, 265, 302, 306, 322, 333, 358, 365, 416
  fever 45 ,
  delirium 371
Denis Browne boots **415**
dental
  care **239**
  caries 247, 379
dentition 4, 5, 7, 74, 292
deodorants 310
dermatomyositis **223**
diabetes **390**
  insipidus **375**
  mellitus **317**, 329, 331
diabetic
  Association 322
  coma **318**
  crisis 246
  diet 319
  playing cards 319
diaphragmatic
  hernia 74, **76**
  pleurisy 267
diarrhoea 268, 273, 276, 279, 314, 333, 343, 371, 376, 416
  and vomiting 171, **258**, 293
diathermy 349
diet
  in burns 445
  in coeliac disease 304
  in constipation 255
  in cystic fibrosis 309
  in diabetes 319
  in eczema 398
  in jaundice 277
  in nephritis 342
  in phenylketonuria 298
  in renal disease 345
  at six months 34
diet—*contd.*
  in Still's disease 221
  in tuberculosis 423
digitalization 191
dinner fork deformity **216**
diphtheria 160, 161, 208, **435**
  immunization **15**, 437
disaccharide deficiency 263
double
  kidney (horseshoe) **347**
  ureters 75, **347**
  vision 379
diuresis 341
diverticulum (Meckel's) **290**
douching, vaginal 332
Douglas operation 183
Down's syndrome **73**, 283, 391
drinking straws 212
drowsiness 343, 361, 374
drug
  addicts, babies born to **60**
  dosage for children 113
duck bill appearance 369
Duhamel's operation 284
duodenal
  intubation **308**
  obstruction 81
  secretions **302**
dwarfism 314, 341, 343
dysentery 267
  bacillus 259
dyspnoea 214, 226, 340
  paroxysmal 197

ear
  mopping 172, **173**
  nose and throat examination **268**
  syringing 172, **175**
Echo virus group 429
ectopia vesicae 75, **352**
ectopic anus **289**, 290
eczema **395**
Ehler Danlos syndrome 235
elbow splints 180, 181, 182
electrocardiogram 200, 313
electroencephalogram 365, 366
electrolyte balance 82, 92, **260**, 266, 267
electrolytes 306, 315, 340
electrolyte estimation 200
electromyogram 223, 382
electromyograph 404
electromyography 405
emboli 208
emotional
  development **8**
  reactions to hospital **111**
  stress 318
emphysema 163

empyema
  thoracic **149**
  drainage of 150
encephalitis
  acute **376**, 391
  hypertensive 338
  lead **377**
  lethargica 376
encephalogram, air (pneumoencephalogram) **363**
encephalopathy 338
  hypertensive 340
encopresis 390
endocarditis 224, 374
  bacterial **208**
endotracheal intubation 180
enema 254, 388, 391
  gastrographin 307
enteritis, infantile **258**
enteric fever 435
entero colitis 283
enuresis 318, **389**
enzymes, pancreatic 308
epidemic diarrhoea 428
epidemic myalgia (Coxsackie) 424
epilation 232
epilepsy 63, **366**, 367
epiphysis 407, 419
epispadias 74
epistaxis 231, 233
Erb's palsy **65**
erythema 220, 223
  marginatum 211
  nodosum **211**, 220
erythrocyte sedimentation rate (ESR) 214, 215, 220, 222, 224, 424
erythroedema (Pink disease) **368**
escharectomy 444
Escherichia coli 72, 176, 259, 269, 332, 370
euphoria, post-operation 204
examining the child patient **121**, **132**
exchange blood transfusion **69**
excoriated buttocks 302
excretion tests 355
exomphalos 74, **352**
expected weight 20
expressed breast milk 264
extra-corporeal circulation **198**
extrasystole 186
eye abnormalities 74

facial palsy 360, 374
facio-scapulo-humeral muscular dystrophy 405
faeces
  collection **258**
  impacted 389
faeces—*contd.*
  incontinence **390**
  observation of 259
Fallot's tetralogy 193, **197**
fasting blood sugar 300
fat
  balance **302**, 305
  intolerance 302
feed bottles **28**, 242
  disinfection **264**
  kitchen 242
  sterilization 28
feeding
  difficulties **31**
  the infant **56**
ferric chloride urine test 318
fetal circulation 193
fibrillation, atrial 186
fibrocystic disease of the pancreas 301, 302, **307**
first year of life **3**
fistula
  recto-vaginal 74, 83, **289**, 354
  tracheo-oesophageal **79**
flatus 267, 270
  tube 190
fluid
  intake chart **110**
  requirements, infants **20**
folic acid 227, 304
  deficiency 376
fontanelles 3, 7, 63, 64, 73, 262, 293, 313, 360, 361, 364
  bulging **371**
food allergies 396
food fads 10
foreskin 326, **349**
foreign bodies
  in the bladder 329
  in the vagina 331
fractures in the newborn 66
fragilitas osseum (osteogenesis imperfecta) **418**
frequency of micturition 423
Friedreich's ataxia **381**
frog
  plaster **409**, 412
  position in abdominal pain 269
frontal bossing 360, 417
furred tongue 210, 247, 255, 268, 276, 280

galactosaemia 276, **299**
galactosuria **300**
gallow type extension 446
gallstones 275
gamma-globulin 301, **342**, 437
gangrene 265, 267
gastric
  lavage 247,249,250,251,**252**,424

gastric—*contd.*
suction, continuous 271, **272**
gastritis **247**, 249, 250
gastro-enteritis 72, 247, **258**, 263, 267, 283, 343
gastroenterostomy 82
Gastrografin enema 307
gastrostomy **80**, 82
Gaucher's disease 301
genetic counselling 74, 310, 382, 388, 406
genito-urinary tract
congenital abnormalities 75
surgical conditions **346**
German measles (rubella) 170, **432**
Ghon focus **426**
giddiness 225
gigantism 314
gingivitis **241**
glandular fever **435**
glomerulonephritis **335**
glossoptosis **183**
glucose
6-phosphate dehydrogenase (G-6-PD) 229
tolerance curve 302
tolerance test 305, 318
gluten 303
free diet **304**
glycogen
disease (van Gierke's) **300**
storage disorder **301**
glycosuria 316, 317
gonococcus 269
gonorrhoea 331, 332
gowns, barrier **47**
granuloma 281
Grommet tube **173**
growth, motor development **11**
Guthrie test 60, **297**

haematemesis 278
haematocrit **208**, 441
haematoma, subdural **64**
haematuria 231, 234, 296, 336, 357, 423
haemoconcentration 260, 441
haemodialysis **344**
haemoglobin 3, 4, 7, 329
estimation 441
levels 179, 181, 220, 221, 225
haemolytic
anaemia **228**, 315
disease of the newborn **68**, 228, 237, 275
streptococcus 165
haemophilia **237**, 238, 329
haemophilus influenzae meningitis 188, **372**
haemorrhage
bowel 281
cerebral 64, 222
retinal 231
subperiosteal 231, 296
in polyarteritis 222
thoracic 204
haemorrhagic disease of the newborn **68**
haemosiderosis 229
haemothorax 204
halitosis 138, 280
harelip (cleft lip) 74, **181**
Harrison's sulcus 293
hay fever 395
headache 210, 223, 225, 231, 246, 336, 343, 361, 363, 365, 366, 370, 376, 416, 430
head
box 85
circumference 2, 3, **361**, 371
injuries in the newborn **62**
measurements **361**, 387, **389**
retraction 333, 361, **371**
rotation test 53
Heaf test **422**
hearing 3
aids 380
heart (see cardiac)
block 186
congenital malformation 188, **194**
disease
inflammatory 188, **208**
types of 188, 193
lesions, cyanotic 197
and great vessels, surgery **198**
–lung machine 200
heel and ear manoeuvre 53
hemiplegia 375
hemispherectomy **375**
Henoch–Schönlein's
purpura 237
syndrome **222**, 237
hepatitis
acute virus 276
complications **278**
epidemic 276
giant cell 276
infectious 276
infective **275**, 276, 329
serum 275
hereditary spherocytosis (acholuric jaundice) **229**
hernia
diaphragmatic **76**
hiatus 75, **77**
inguinal **289**
irreducible 289
strangulated **289**

hernia—*contd.*
  supra-umbilical **288**
  umbilical **288**
herpangina (Coxsackie) 428
herpes 145, 239, **240**, 241
hiatus hernia 75, **77**
  chair 78
Hirschsprung's disease 75, 254, 281, **282**
Hodgkin's disease **234**
hoop traction 410
Horner's syndrome 204
horseshoe kidney 75, **347**
hospital routine 98
hot cross bun skull **293**
hot fomentations 270
household dust 395
humidity, room 54
humidifier 205
hunger stools **249**
hyaluronidase (Hyalase) **92**
hydramnios in pregnancy 81
hydrocele 74, **353**
hydrocephalus 63, 74, 363, 371, 372, 376, **382**, 387, 389
  communicating **382**
  non-communicating 364, **382**
  nursing care 384
hydronephrosis **347**, 348, 349, 355
hydrops fetalis 69
hydrothorax 340
hydro-ureters **333**, 347, 349, 355
hyperactivity 392
hyperflexion of wrist 216
hyperglycaemic coma **322**
hyperpyrexia 416
hypertension 223, 224, 235, 316, 336
  portal 278
hypertensive encephalopathy 338, 340
hypervitaminosis 295
hypertrophy of right ventricle 197
hypogammaglobulinaemia 301
hypoglycaemia 17, 53, 300, 365
hypoglycaemic
  coma 321, 322
  convulsions 300
  reaction 321
hypoplastic anaemia 228
hypospadias 74, **351**
hypostatic pneumonia 384
hypotension 446
hypothermia 198, **206**
hypothyroidism 240, 254, **312**
hypoxia 193

ice bag 289
icterus gravis neonatorum **69**
idiopathic thrombocytopenic purpura 210, **235**, 236, **237**
ileal loop **354**
ileostomy bag 353
immune deficiency disease 301
immunity to tuberculosis 421
immunization and vaccination **14**, 15
  contra-indications **437**
  and eczema **398**
  for tetanus **429**
imperforate anus 74, **82**
impetigo contagiosa 117, **399**
incontinence 348, 349, 367, 373, 388, 390
  with overflow **388**
incubators 53, **55**, 85
indwelling urinary catheter 346, 351, 446
infant feeding **16**–35
infantile
  eczema **395**
  gastro-enteritis **258**
  paralysis (poliomyelitis) **430**
infected tonsils 416
infection
  prevention in baby units **45**
  in the newborn **72**
infectious
  babies **48**
  mononucleosis (glandular fever) **435**
  precautions in tuberculosis 423
infective hepatitis 275, **276**
infested head 121, 399, **402**
influenza 434
infra-red ray therapy 221
inhalations (asthma) 152
injuries
  at birth **62**, 315
  intracranial 63
  local nerve **64**
insulin
  coma **322**
  reaction 321
  therapy 319
intercostal drainage 203, **207**
intercurrent infection 310
intertrigo 43
intestinal
  atresia 254
  obstruction **264**, 290, 307
  parasites 226, **278**, 390
  worms **390**
intracranial
  bleeding 52
  injuries **63**
  pressure 344, **361**, 371, 373, 377
  tumours 368, **375**
intradermal tests 396
intrapericardial injection 200
intraperitoneal fluid **270**

intravenous
  infusion **86**, 265, 266, 271, 284, 287
  pyelography **328**, 333, 355
  therapy 306
intubation, endotracheal 54, 77, 136, 429
intussusception 222, **265**, 290
ion exchange resin 341
iridocyclitis 221
iron 227, 234, 304, 358
  additional to diet 24
  and deficiency anaemia 226
  requirements for babies 57
  therapy 182

jaundice 69, 230, **274**
  acholuric **229**, 275
  acute virus **276**
  in atresia of bile duct **83**
  catarrhal **276**
  diet 277
  in haemolytic disease 68, 228, 237, **275**
  in infective hepatitis **275**
  in leukaemia 230
  obstructive 273, **275**, 301
  physiological **276**
  in sepsis 275
  severe neonatal **69**
  transfusion 275
jejunal biopsy **305**
jugular vein puncture **198**

Kaposi vericelliform dermatitis **398**
kernicterus 52, **69**
Kernig's sign 430
ketone bodies 246
ketonuria 260, 300
ketosis 300, 317, 318
knee chest position 197
kidney, horseshoe 74, **347**
Klippel-Feil syndrome 407
kyphosis 405

lactation, stimulation **19**
lamblia intestinalis 302
laparotomy 84, 267, 284, 290
laryngeal
  oedema **160**
  papilloma 158, 160
  spasm 158
  stridor 160
  web 160
laryngismus stridulus **158**
laryngitis stridulosa **158**
laryngoscopy 54, **157**
laryngo-tracheitis **158**, 160, 164
last offices 459
lateral sinus thrombosis 176

lead encephalopathy **377**
leucocytosis 232, 435
leucopenia 224
leukaemia, acute **230**, 241, 329
lipoid nephrosis 339
lipoidosis 301
lipoid
  pneumonia 254
  storage disorder 301
liver
  damage 278, 447
  enlarged 299, 300
  failure 229
  necrosis 278
lobar pneumonia **144**
lobectomy **144**
lock jaw (tetanus) **429**
Logan's bow **180**
lordosis 335, 405
low birthweight baby **50**, 377
lumbar puncture 268, **362**, 371, 376, 424
lung
  collapse 147, 280
  infection, chronic 307
  resection 144
Lundt and Browder method (burns) 440
lupus erythematosus **224**

major epilepsy **366**
malabsorption 227
  syndrome 227
maladie de Roger 195
malaise 430, 434
malar flush 269
malformation of vagina 354
malignancy 316, 357
malnutrition 273, 379
Malta fever (brucellosis) 436
Mantoux test 139, 148, 302, **422**
masculinization 315
masks **46**, 157
  technique for use of 46
mastitis 61, 434
mastoidectomy 170
mastoiditis **176**, 263
masturbation **10**
measles 138, 318, 342, **431**, 432
  vaccination **15**
meatotomy 351
Meckel's diverticulum 290
meconium **44**, 256, 283
  ileus **74**, 307
mediastinal lymph nodes 426
medicines
  giving of **112**
  dosage **113**
megacolon **281**
megaloblastic anaemia 376

mega ureters **347**
melaena **257**
  in the newborn **66**
  stools 222
meningeal cry 361, **370**
meningismus 333
meningitis 72, 73, 144, 246, 259, 267, 365, **370**, 387
  aseptic (Echo) **428**
  benign lymphocytic **428**
  complications 371
  haemophilus influenzae **372**
  meningococcal 237, **372**
  nursing care **373**
  subacute 371
  tuberculous **426**
meningocele 76, **386**, 389
meningomyelocele **386**
mental
  deficiency 371, 376, **391**
  handicap 254, 255, 273, 275, 297, 299, 377, **391**, 404
  subnormality **368**, 390
mercury 368
mesenteric
  adenitis 267, 301
  lymphadenitis **290**
  lymph nodes 290
metabolic disorders **292**–311
metastases **357**, 358
methaemoglobinaemia, acquired 235
microcephaly 74, 391
micrognathia 74
microphthalmia 73
microstoma **183**
micturition, frequency of 268
midstream specimen of urine **327**
migraine 246
milestones **1**–12, 391
milia 59
miliary tuberculosis **423**
milk
  constitution of 21
  cow's 21, 24
  dried 22
  evaporated 23
  modification 22
  room **25**
mitral stenosis **196**, 214
mittens 61, 190, 279, 397
mongolism (Down's syndrome) **73**
moonface 316
morbilli (measles) **432**
moro reflex **53**
mother–baby relationship **36**
moulding of head 61
motor development **11**
mouth breathers 168, 239
mucolytic agents 162
mucoviscidosis (cystic fibrosis) **307**
mucus extractor 54, 55
mumps **434**
muscle biopsy 223, 382, **405**
muscular
  dystrophy 254, **404**
    pseudo-hypertrophic 404
mustard procedure 198
myalgia, epidemic 428
myelomeningocele 74, **386**
myocarditis **208**, 223
myopathies **405**
myotonia congenita 405
myringoplasty **176**
myringotomy **172**

naevi **74**
  cavernous 74
  portwine 75
  strawberry 74
  Sturge-Weber **375**
nails of the newborn 73, 74
napkins
  disinfection **48**
  disposal in gastro-enteritis 264
  method of folding **40**
  preparation for inspection **44**
nasal drops 141, **142**, 172
naso-gastric
  tube **81**, 115, 202, 265, 271, 284, 286, 445
  feeds **190**
nebulizer 310
necrosis of the liver 278
neonatal jaundice **69**
nephrectomy **355**
nephritis 166, 222, 210, 254, 315, 329, **335**
  classification **335**
  Ellis type I 335
  acute haemorrhagic **335**
  post-streptococcal **335**
nephroblastoma (Wilm's tumour) **357**
nephrosis 210, 335, **338**, 390
nephrostomy 347, **355**
nephrotic syndrome 335, **338**, 339
nervous system, the **360**–93
neuritis 377
neurological
  bladder **348**
  examination 268
  observations **352**
neuromuscular
  disease 391
  incoordination, bladder **348**
newborn babies
  abnormalities **59**–85
  bathing **39**
  general care 36

newborn babies—*contd.*
stools **44**
nursing the **36**
Niemann-Pick disease **301**
nipple shields 178
nits **403**
non-accidental injury **93**
non-protein nitrogen in the blood 249
notifiable diseases **372**, 432–6

obesity 316
obliteration of bile duct, congenital 62, 74, 75, **83**, **275**, 329
obstruction, intestinal 246, **307**
occult blood 296
occupational therapist 221, 374
odours, significance of **240**
oedema 214, 299, 306, 336, 338, 339, 340, 341, 342, 444
in heart failure 189
in the newborn **70**
oesophageal
atresia 74, **78**
graft **80**
temperature **80**
oesophagoscopy 78
oliguria 446
oophoritis 434
operations in childhood **103**
ophthalmia neonatorum 84
ophthalmitis 281
opisthotonos **370**
oral
hygiene 233
toilet 270
orchidopexy **289**
orchitis 434
orthodontic treatment 181
ornithosis (psittacosis) 436
orthostatic albuminuria 329, **334**
Ortolani sign **409**
oscillator 115
osteochondritis **407**
osteogenesis imperfecta 74, **418**
osteomyelitis 72, **415**
osteoporosis 220, 303, 317
osteotomy 353
otitis media 138, 156, 157, 167, 170, **171**, 259, 261, 263, 374
otorrhoea **173**
oxycephaly 74
oxygen
dangers of **54**, 85
methods of administration 85
requirements, low birthweight babies, 53
tent 200
therapy **135**, 137, 147, 197, 310
in tracheostomy patients 136
oxymist tent **189**
oxyuris vermicularis **278**

pace maker 198
packed cell transfusion 228, 330
Palmer mechanical injector 320
palsy
cerebral 63, 170, 368, **377**, 378, 380, 391
Erb's **65**
facial 360, 374
pancreatic
deficiency 308
enzyme 308
insufficiency 307
medication 308
pancreatitis 434
papilloedema 361, 371, 375
papilloma 160
paracentesis
abdominis **340**
thoracis **134**, 149
paralysis 371, 372, 381
correction of deformities 419
facial 64
intestinal **270**
paralytic ileus **271**
paraphimosis **350**
parasites, intestinal 262, **278**, 390
parasympathetic ganglia 282
parathyroid gland **317**
paratyphoid 435
parenteral fluids 262
parotitis epidemic (mumps) **434**
patent ductus arteriosus **193**
patient assignment 101, **109**
pathological fractures 220
Paul Bunnell test 435
Paul's tubing 325, 446
pediculosis capitis **402**
Pel Ebstein's fever **234**
pelvic
abscess **271**
appendix 268, **269**
perforated 269
pemphigus 73
penile clamp 388
percentile of average milestones 1
peri-anal irritation 278, 287
periarteritis nodosa **223**
pericarditis 208, 214, 220
peristalsis, visible 81, 249, 283
peritoneal dialysis 344, **345**
peritonitis 268, 269, 342
peritonsillar abscess (quinsy) **167**
Perthe's disease **407**
pertussis **433**
immunization 14, 437
pes cavus 381
petechiae 209, 231, 325

petechial haemorrhages 228, 372
petit mal **366**
Peyer's patches 435
phenistix 298
phenylketonuria 60, **297**
  diet in **298**
phenylalanine 297, 298, 299
phimosis 349
phosphorus
  levels 317
  metabolism 292
photophobia 370
phototherapy **52**
physiological jaundice **52**, **61**, 83
physiotherapy 310, 388, 389, 392, 413, 449
pica 224
Pierre Robin syndrome **183**
pillows, use and abuse 37, **119**, **146**, 217, 270, 384
pilocarpine iontophoresis 308
Pink disease **368**
pituitary gland **314**
pin worms 278
plantar creases 53
plasma
  bicarbonate 249
  protein 340
plaster of paris, care of children in **419**
plastic surgery 317, 351
platelet
  deficiency 235
  transfusion 235
play **106**, 193, 306, 374
pleural
  effusion 148
  rub 429
pleurisy 147, **148**, 214, 224
  diaphragmatic **267**
pneumo-encephalogram **363**
pneumonia 72, 183, 196, 263, 267, 405, 447
  aspiration 242
  broncho **146**, 147, 426
  consolidation 428, 429
  inhalation 64
  lipoid 254
  lobar **144**
pneumothorax **204**, 205
poisoning 243, 244, 247
poliomyelitis **430**
  bulbar involvement 431
  immunization 14
polyarteritis nodosa 223
polycystic kidneys 329
polymorphonuclear leucocytosis 223
polyneuritis (Pink disease) **368**
polyuria 343
portal hypertension 278
possetting 32
postural
  albuminuria 334
  drainage 140, 142
potassium citrate 201
potting **99**
precocity 315
premature babies **50**–8, 226, 227, 377
premaxilla 178
pre-menstrual pain 267
pressure
  areas 214, 270
  sores 306
primary
  bleeding 356
  complex 426
  focus 426
  tuberculosis 426
procaine, intrapericardial 201
progressive spinal muscular atrophy 381
protein bound iodine level 313
proteinuria 223, 224, 338, 341
projectile vomiting 249
prothrombin 235
pseudohermaphroditism 74
pseudohypertrophic muscular dystrophy **404**
pseudo rubella (roseola infantum) 434
psittacosis 436
psychiatrist 255, 281
psychological disturbances 273, 396
puberty 320
pulmonary stenosis 197
pulse 185
  abnormalities **185**
  apical beat 186
  in cretinism 312
  extrasystole 186
  in heart block 186
  sinus arrhythmia 186
  sleeping **185**
  sluggish 276
  taking of **38**
punishment 9
purpura
  anaphylactoid 222
  familial thrombocytopenic **237**
  Henoch-Schönlein's **222**
  idiopathic 235
  symptomatic **235**
pyelitis 144, 246, 261, **332**
pyelography 347
  intravenous **328**, 355, 357
  retrograde 330, 335
pyelonephritis 329, **332**

pyeloplasty 347
pyloric
stenosis, congenital hypertrophic 7, **247**–52, 254
ladder diet 250, 251
schedule 267

quinsy 167

radioactive iodine 312
radium therapy 75, **358**
Ramstedt's operation **250**
Rashkind's
balloon 198
procedure 208
ready-feed concept **26**
rectal
biopsy **284**, 301
examination 268
procidentia **273**
prolapse 273, 302, 306, 369
causes 273
operation 274
swabs **260**, 268
temperature 263
recto-urethral fistula **83**
recto-vaginal fistula 74, 83, **289**, 354
Redivac bottle 207
red currant jelly stool **266**
reflex
conditioned 390
nervous system 361
regurgitation 32
relatives, care of **232**
religious rites **465**
renal
biopsy **340**
complications 446
damage 447
dwarfism 343
failure 222, 223, 295, **343**
infections 390
rickets 343
transplant 344
resection of bowel 265, 266, **284**
resident mothers 96, **102**
respirations
in asthma 154
changes in 131
failure 204
inverted **145**
obstruction 158, 314
sighing 211
rates 3, 4, 5, 7
respiratory distress syndrome **67**
restrainers **116**
resuscitation 114, 201
retention of urine **327**
retinal haemorrhage 344
retrognathia 183
retrograde pyelography **330**, 335
retrolental fibroplasia 85
retropharyngeal abscess 166
rheumatic
carditis 209, **210**
fever 166, 196, **210**, 315
nodules **211**, 220
rheumatoid arthritis **219**, 315
Rhesus incompatibility **68**
rib resection 200
rickets **292**, 306, 343
diet in 293
rickety rosary 293
rigor 333, 416
ringworm **402**
risus sardonicus **429**
roseola infantum (pseudo rubella) 434
Rose Waaler test 220
Rothera's urine test **318**
roughage in diet 255
round worms 275, **280**
rubella 170, 391, **432**
vaccination **15**
ruminating 32

saccharine 264
safeguarding health **12**
safety
in the home **125**
measures in hospital **116**
St Vitus' dance (chorea) **215**
salmonella 259
salicylates 211, 221
salt in nephritis diet 338
scabies **401**
scalds, classification **440**
scalp vein infusion **92**
scarf sign 53
scarlet fever (scarlatina) 432
Schick test 435
schooling 221, 306
schools
special 13, 215
for epileptics 367
for mentally handicapped 393
open air 143
for physically handicapped 389
Schüller–Christian syndrome **301**
sclerema (cold baby) **71**
scleroderma 223
sclerosis of bladder neck **349**
scurvy 237, 241, **296**
diet in 297
second year, the 6
septicaemia 208, 266, 271, 371, 389, 416
septostomy, atrial **198**

serum
  bilirubin levels 52
  calcium 365
  cholesterol 340
  glucose 53
  lipid levels 313
  potassium 341
  protein 222, 260, 306
sex
  determination **316**
  questioning 9
sexual precocity 316
shaving 361
shock 204, 266, 316, 322, 343
shunt 208
shunting operation 198
sick children
  calling the doctor 125
  at home **124**
  safety 125
  toys 126
sickle cell anaemia **230**
sighing respirations 211
'Signe de Dance' 266
silver swaddler 72
sinus arrhythmia 186
sinusitis 138, 156, 167, 170, 247
sixth disease (roseola infantum) 434
skimmed milk 264
skin
  diseases **395**
  grafting 418, 443, **444**
  in hepatitis 274, 276
  infections in the newborn 73
sleep 3, 4, 5
sleeping pulse **185**, 213, 217
sleep walking 246
smallpox vaccination 15, **398**, 433
social worker 388
sodium
  intake 191
  levels 307, 341
  replacement 309
somnolence syndrome 232
sore buttocks 43, 262, 263
sore throat 213
Southey's tubes 340
soya bean milk 300
spasmo-episthotonos 429
spastic paralysis 407
spasticity 275
special care nurseries 58, 60
special schools 13, 143, 215, 367, 389, 393
speech
  difficulty 216, 378, 381
  therapy **182**
spherocytosis, hereditary 229
spina bifida 75, **385**, 390, 391, 407, 413
Spitz–Holter valve **382**, 384
splenectomy 229, 237
splinting 87, 401
splints 397
sputum
  in asthma 151
  in bronchiectasis 138, 140, 141
  in tuberculosis 424
squatting 197
status asthmaticus 154
steam
  inhalations 141, 172
  tent 135, **159**
  therapy 54, **135**, 137
steatorrhoea **301**
Steindler's operation **415**
sterilization of feeding equipment **29**
sterno-mastoid tumour 65, **406**
steroids 211, 221, 222, 223, 224, 228, 231, 341, 376
sticky eyes 84
Still's disease **219**
stomatitis 231, 241, 369
  aphthous 240
  catarrhal 240
  ulcerative 240
stools
  in coeliac disease 303
  collection of specimens **258**
  in cystic fibrosis 307
  in gastro-enteritis 259
  impacted 283
  jaundice 275
  in the newborn 3, 44
  in obliteration of the bile duct 83
  pea soup 257
  red currant jelly 257
  types **256**
stork beak marks 60
strabismus 74, 85, 361
strangulated hernia 265
stridor 158
Sturge-Weber syndrome 364, **375**
subcutaneous infusion **92**, 261
subdural tap 371
sub-periosteal bleeding **296**
subphrenic abscess **271**
supplementary feeds **36**
suppositories 314
supra-renal gland 315
surgical emphysema 162
separation of cranial sutures 361
sweat test 302, 307
sweating 210, 266, 369
Swenson's operation **284**
symptomatic thrombocytopenic purpura **236**

syndactyle 74, **417**
Synder sling 407
syphilis 391
  congenital 276
syringing ears 172, 173, **175**
systolic murmur 196

taches cérébrales **372**
tachycardia 185, 220, 223, 416
taenia saginata 280
talipes 74, 413
  calcaneo valgus 413
  calcaneo varus 414
  equino valgus 414
  equino varus 388, 415
tapeworm **280**
teats **30**
teething **242**
  order of eruption 4
telangiectasis 375
temper tantrums 7
temperature 44
  in the newborn 44
  maintaining the 44
  oesophageal 206
  taking the 7
temporal arteritis 223
tendon, Achillis 413
tepid sponging 333
terminal illness 455
testes
  malignant 352
  migration of 352
  undescended 252
tetanus **429**
  antitoxin 429
  neonatal 429
  passive immunization 430
  toxoid 429, **437**
tetany 17, **293**, 302, 306, 317, 365
thalassaemia 229, 230
thermometers
  bath 119
  lotion 119
  rectal 119
thirst 292, 333
thoracic empyema **149**
  drainage of 150
thoracotomy 77, 78, 80, 198, 200
thread worms **278**
  infestation 331
thrombocytopenic purpura 69
thrombosis 223
  cerebral 204
  in polyarteritis nodosa 223
thrush 57, 233, **242**, 243, 262
thumb sucking 10
thyroid
  gland **312**
  therapy **313**
thyrotoxicosis **312**
tinea interdigitalis **402**
tinnitus 211
toilet training 273
tongue
  enlarged 74, 240, 301, 313
  tie **243**
tonsils 152, 241, 380
tonsillectomy **167**, 241, 320, 437
  position 168, 181
tonsillitis **165**, 167, 171, 267, 318, 336, 380
torticollis **406**
toxaemia 269, 374, 416
toxocariasis **280**
toxoplasmosis 376
toys 8, 217
tracheal intubation 429
tracheitis 138
tracheo-oesophageal fistula **78**
tracheostomy 159, **160**, 190, 429, 437
transfusion
  apparatus 86
  jaundice 275
  procedure 86
  splinting **87**
transplant
  renal 343
  ureters 353, **354**
transposition of great vessels 198
trauma 329
triple arthrodesis (Steindler's operation) **415**
tripod sign 430
trismus 429
trocath 345
trophic ulceration 389
tube feeding 148, 253, 373
tuberculosis **420**–7
  kidney 329, 355
tuberculous
  meningitis 254, 370, 423, 424
  peritonitis 301
tumours 265, 315, 316, 365, 375
twitching 235

ulceration
  of bowel 302
  of meatus (penis) 349
  of oesophagus 77, 79
ulcerative
  colitis 210, 269
  stomatitis 240, 241
ulcers of mouth 232, 240, 241
umbilical
  cord 42, 61, 69
  hernia 74
  vein 70, 88

umbilicus 267, 275
  eversion 283
undescended testicle 74, 289
undulant fever (brucellosis) 436
unguentum emulsificans 396
upper respiratory tract infection 226
uraemia **343**, 346, 347, 357
urea clearance test 331
ureterocele 349
ureters
  double 74, **347**
  stenosis **347**
  transplantation **348**
ureteric valves 347
urethra
  congenital abnormalities 347
  dilatation of 348
urethral
  stricture 349
  valves 348
urethrogram **348**
urethrostomy 348
urinary
  diseases **324**
  diversion 388
  infections 72, 73, 267, 321, 332, 347
  investigations 328
  tract abnormalities **75**, 332, 334, 353, 390
urine
  abnormalities **329**
  back pressure 348, 349
  collecting bag 326
  collection of **325**
  early morning specimen **326**, 334, 337
  midstream **327**
  in congenital obliteration of the bile duct 83
  jaundice 276, 277
  retention 327, 334, 348, 371
  supra pubic aspiration **327**
  suppression 357
  twenty-four hour specimen **327**
  vitamin C test 296
urticarial rash 222, 223

vaccination 14, 398
  BCG 15, 398, **422**
  in eczema **398**
vaginal douching 332
valvotomy 196
varicella (chickenpox) **433**
varicose veins in oesophagus 278
variola (smallpox) **433**
venepuncture in infants **199**
venous pressure, central 202
ventilation, mechanical artificial 204, 206
ventilator 85, 202
ventricular
  fibrillation 187
  septal defect **195**
  stenosis 197
ventriculography **364**, 374
vernix caseosa 60
vesico-ureteric reflex **347**
Vincent's angina **241**
virilism 316
visceral larvae migrans 280
visiting **105**, 193
visual disturbances 344, 374, 376, 406
vitamins 25, 286
vitamin
  A 304
  absorption 254, 267
  B deficiency 365
  C 296
  D 292, 293, 304, 309, 317, 343
  K 52, 70, 84
  requirements 57
vitello intestinal duct 290
voiding urethrogram **348**
volvulus **265**
vomiting 31 ff.
von Gierke's disease 300
vulvo-vaginitis 279, **331**

Waller's rule of nine **440**
Waterston's operation **197**
wax baths 221
weaning 32
weighing 262, 446
weight in disease 215, 217, 336, 337
weight of the newborn 45
Weil's disease **275**
Werdnig-Hoffman's disease **382**
Whitehead's varnish 181
whooping cough (pertussis) 138, 273, 433
  protection **14**
wigs 375
Wilm's tumour 329, 355, **357**
wind, bringing up 30
witch hazel ointment 255
wrist and ankle restrainers 53, 162
woollie rash 61
Wood's glass **402**
wry neck **406**

xanthomatosis 301
xylose excretion test 305